FUNCTIONAL NEUROANATOMY

FUNCTIONAL NEUROANATOMY

Including an atlas of the brain stem, and of the whole brain in coronal and horizontal sections.

By N. B. EVERETT, Ph.D.

Professor and Chairman, Department of Biological Structure, University of Washington School of Medicine, Seattle, Washington

With the Assistance of

JOHN W. SUNDSTEN, Ph.D.

Associate Professor, Department of Biological Structure, University of Washington School of Medicine, Seattle, Washington

and

RAYMOND D. LUND, Ph.D.

Assistant Professor of Biological Structure and Neurosurgery, University of Washington School of Medicine, Seattle, Washington

Sixth Edition, Thoroughly Revised, 297 Illustrations, 39 in Color

LEA & FEBIGER   Philadelphia

First Edition, 1948 by A. R. Buchanan
Second Edition, 1951 by A. R. Buchanan
Third Edition, 1957 by A. R. Buchanan
Fourth Edition, 1961 by A. R. Buchanan
Fifth Edition, 1965 by N. B. Everett
Sixth Edition, 1971 by N. B. Everett

Reprinted, February, 1972
Reprinted, June, 1973

ISBN 0-8121-0324-6

Published in Great Britain by Henry Kimpton, London

Library of Congress Catalog Card Number: 70-135680

Printed in the United States of America

Preface

In this thoroughly revised edition of *Functional Neuroanatomy* an effort has been made, as previously, to present the material necessary for understanding the structure and function of the nervous system in the minimal number of pages. This approach has been extended by eliminating specific references in the body of the text, by combining material of certain chapters, and by deleting unnecessary details. An appropriate list of references, however, is given at the end of each chapter to serve as a guide to further reading. Recent, as well as earlier and more traditional, references are included.

Chapter 3, Histology and Cytology of Neurons and Neurolgia, is a new chapter that includes an appropriate account of the fine structure of nerve cells and of glial elements.

Thirty-nine new figures have been added to this edition and many of the previous illustrations have been improved. Where necessary, changes in labeling of structures have been made to coincide with the Paris Nomina Anatomica (PNA).

Several new and well-labeled photographs of the gross brain and of horizontal and coronal sections of the brain are included. In addition, a new atlas section has been added that includes photographs of three series of sections: (1) Weil-stained transverse sections of the brain stem; (2) a series of coronal sections of the brain stained by the ferric ferrocyanide method of Tompsett; and (3) a series of horizontal sections of the brain, alternately stained for cells and fibers.

The author has been fortunate in having the assistance of Doctors John W. Sundsten and Raymond D. Lund throughout all phases of the revision. Special recognition is accorded Dr. Sundsten for the reorganization and rewriting of Chapters 21 and 24, The Diencephalon and The Rhinencephalon; and to Dr. Lund for contributing Chapter 3, Histology and Cytology of Neurons and Neuroglia.

It is a privilege to acknowledge the contributions of Mr. Thomas Stebbins, Director of the Division of Health Sciences Illustration, and his staff to this revision, and again to Mr. George W. Reis for many of the photographs. Mrs. Doris E. Ringer, Publications Editor within the department and personal secretary to the author, is accorded a sincere and special note of appreciation for her valuable contributions throughout all aspects of this revision.

Acknowledgment is made to many teachers and students of neuroanatomy, who have used the previous edition, for their suggestions, many of which have been incorporated in this revision.

It is again a pleasure to acknowledge the support, patience, and cooperation of the publishers, Lea & Febiger, in making this revision.

N. B. EVERETT

Seattle, Washington

v

Preface to Fifth Edition

The four previous editions of *Functional Neuroanatomy* were prepared by Dr. A. R. Buchanan, Professor of Anatomy at the University of Colorado School of Medicine. Dr. Buchanan having recently retired from teaching has turned over the book to me. It is indeed a pleasure to revise this book in its fifth edition.

In this edition I have continued the policy of presenting the material necessary for understanding the structure and function of the nervous system in the least number of pages. Additionally, as in previous editions the longitudinal approach has been used in the presentation. For example, ascending and descending tracts are traced from origin to termination at the time they are first mentioned in the text. This approach, in my experience, has made the subject of neuroanatomy more stimulating and comprehensible to the student. A particular advantage of treatment in this way is to provide for an effective correlation with the study of neurophysiology which students often study concurrently with neuroanatomy. The practice of many schools, as has been the case here for many years, is for the anatomist and physiologist, with some support from the clinical neurologist, to join forces in offering a conjoint course in neuroanatomy and neurophysiology for medical and graduate students. Within this framework the longitudinal approach is par-

ticularly valuable to students and faculty in making the appropriate structural and functional correlations. The importance of regional considerations of the central nervous system is recognized, however, and in this edition a number of photographs of the various levels of the brain stem and spinal cord are interspersed throughout the text along with diagrams of the corresponding levels to provide more adequately for regional study. These photographs of sections, primarily of Weil-stained preparations, are well labeled and may be used in conjunction with the accompanying diagrams of sections. This combination allows for considerable flexibility in using the text in accord with varying needs for detailed study of the nuclei and fiber tracts of the brain stem and spinal cord. In addition to these photographs a number of new and improved drawings and diagrams have been added. These include several new half-tone and pen and ink drawings, line diagrams and 21 new color illustrations.

Major changes have been made in much of the text material. The chapter on development has been completely rewritten and a new chapter has been added on the genesis and histology of the neural elements which includes a consideration of nerve degeneration and regeneration. Treatment of tactile, pain, thermal, visceral, afferent and proprioceptive pathways has been combined into one chapter. The chapters on the motor systems have been rewritten and rearranged, bringing together the considerations of the extrapyramidal system and basal ganglia. The chapter on the cerebellum has been thoroughly revised, as well as the chapter on the diencephalon which includes a more complete treatise of the thalamus and hypothalamus. Another major change concerns a revision and expansion of the chapter on the rhinencephalon.

I gratefully acknowledge the contributions of three departmental associates to this edition. Chapter 2, "Development of the Nervous System," and Chapter 3, "Genesis and Histology of Neural Elements: Degeneration and Regeneration of Nerves" are the contributions of Dr. Bodemer. The rewriting and reorganization of the material incorporated in Chapter 5, "Somatic Tactile, Proprioceptive, Pain and Thermal Pathways: Visceral Afferent Pathways" are the contributions of Dr. Rieke. In addition, both Drs. Bodemer and Rieke have given general assistance throughout all phases of this revision. Dr. John W. Sundsten contributed significantly to Chapter 20, "The Diencephalon," particularly the section on the hypothalamus. He also made important suggestions for Chapter 23, "The Rhinencephalon."

I am grateful for the contributions made by the medical artists to this revision, particularly those of Miss Jessie Phillips, Director of Health Sciences Illustration and of Marjorie L. Domenowske who made many of the new drawings. The careful and efficient preparation of the manuscript and the valuable contribution to proofreading made by my secretary, Mrs. Doris E. Ringer, are deeply appreciated. Acknowledgment is made to Mr. George W. Reis for the newly added photographs of the brain stem and spinal cord sections.

Finally, I acknowledge the full cooperation of the publishers throughout the course of this revision.

N. B. EVERETT

Seattle, Washington

Contents

Chapter 1

Introduction to the Central and Peripheral Nervous Systems

The nervous system is responsible for maintaining contact between the individual and his external and internal environments and for the individual's proper adjustment to these environments. Contact with the external environment is maintained through receptors at the surface of the body and with the internal environment through receptors in muscles, joints, ligaments, and the visceral organs of the thorax and abdomen. Adjustments to the environment are facilitated by reflex arcs consisting of afferent neurons, centers within the spinal cord or brain, and effer-ent neurons. The efferent neurons carry motor impulses from the central nervous system to effector mechanisms including smooth and striated muscle (cardiac and skeletal) and glandular structures.

The adult nervous system may be divided into *central* and *peripheral divisions*. The **central nervous system** includes the spinal cord and brain (Figs. 1, 2, 3, 4). The main subdivisions of the brain are *cerebrum, cerebellum,* and *brain stem.* The brain stem consists of the *diencephalon, mesencephalon, pons,* and *medulla oblongata.*

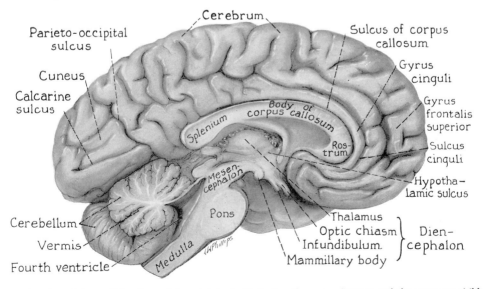

FIG. 1. Drawing of the medial surface of the adult brain illustrating the major divisions and the structures visible in a sagittal section.

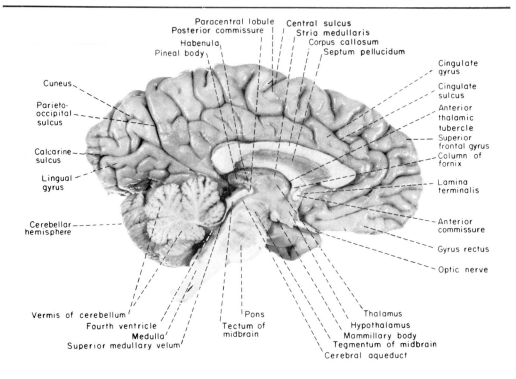

FIG. 2. Photograph of the medial surface of the adult brain cut in sagittal section.

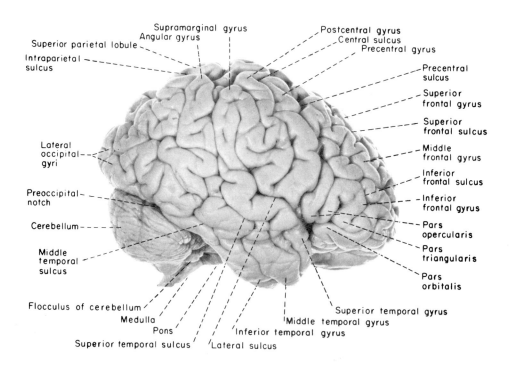

FIG. 3. Photograph of the lateral surface of the adult brain.

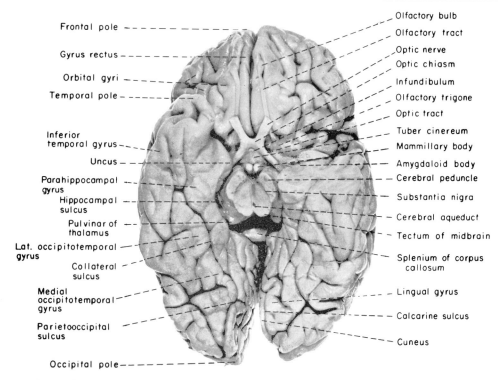

Frontal pole
Gyrus rectus
Orbital gyri
Temporal pole
Inferior temporal gyrus
Uncus
Parahippocampal gyrus
Hippocampal sulcus
Pulvinar of thalamus
Lat. occipitotemporal gyrus
Collateral sulcus
Medial occipitotemporal gyrus
Parietooccipital sulcus
Occipital pole

Olfactory bulb
Olfactory tract
Optic nerve
Optic chiasm
Infundibulum
Olfactory trigone
Optic tract
Tuber cinereum
Mammillary body
Amygdaloid body
Cerebral peduncle
Substantia nigra
Cerebral aqueduct
Tectum of midbrain
Splenium of corpus callosum
Lingual gyrus
Calcarine sulcus
Cuneus

FIG. 4. Photograph of the inferior surface of the adult brain. (The rostral portion of the left temporal lobe crd the brain stem caudal to the midbrain have been removed.)

The **peripheral nervous system** includes the spinal and cranial nerves and the numerous ganglia and plexuses concerned with visceral innervation. Each **spinal nerve** is attached to the spinal cord by two roots—a ventral, or anterior, and a dorsal, or posterior; these roots unite to form the spinal nerve which then divides into ventral and dorsal rami (Fig. 5). The anterior or ventral rami of the spinal nerves form the cervical, brachial, lumbar, sacral, and coccygeal plexuses and, in the thoracic region, the intercostal and subcostal nerves. The posterior or dorsal rami are distributed to the skin on the dorsal aspects of head, neck, and trunk and to the erector spinae group of muscles.

The *ventral roots* of all spinal nerves contain somatic efferent (motor) fibers which innervate skeletal muscles (Fig. 5). Those of the thoracic, upper lumbar, and middle sacral nerves also contain general visceral efferent fibers which end

in relation to ganglionic cells of the autonomic system and innervate visceral organs. The somatic efferent fibers arise from cells in the anterior (ventral) gray columns of the cord, and the general visceral efferent fibers arise from the lateral gray columns.

The *dorsal roots* contain general somatic afferent (sensory) and general visceral afferent fibers which originate in dorsal root ganglia cells. The single processes of these cells divide into peripheral and central divisions. The peripheral divisions of the processes of general somatic afferent neurons are distributed to somatic receptors by way of the spinal nerves; those of general visceral afferent neurons to visceral receptors by way of the spinal nerves and the various plexuses of the visceral nervous system. The central divisions of the processes of both somatic and visceral afferent neurons enter the spinal cord through the dorsal roots (Fig. 5).

The **cranial nerves** (Fig. 6) are less

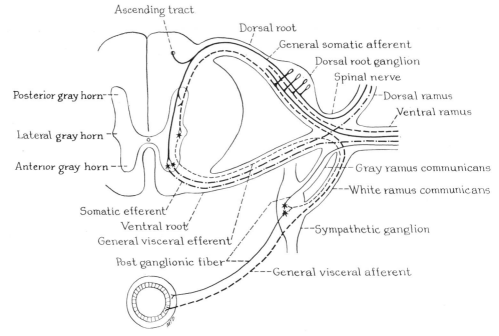

FIG. 5. Cross-section diagram of the thoracic spinal cord with a spinal nerve attached. The component fibers of the nerve are shown.

regular in their arrangement than the spinal nerves. Some have motor and sensory roots; some are entirely sensory in function; and at least one—the hypoglossal—is purely motor. Sensory ganglia, structurally and functionally analogous to the dorsal root ganglia of the spinal nerves, are associated with the sensory roots of cranial nerves. Sensory fibers terminate in and motor fibers originate from gray areas in the brain stem which are functional analogues of the gray columns in the spinal cord.

The *cranial* (or cerebral) and *spinal nerves* contain seven functional types of fibers: general somatic afferent, special somatic afferent, general visceral afferent, special visceral afferent, somatic efferent, general visceral efferent, and special visceral efferent. There are no special somatic efferent fibers and, as will be noted below, no given nerve contains all seven types of fibers.

General somatic afferent fibers are present in all the spinal nerves (except Cl which usually has no sensory root) and in a number of cranial nerves. Their cell bodies are in sensory ganglia, and they conduct impulses to the central nervous system from receptors in skin, muscle, and connective tissues.

Special somatic afferent fibers are found only in the optic and vestibulocochlear nerves. The fibers in the optic nerve conduct visual impulses from the retina to the brain and arise from cell bodies within the retina (Chap. 9). The vestibulocochlear nerve is composed of the axons of neurons whose cell bodies are in the spiral and vestibular ganglia (Chap. 9). The dendrites of these neurons are distributed to special receptors in the internal ear.

General visceral afferent fibers are present in the spinal nerves and in some of the cranial nerves. They are distributed to receptors in the visceral structures of the neck, thorax, abdomen, and pelvis, and to blood vessels and glandular structures everywhere. Their cells of origin are in the sensory ganglia of spinal nerves (Fig. 5, dorsal root ganglia) and in the ganglia

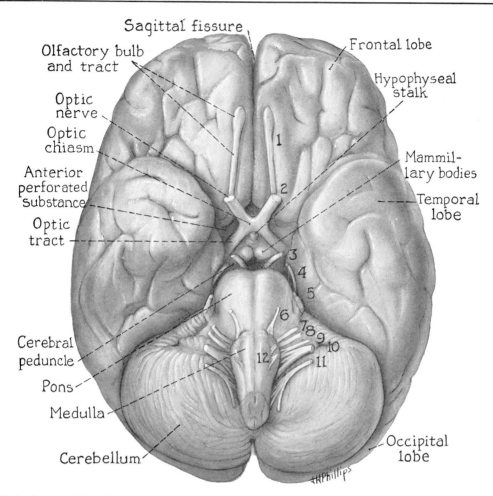

Saqittal fissure

Olfactory bulb
and tract

Optic
nerve

Optic
chiasm

Anterior
perforated
substance

Optic
tract

Frontal lobe

Hypophyseal
stalk

Mammil-
lary bodies

Temporal
lobe

1

2

3
4
5

6
7
8
9
10

12
11

Cerebral
peduncle

Pons

Medulla

Cerebellum

Occipital
lobe

FIG. 6. Drawing of the inferior surface of the brain.

of certain cranial nerves. General visceral afferent neurons function as afferent limbs of visceral reflex arcs and conduct impulses (particularly pain impulses) to the conscious level.

Special visceral afferent fibers are concerned only with the special senses of smell and taste; we therefore find them in the olfactory, glossopharyngeal, vagus, and facial nerves (nervus intermedius). The cell bodies of the olfactory nerves are in the olfactory mucous membrane, those of the facial nerves in the geniculate ganglia, and those of the glossopharyngeal and vagus nerves in the inferior ganglia of these nerves. The *inferior ganglion* of the glossopharyngeal nerve is located in a groove on the posterior aspect of the

petrosa of the temporal bone at the upper limit of the jugular foramen. The *inferior ganglion* (nodose) of the vagus is manifested by an ovoid enlargement on the nerve immediately inferior to its emergence from the jugular foramen. The geniculate ganglion is in the facial canal within the petrosa of the temporal bone (Chap. 8) and is so designated because of its association with the external genu of the facial nerve.

Somatic efferent fibers arise from motor nerve cells in the spinal cord and brain stem. They are distributed to striated muscles of mesodermal somite origin and are found in all spinal nerves and in the oculomotor, trochlear, abducens, and hypoglossal nerves. Their occurrence in these four cranial nerves is due to the presence of head and occipital somites in the embryo.

General visceral efferent fibers are present in the oculomotor, facial, glossopharyngeal, and vagus nerves, in all the thoracic nerves, in the upper two or three lumbar nerves, and in the middle three sacral nerves. They arise from cell bodies in certain nuclei of the brain stem and in the lateral gray columns of the spinal cord; they are distributed to the peripheral ganglia of the autonomic system (Fig. 5). The axons of the ganglion cells, on which they synapse, are then distributed to smooth muscle, cardiac muscle, and glands throughout the body.

The term *"special visceral efferent"* is unfortunate in that these fibers are distributed to striated or voluntary muscles, but only to those which originate from the mesoderm of the branchial or *visceral* arches. A more appropriate characterization would be *"branchial motor fibers."* The muscles supplied by these fibers include those of the larynx, pharynx, and soft palate, the muscles of mastication, and the muscles of expression. Special visceral efferent fibers are, therefore, found in the vagus, spinal accessory, glossopharyngeal, trigeminal, and facial nerves. The spinal accessory also supplies the trapezius and sternocleidomastoid muscles which are believed to be at least partly of branchial arch origin.

BIBLIOGRAPHY

Herrick, C. J., 1918: *An Introduction to Neurology,* W. B. Saunders Co., Philadelphia. (Re nerve components.)

Chapter 2

Development of the Nervous System

The human nervous system begins to develop during the third week of embryogenesis as an induced hyperplasia in the superficial ectoderm in the midline cephalic to Hensen's node (Fig. 7). This structure, the *neural plate,* gives rise to all divisions of the adult nervous system. Soon after its formation the neural plate is converted into a trough, the *neural groove;* the neural groove is bounded by prominent *neural folds,* which are most clearly defined in the extreme cranial end of the neural plate. During the first month of development, the neural folds grow from their dorsal borders, and continued overgrowth results in the approximation of the free edges of the folds. An apparent selective affinity of the constituent epithelial cells produces a fusion of the two neural folds with the consequent formation of a *neural tube.* The *neural crest* is a differentiation of cells at the lateral edge of each neural fold in a zone intermediate between the neural plate and skin ectoderm, which separates from the latter at the time the neural folds fuse. Closure of the neural groove does not occur simultaneously along the length of the embryo, but begins in the future thoracic region, progressing cranially and caudally. The ends of the neural tube remain open for some time at the *anterior* and *posterior neuropores.* The anterior neuropore finally closes at the 20-somite stage of development; the caudal end of the tube

is completely closed with obliteration of the posterior neuropore at the 25-somite stage. With completion of the neural tube, the neural epithelium is completely dissociated from the superficial ectoderm, and the tube lies bounded dorsally by the epidermis, ventrally by the notochord, and laterally by the mesodermal somites (Fig. 7). The neural crest cells form ear-like clusters at the dorsolateral borders of the neural tube, occupying the angle formed by the neural tube, superficial ectoderm, and mesoderm (Figs. 7, 8).

From the outset of development the cranial portion of the neural tube expands faster than the more caudal portions, and consequently, the prospective brain is clearly visible even before closure of the neuropores. Soon after the neural tube has closed, the brain is divisible into three prominent hollow swellings. These initial cavities are designated the *primary brain vesicles* (Fig. 9). The most cephalic vesicle is the *prosencephalon,* the middle vesicle is the *mesencephalon,* and the large caudal chamber is the *rhombencephalon.* The latter vesicle continues insensibly into the *myelon,* or future spinal cord. The three primary brain vesicles soon divide further into five *secondary brain vesicles* (Fig. 10). Thus, the prosencephalon is subdivided into the *telencephalon* and *diencephalon;* the rhombencephalon constricts to form the *metencephalon* and

2

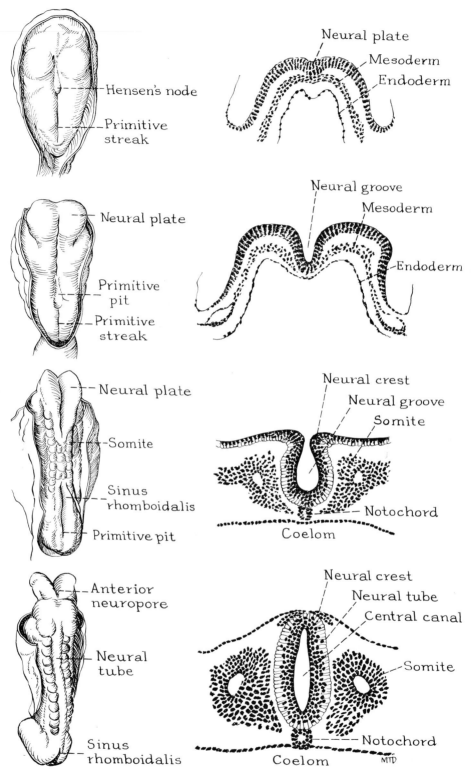

FIG. 7. Stages in the early development of the human nervous system from the presomite stage to closure of the
neural tube, except at the anterior and posterior neuropores (after Streeter). At left, the embryo is illustrated in
external view; at right, the same stage is shown in transverse section.

myelencephalon. The mesencephalon does not undergo further division.

Establishment of the five secondary brain vesicles completes the initial stages of development preparatory to differentiation of the various regions of the brain, and the derivatives of these several vesicles soon begin to form. The telencephalon gives rise to the *cerebral hemispheres, rhinencephalon,* and *corpus striatum,* and encloses the *lateral ventricles* and the fore-

most part of the third ventricle. The diencephalon gives origin to the various components of the *epithalamus, thalamus,* and *hypothalamus* in the adult brain, and encloses the major part of the third ventricle. The mesencephalon, containing the cerebral aqueduct, differentiates into the *corpora quadrigemina* and the *crura cerebri.* The *cerebellum* and *pons* arise from the metencephalon. The myelencephalon is represented in the adult by the *medulla*

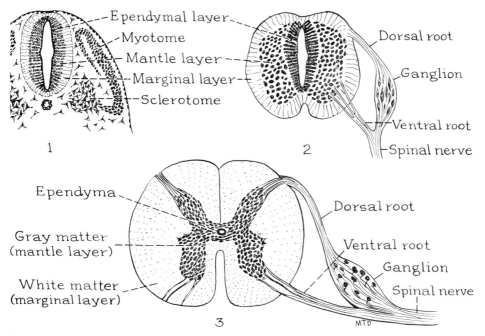

FIG. 8. Semidiagrammatic transverse sections of developing embryo illustrating the early development of the neural tube and formation of a spinal nerve.

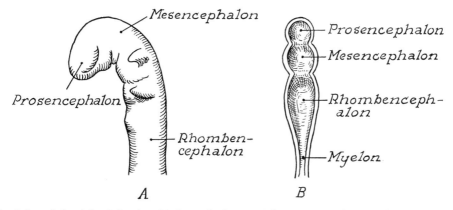

FIG. 9. A, Lateral view (after Pölitzer) and B, longitudinal section (after Arey) of early human brain. The three primitive brain vesicles are indicated.

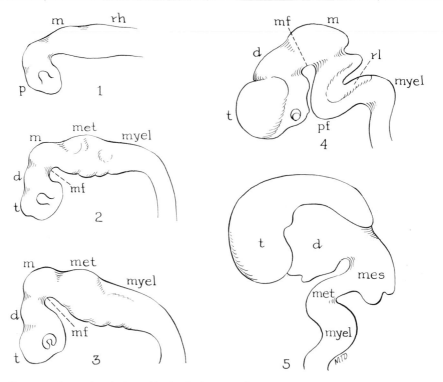

FIG. 10.   Flexures and secondary brain vesicles in the human embryo.

oblongata. The *fourth ventricle* extends through both metencephalon and myelencephalon. The boundaries between the secondary brain vesicles, never distinct, are further obscured in the adult brain by growth shiftings, elaboration of various structures from the ventricular walls, and the development of large fiber tracts, such as the *middle cerebellar peduncle* (*brachium pontis*) and *pyramids*. The original longitudinal continuity of the brain vesicles is indicated in the adult, however, by the brain *ventricles,* and the secondary vesicles of the embyronic brain provide a useful and commonly used frame of reference for analysis of the adult brain.

Mechanical factors are important determinants in the development of the nervous system. Thus, following closure of the neuropores, the neural tube is the most rapidly expanding element in the relatively enclosed cranial area. This expansion derives from growth, changes in vol-

ume attendant on cellular proliferation, growth in mass, and increased intraventricular pressure caused by accumulation of fluid secreted by the ependyma and the developing choroid plexuses. Between the fifth and sixth weeks of development an imbalance between the rate of neural expansion and available space manifests itself in the development of *flexures* of the brain (Fig. 10). During the fifth week, primarily because of increased cellular proliferation and intraventricular pressure, the growth rate of the cranial end of the embryonic brain greatly exceeds the growth rate of the mesenchyme condensed to form the skull resulting in the formation of a bend in the neural tube at the level of the mesencephalon, the *mesencephalic* (cephalic) *flexure* (Fig. 10). Increased pressure inside the loop of neural tube tends to displace the mesencephalon caudally, and in this way the mesencephalic flexure contributes to the formation of the dorsal *pontine flexure*

(Fig. 10). Rapid expansion of the cerebral hemispheres results in an accentuation of the pontine flexure. In the later stages of development both flexures are less prominent; retention of the mesencephalic flexure, however, explains the fact that, in the adult, the telencephalon and diencephalon are aligned perpendicularly to the longitudinal axis of the lower brain stem (Fig. 10). It also may be noted that the approximation of the free edges of the pontine flexure provides a favorable situation for the incorporation of the *rhombic lip* into the developing cerebellum.

The *myelon,* or spinal cord, is the least modified of the primary brain vesicles in the adult; it is valuable, therefore, in analysis of the fundamental organization of the central nervous system. Initially the spinal cord is an unsegmented tube, extending from the caudal end of the rhombencephalon to the tip of the embry-

onic tail. As the somatic mesoderm lateral to the neural tube segments into somites, a faint segmentation of the myelon becomes apparent. A fundamental metamerism is thus imposed on the myelon by segmentation of the mesoderm, and for each mesodermal somite there is a corresponding *neuromere,* or spinal cord segment. Each neuromere gives origin to a pair of spinal nerves which grow out on either side into the surrounding mesoderm and ectoderm. Once established, the relation of a nerve with peripheral structures, e.g., muscle, is thenceforth retained. Thus, although various distortions of the original neural metameric pattern often obscure them, the original neuromere-somite relation remains apparent through patterns of muscle innervation and the strips of cutaneous innervation designated as *dermatomes.* In the latter case the original segmental innervation pattern is modified greatly by the devel-

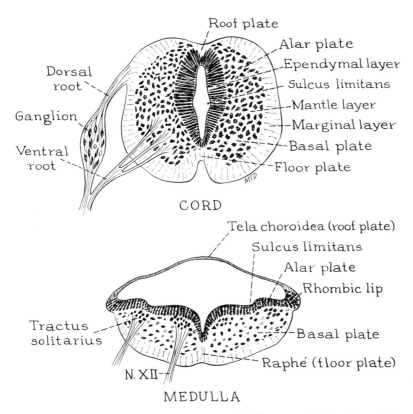

FIG. 11. Transverse sections of embryonic spinal cord and medulla illustrating similarity of organization.

opment and torsion of the limb buds and regression of the embryonic tail; the pattern is clearly apparent, however, in the band-like dermatomes of the trunk.

Early in its development the organization of the myelon permits analysis of its functional areas and the structural characteristics of the brain stem. A bilateral longitudinal furrow develops along the inner, luminal surface of the neural tube which is designated the *sulcus limitans* (Fig. 11) which divides each half of the neural tube into dorsal and ventral portions. That portion of the lateral wall of the neural tube located dorsal to the sulcus is called the *alar plate;* the lateral wall of the neural tube ventral to the sulcus limitans is designated the *basal plate.* The alar plates are connected across the dorsal midline by the *roof plate,* and the basal plates interconnect through the *floor plate.* These primary regions of the neural tube provide a means for analysis of the early topographical and functional organization of the spinal cord. The alar plate comprises the future sensory area of the spinal cord; the basal plate gives rise to the motor elements of the spinal cord. The roof plate and floor plate generally do not give origin to any prominent neural structures. The roof plate disappears with the formation of the *posterior median septum* of the spinal cord; the floor plate persists above the *anterior median fissure.* The basal and alar plates each differentiate into three layers: an inner *ependymal layer,* an intermediate *mantle layer,* and an outer *marginal layer* (Figs. 8, 11). The embryonic ependymal layer contains the germinal cells and, in the adult, forms the lining of the *central canal* of the spinal cord and the ventricles of the brain. The mantle layer becomes the *gray matter* of the spinal cord as cells accumulate from the proliferating ependymal elements. The marginal layer becomes the *white matter* of the spinal cord; it is formed by ascending and descending processes of nerve cells in the gray matter and nerve fibers entering from the dorsal root ganglia.

The relationship of gray and white matter in the adult spinal cord corresponds to that of the mantle and marginal layers in the developing neural tube. There is, however, considerable modification of the arrangement in the brain, as will become apparent in a later discussion of that part of the central nervous system.

As the free edges of the neural folds fuse to close the neural tube and the neural epithelium separates from the superficial ectoderm, the cells comprising the neural crest begin to migrate from the dorsolateral surface of the neural tube. Initially, neural crest cells are aligned as an unsegmented, loosely organized cellular sheet along the dorsolateral border of the myelon in the angle between the neural tube, the ectoderm, and the somites (Figs. 7, 8). The neural crest soon undergoes segmentation into discrete cellular condensations, corresponding to the neuromeres and mesodermal somites. These early cellular condensations are the primordia of the *dorsal root ganglia* of the spinal nerves. In addition to forming the spinal ganglia, neural crest cells also migrate ventrally and medially to contribute to the autonomic ganglia and the medulla of the adrenal gland. Neural crest cells also participate in formation of certain cranial nerve ganglia and, by inward migration, the mesencephalic nucleus of the trigeminal nerve.

The **spinal nerve** develops from cells located inside and outside the neural tube. The neurons formed in the spinal ganglia develop into pseudounipolar neurons; from the cell body a proximal fiber passes into the alar region of the developing spinal cord, and a distal fiber process proceeds laterally and ventrally to become part of the spinal nerve. The processes of the pseudounipolar neurons with cell bodies located in the spinal ganglia thus form most of the dorsal root of the spinal nerve. The dorsal root of a spinal nerve is therefore sensory in nature. The ventral root of the spinal nerve forms as the accumulation of nerve fibers emerging from the basal plate of the neural tube. These fibers represent the axis cylinders of multipolar motoneurons with cell bodies in the future anterior column of the spinal cord gray matter. The ventral root of a spinal nerve is thus motor in nature. The union of the dorsal and ventral roots effects the formation of the spinal nerve (Fig. 8). The *rami communicantes* are formed by nerve fibers emerging from cells located in the *intermediolateral column* of the spinal cord gray matter, the autonomic ganglia, and sensory neurons in the spinal ganglia. The connective tissue sheath of the nerve forms from mesodermal cells.

The organization of the neural tube according to alar and basal plates connected by roof and floor plates, respectively, is apparent in the brain as well as the spinal cord. The *sulcus limitans* is well developed in the myelencephalon (Fig. 11), separating basal plate from the laterally displaced alar plate. The greatly attenuated roof plate participates in formation of the choroid plexus; the floor plate is incorporated into the midline raphé. The distinction of the alar and basal plates according to sensory and motor function is valid also in the brain, and the disposition of sensory and motor nuclear groups in the brain stem may be thus ascertained. The basal plate probably does not extend rostral to the mammillary recess of the diencephalon, and the correlation of motor and sensory function according to the embryonic plates is not unreservedly applicable to the derivatives of the prosencephalon. The neural structures associated with the telencephalon and diencephalon appear to originate primarily from the embryonic alar plate.

The *myelencephalon* develops into the medulla oblongata of the adult brain. It is modified only slightly from the fundamental structure of the spinal cord. As in the medulla, the sulcus limitans forms the boundary between the dorsal, sensory region and the ventral, motor region of the metencephalon. The *tegmentum* of

the pons derives from the basal plate; the fibrous portion of the pons is an addition to the primary metencephalon consequent to the development of the cerebrum and cerebellum, and the development of large fiber tracts in the medulla and pons. The cerebellum is of bipartite origin. Part of the cerebellum develops from the rhombic lips located on each side of the fourth ventricle. Each *rhombic lip* is a thickened portion of the alar plate of the rhombencephalon developed at its junction with the roof plate. The pontine flexure causes the approximation of the rhombic lips (Fig. 10), enabling their fusion and growth to form the *flocculonodular lobe* of the cerebellum. The larger, phylogenetically younger, *corpus cerebelli* develops through fusion of the alar plates of the metencephalon cranial to the rhombic lips and the flocculonodular lobe. The *posterolateral fissure* is the line of demarcation between these two, embryologically distinct, portions of the cerebellum. The *tectum,* or *corpora quadrigemina,* of the mesencephalon develops from the alar plates of the embryonic mesencephalon; the tegmentum of the mesencephalon develops from the basal plates. The peduncular portion of the mesencephalon, like the fibrous pons, is added to the embryonic mesencephalon consequent to the development of large fiber tracts associated with the cerebral hemispheres. The diencephalon develops into three distinct regions. The epithalamus derives from the roof plate and upper ends of the alar plates; the choroid plexus of the third ventricle forms from the roof plate. The (dorsal) thalamus is formed from the alar plates of the diencephalon; its ventral border is defined by the hypothalamic sulcus. Although the *hypothalamic sulcus* is probably not homologous with the sulcus limitans, the hypothalamic nuclei develop inferior to it in the basal portion of the diencephalon. It may be questioned, however, whether this region represents the embryonic basal plates. The large cerebral hemispheres develop as

CORD

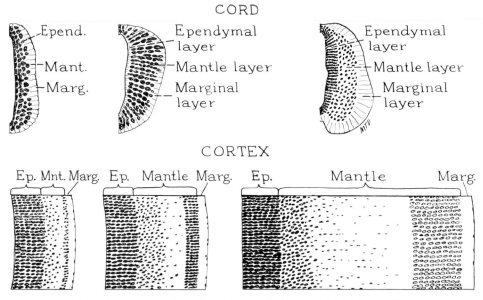

CORTEX

FIG. 12. Diagrams illustrating formation of spinal cord and cerebral cortex in the human embryo.

lateral evaginations from the telencephalon; they are derived from the alar plates. The *corpus striatum* arises from the inner walls of the telencephalic vesicles; and the *internal capsule* develops at the site where the corpus striatum undergoes a secondary fusion with the lateral walls of the diencephalon.

The **cerebral and cerebellar cortices** develop according to a distinctive pattern. It will be recalled that in the spinal cord proliferation of cells from the ependymal layer results in formation of the cellular mantle layer, and fibers elaborated by cells in the mantle layer accumulate to form an external marginal layer (Fig. 12). In the formation of the cerebral and cerebellar cortices, however, cells derived from germinal elements in the ependymal layer of the telencephalon and metencephalon, respectively, migrate centrifugally to establish a layer of cell bodies (gray matter) near the surface of the vesicle. Thus, in the cerebral cortex, cells migrate external to the mantle layer during the second month of development, establishing thereby a prominent layer of *pyramidal cells*. The primitive cortex therefore consists of an ependymal

layer, a relatively diffuse intermediate layer, a primitive pyramidal layer, and an outer marginal layer. During succeeding months, the innermost portion of the intermediate layer develops into the prominent central white mass of myelinated fibers. The external portion of the intermediate layer, the subdivided pyramidal layer, and the insignificant marginal layer comprise the definitive six-layered cerebral cortex of the adult brain (Fig. 12).

The developing nervous system is influenced by many factors, and its final configurations are the results of external, as well as internal, factors. Thus, the segmentation of the spinal cord and the metameric pattern of spinal nerve ganglia is essentially an imposed pattern, the result of segmentation of the mesoderm into somites. The size of certain areas of the spinal cord may depend also on external factors. The cervical and lumbosacral enlargements of the spinal cord are, for example, the direct expression of the large peripheral innervation derived from these segments of the cord and relate to the development of the limb buds at these levels. It should be noted further that an important factor in the final form assumed by the developing nervous system is a result of patterns of cell deaths during ontogeny.

BIBLIOGRAPHY

Arey, L. B., 1965: *Developmental Anatomy.* 7th ed. W. B. Saunders Co., Philadelphia.

Barron, D. H., 1948: Some effects of amputation of the chick wing bud on the early differentiation of the motor neuroblasts in the associated segments of the spinal cord. J. Comp. Neurol., *88,* 93–127.

Bergquist, H., and Källen, B., 1954: Notes on the early histogenesis and morphogenesis of the central nervous system in vertebrates. J. Comp. Neurol., *100,* 627–659.

Bodemer, C. W., 1968: *Modern Embryology.* Holt, Rinehart and Winston, Inc., New York.

Detwiler, S. R., 1936: *Neuroembryology.* The Macmillan Co., New York.

Hamburger, V., and Levi-Montalcini, R., 1949: Proliferation, differentiation and degeneration in the spinal ganglia of the chick embryo under normal and experimental conditions. J. Exp. Zool., *111,* 457–501.

Hamburger, V., and Levi-Montalcini, R., 1950: Some aspects of neuroembryology. In *Genetic Neurology,* Paul Weiss, Ed. University of Chicago Press, Chicago, pp. 128–160.

Hamilton, W. J., Boyd, J. D., and Mossman, H. W., 1964: *Human Embryology,* 3rd ed., rev. Williams & Wilkins Co., Baltimore.

Hammond, W. S., and Yntema, C. L., 1947: Depletions in the thoraco-lumbar sympathetic system following removal of neural crest in the chick. J. Comp. Neurol., *86,* 237–265.

Horstadius, S., 1950: *The Neural Crest.* Oxford University Press, London.

Kingsbury, B. F., 1922: The fundamental plan of the vertebrate brain. J. Comp. Neurol., *34,* 461–491.

Langman, J., 1969: *Medical Embryology,* 2nd ed. Williams & Wilkins Co., Baltimore.

Larsell, O., 1947: The development of the cerebellum in man in relation to its comparative anatomy. J. Comp. Neurol., *87,* 85–129.

Patten, B. M., 1968: *Human Embryology,* 3rd ed. Blakiston Div., McGraw-Hill Book Co., New York.

Sauer, F. C., 1935: Mitosis in the neural tube. J. Comp. Neurol., *62,* 377–405.

Sidman, R. L., Miale, I. L., and Feder, N., 1959: Cell proliferation and migration in the primitive ependymal zone; an autoradiographic study of histogenesis in the nervous system. J. Exp. Neurol., *1,* 322–333.

Weiss, P. A., 1955: Nervous system (neurogenesis). In *Analysis of Development,* B. H. Willier, P. A. Weiss, and V. Hamburger, Eds. W. B. Saunders Co., Philadelphia, pp. 346–401.

Chapter 3

Histology and Cytology of Neurons and Neuroglia

The nervous system is composed of two cell types, *nerve cells (or neurons)* and *neuroglial cells* (often simply called glial cells), both derived from the ectoderm. The neurons are concerned with conduction whereas the neuroglial cells perform a variety of secondary functions.

Both cell types differentiate from a basic cell type—the *matrix cell* (Fig. 13). Initially the matrix cells line the ventricular canal as neurectodermal cells. In the first stage of histogenetic development, these cells divide and migrate away from the central canal. In the second stage,

some cells differentiate into *neuroblasts,* or primitive neurons, which lose the capacity to divide, but still are capable of migration. In the third stage which can continue postnatally for a short period in some animals, matrix cells differentiate into *glioblasts*. These cells (sometimes called spongioblasts) differentiate into the mature neuroglial forms. Some of these cells may persist in the adult brain.

Most neurons are specialized for receiving information, for computing it, and then transmitting it to other cells. If the information is received directly from

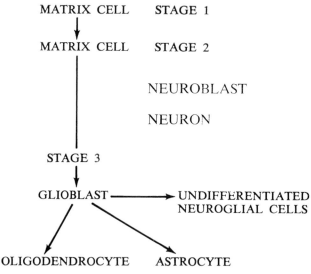

FIG. 13. Cell lineage in the central nervous system.

the external or internal environment, the cell is called a *receptor neuron;* if it directly influences cells other than nerve cells—glandular or muscle cells—the neuron is called an *effector neuron.* The general organization of receptor and effector neurons is, however, similar to that of the regular neurons of the central nervous system.

A typical neuron (Fig. 14a) has a central region where the nucleus is situated called the *cell body* or *soma* (sometimes rather carelessly called the *cell*). The term perikaryon refers to the cytoplasm around the nucleus rather than the whole region. One or more processes—*dendrites*—extend from the cell body. They are characteristically wide at their origin becoming gradually narrower farther away. They often have small outpouchings—*dendritic spines*—and these outpouchings as well as regions on the surface of the rest of the dendrite (and of the cell body) are the sites where the neuron receives most of its information from other cells. Receptor cells also have a process which can be equated with the dendrite whose primary function is to transduce physical parameters into electrical events which can be recognized and handled at the computing center of the cell. This results in some specializations in its morphology and relations. Further, there is often a considerable distance from the site where the receptor (dendritic) process is effective to the cell body, which means that the dendrite must be considerably elongated. Such is the case with the cutaneous receptor processes, there being as much as 1 meter from the peripheral processes (often misleadingly called nerve endings) to the cell body situated in the dorsal root ganglion adjacent to the spinal cord. The conduction process

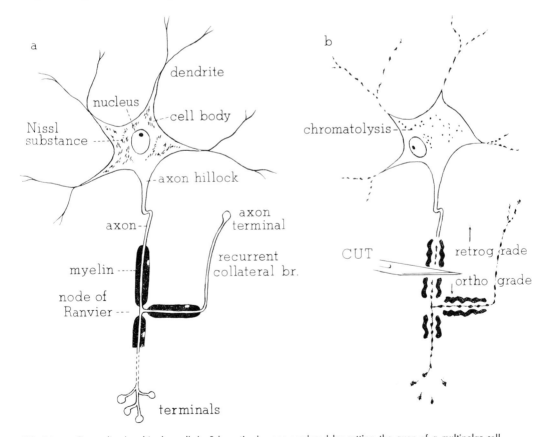

FIG. 14. a, Generalized multipolar cell. b, Schematic changes produced by cutting the axon of a multipolar cell.

characteristic of dendrites decays with distance, so that the peripheral processes of such sensory neurons, to be effective, show many of the characteristics of axons, in transmitting action potentials and having a myelin wrapping.

One further process, the *axon,* arises from the cell body at a region called the *axon hillock.* The axon is distinguished from the dendrites by being narrower at its origin and by being much longer. It branches copiously and forms contacts with other neurons at *synapses* or with muscles at *motor end plates.*

Nerve cells are classified according to the number and pattern of processes arising from the cell body. The first type of

nerve cell is the *unipolar cell* (Fig. 15a) with only one process arising from the cell body. It is found quite commonly during development, but in the adult mammalian brain it is restricted to certain sites. For example, many of the amacrine cells of the retina fall in this category; the single process divides into a number of smaller branches. Each branch may function both as an axon and a dendrite because it both receives and transmits information. Since the cell has no definitive axon it is called an *anaxonic cell.*

The second type of nerve cell is the *bipolar cell* (Fig. 15b). This cell has one axon and one primary dendrite. Again, it is not common in the adult mammalian

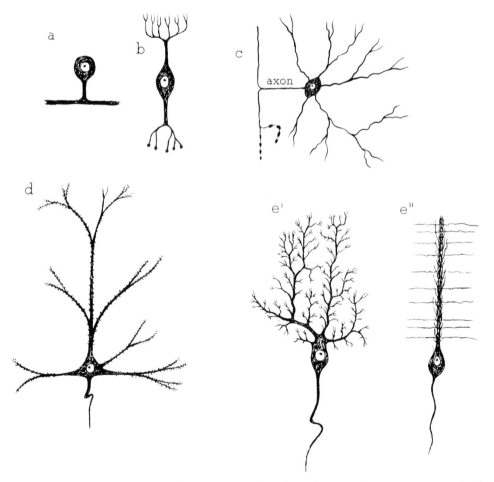

FIG. 15.   Generalized cell types: a, Unipolar (or pseudounipolar); b, Bipolar; c, Multipolar—stellate; d, Multipolar—pyramidal; e', Purkinje cell of cerebellum cut in a plane perpendicular to the parallel fibers; e", Purkinje cell of cerebellum cut in the plane of the parallel fibers.

nervous system. It includes many receptor neurons and some of the neurons connected with them. One example of the latter is the bipolar cell of the retina. Two types of bipolar receptor neurons can be defined, one in which the receptor process itself is modified for transducing a specific physical parameter of the environment into an electrical event, and the other in which the tissue around the sensory process is modified for this purpose. In the former group are the retinal receptor cells, the rods and cones. Here the outer part of the receptor process, the outer segment (a modified cilium), has an elaborately invaginated surface membrane forming plates which increase the chance of small amounts of light activating the cell. In the latter group are the cutaneous receptors. The peripheral processes of the cutaneous nerves (whose cell bodies lie in the dorsal root ganglion) may lie in the dermis or epidermis with no special investing tissue (Fig. 16A) and in this site may be activated by a variety of stimuli. The processes instead may lie around special structures such as hair roots (Fig. 16F) and are excited only when the hair is displaced. The third possibility is that the terminal part may be *encapsulated* with a special cell type, and this capsule, in some cases at least, may be responsible for specifying the effective input. One obvious type, the Pacinian corpuscle (Fig. 16H), consists of laminae of epithelial cells about 1 μ thick wrapped over the terminal part of the nerve to give the appearance of an onion skin. This type is specific for deep pressure. A further type, Merkel's disc (Fig. 16E), consists of an association of a group of terminal processes of a nerve and

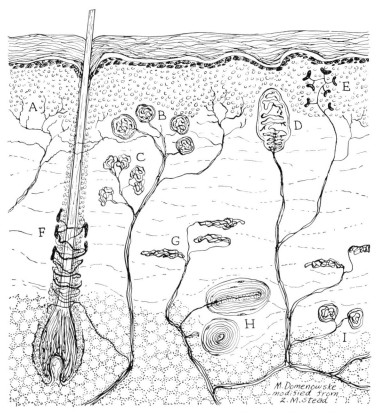

FIG. 16. Composite diagram showing various receptors associated with human skin. Modified from Stead (Wollard, Weddell, and Harpman). A, "Free" nerve endings; B, Krause's end bulbs; C, Ruffini's endings; D, Meissner's corpuscles; E, Merkel's discs; F, nerve fibers and endings on hair follicle; G, Ruffini's endings; H, Pacinian corpuscles; I, Golgi-Mazzoni endings.

of epithelial cells. Its specific physiological characteristics are unclear, and its relation to a series of quite similar formations—Krause end bulbs (Fig. 16B), Ruffini corpuscles (Fig. 16C)—is far from settled. It is apparent that each does not necessarily carry a specific modality, such as touch, heat, pain, and, possibly, that each may represent different stages of the same structure.

Some cells which are bipolar during development, later become unipolar, the dendrite and axon moving around from opposite poles and fusing to form one process leading from the cell body, which divides shortly afterwards. This type, a modification of a bipolar cell type which appears more like a unipolar cell type, is called a *pseudounipolar cell*. The major example of this type is the primary sensory neuron with its cell body in the dorsal root ganglion.

The third class of neurons (and this comprises the largest number of nerve cells) is termed a *multipolar cell*. The cells have one axon and more than one dendrite arising from the cell body. A number of different varieties are classified according to the configuration of the dendrites.

Neurons in which the dendrites radiate from all sides in a roughly symmetrical pattern are called multipolar. (This is somewhat confusing, being the same term as that applied to the whole class.) Effector cells, such as the anterior horn cells of the spinal cord or the cells of autonomic ganglia, fall in this category. Cells of similar appearance but usually of smaller size occurring in areas such as the cerebral cortex are termed *stellate (or star) cells* (Fig. 15c).

Another multipolar cell of some significance is the *pyramidal cell* (Fig. 15d). This cell has a pyramidally shaped body with a large dendrite as much as 2 mm long arising from the apex of the pyramid. This is the *apical dendrite* as opposed to smaller dendrites arising around the base of the pyramid called *basal dendrites*.

Such cells are found particularly in the cerebral cortex and hippocampus.

The significance of cell shape is related closely to the functional requirements of the cell and the organization of the inputs. The anaxonic cell appears to correlate series of paralleled units. The bipolar cell integrates the activity from one paralleled group and transmits it to the next paralleled group. The multipolar cell receives large numbers of inputs from widely different sources. The branching patterns of the cells may determine how the inputs are integrated. In other cases one major input may run in a specific direction, and the dendritic field may be specially oriented to receive a maximum number of contacts from that input. This is especially clear for the Purkinje cells of the cerebellum. Here a major input to the apical dendrites—the parallel fibers—runs in one plane while the dendrites are fanned out perpendicular to the fibers. When viewed perpendicular to the fibers, the dendritic field appears very extensive (Fig. 15e'), but when viewed in sections cut in the plane of the fibers, a single bundle of apical dendritic branches is seen (Fig. 15e'').

Electron microscopic studies reveal that nerve cells have many of the components of other cells. In the perikaryal region are large clumps of granular reticulum as well as free polyribosomal complexes. These regions often are separated by areas containing microtubules (called neurotubules in nervous tissue) and other protein strands about 90 Å in diameter called neurofilaments. The granular reticulum extends into at least the proximal parts of dendrites but not into the axon hillock or axon proper. Microtubules occur throughout most parts of the neuron, whereas the presence and distribution of neurofilaments are extremely variable depending on the cell. Neurofilaments frequently occur in the axon and sometimes in the axon terminal, where they form a ring. There are areas of Golgi apparatus in the cell body and larger dendrites. One

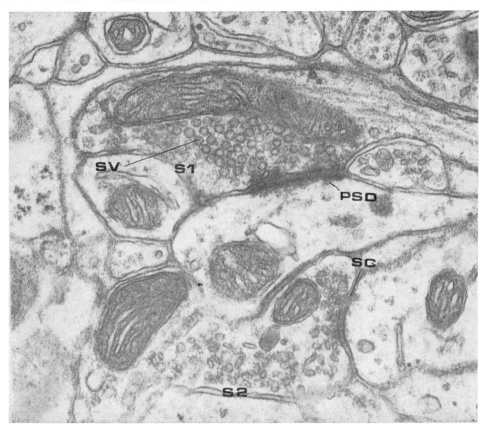

FIG. 17. An electron micrograph of synapses in the central nervous system. SV, synaptic vesicles; SC, synaptic cleft; PSD, postsynaptic density. Synapse S1 has round vesicles in the axon terminal and a well-pronounced postsynaptic density; synapse S2 has flattened vesicles in the axon terminal and a poorly defined synaptic density.

group of specializations not shared by non-nervous cells are the features of the synapse (Fig. 17). In the axon terminal, the presynaptic process, are vesicles of transmitter substance. These may be round and about 500 Å in diameter, or (with some fixatives) flattened and about 150 Å by 300 Å. These vesicles may have no contents visible with regular stains. Correlative studies have shown that round vesicles in some terminals contain acetylcholine (often an excitatory transmitter), while flattened vesicles in other terminals contain γ-aminobutyric acid (GABA) (an inhibitory transmitter). In addition, some terminals also contain vesicles with granular centers which often can be correlated with the presence of norepinephrine.

A special contact site occurs between the presynaptic and dendritic, or other postsynaptic, process. This site allows for adhesion of the two processes and functions as a site for release and reception of transmitted substance. The site consists of a cleft of 100 to 250 Å, containing filaments in some instances and a density on the cytoplasmic aspect. This is often particularly pronounced on the postsynaptic side when the presynaptic vesicles are round, but less clearly defined when they are flattened. In the process of chemical transmission at axon terminals, the contents of the synaptic vesicles are released at the presynaptic membrane, cross the synaptic cleft, and cause membrane permeability changes at the postsynaptic site. Local enzymes produced by the postsyn-

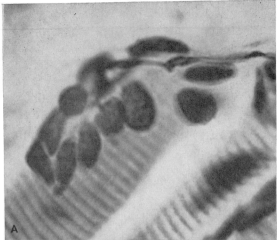

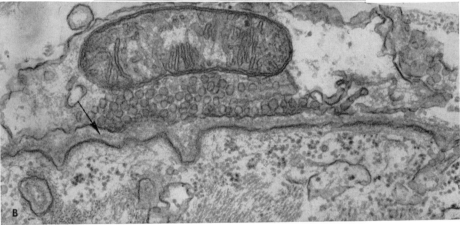

FIG. 18. A, Motor end plate on striated muscle (courtesy of Dr. C. E. Blevins). B, An electron micrograph of a neuromuscular junction. In addition to the features of the central nervous synapse, note the presence of a basal lamina (arrow) in the synaptic cleft. (Courtesy of Dr. D. E. Kelly.)

aptic cell deactivate the transmitter so that its effect will not spread beyond the required site. The connection made between axon terminals and striated muscles, the motor end plate (Fig. 18A, B), is comparable to the synapses between neurons. The difference is that a basal lamina exists between the ectodermal axon terminal and the mesodermal muscle cell, thus widening the synaptic cleft to 650 Å. The muscle membrane is invaginated by junctional folds, and it is generally opposite each of these folds that a specific aggregation of synaptic vesicles may be found in the axon terminal. The termination of an axon on a smooth muscle cell resembles more closely the synapse of nerv-

ous tissue; the presence of a basal lamina interposed between the pre- and postsynaptic membranes being variable.

The appearance of nerve cells under the light microscope is dependent on the techniques used, and, since many staining methods are specific for certain components, they often give a very limited view of nerve cells. One method of particular value, the Golgi technique, stains all parts of single neurons but only a small percentage of the total number of neurons. This allows visualization of single cells without interference from adjacent cells and permits classification of neurons as described above.

The most widely used stains, cresyl

violet and thionine generally termed Nissl stains, show granular reticulum and polyribosomal complexes of the cell body and proximal dendrites. Such material in the cell body is termed Nissl substance, and in degenerative states may break down (a feature which is termed *chromatolysis*).

Another set of stains, the neurofibrillar methods, shows the neurofilaments of electron microscopy. They include the Bielschowsky, Cajal, Bodian, Holmes and Glees techniques. They show axonal patterns, some dendritic formations, and some normal axonal terminals. Axonal terminals are also shown by some Golgi methods as well as by techniques which are particularly sensitive to the mitochondria of terminals such as the Rasmussen method.

The second cell type of the nervous system is the neuroglial cell. With the light microscope these can be shown sometimes by Golgi methods, and specifically by modifications of Cajal methods such as that of Río Hortega. The nuclei and cytoplasm can be shown to some extent by Nissl methods, but since this stain shows little of the total extent of the cell, use of the method often leads

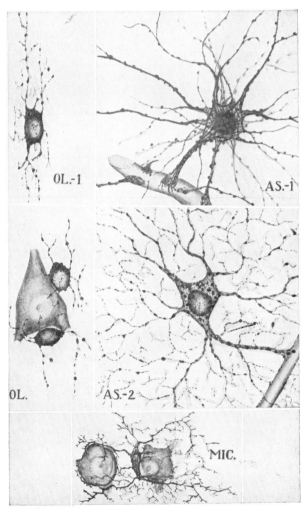

FIG. 19.   Interstitial cells of the central nervous system. AS-1, Fibrous astrocyte with perivascular feet on vessel; AS-2, Protoplasmic astrocyte; MIC., Microglia; OL., Oligodendroglia. (Penfield and Cone, in Cowdry's *Special Cytology*, courtesy of Paul B. Hoeber, Inc.)

3

to ambiguities of identification. The variability inherent in the other methods for showing neuroglia has led to much confusing and contradictory literature stemming from light microscope studies of their form, classification, and behavior. The use of the electron microscope has helped considerably although there are still basic problems which need to be resolved.

Two glial types are usually defined—macroglia and microglia (Fig. 19). The macroglia are of three types: astroglia (astrocytes), oligodendroglia (or oligodendrocytes) of the central nervous system, and Schwann cells of the peripheral nervous system.

The astrocytes (Figs. 19, 20A) have a series of radiating processes in a star-like configuration. They are often the size of

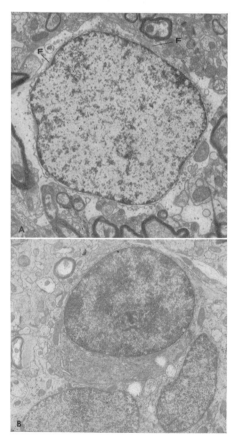

FIG. 20. A, Electron micrograph of an astrocyte showing astrocytic filaments (F) in the cytoplasm. B, Electron micrograph of an oligodendrocyte.

neurons, but are distinguished by the irregular outline and extensive branching of processes. With the use of the electron microscope, processes of astrocytes can be seen ramifying between neuronal profiles in a completely erratic manner. The cytoplasm stains palely and has few microtubules or ribosomes. In some cases (particularly in reactive states), it may contain bundles of fine filaments which are thinner than neurofilaments and do not stain with the usual neurofibrillar methods. Their presence has produced classification of astrocytes into protoplasmic (without filaments) and filamentous (with filaments), but since their presence in any one cell may depend on the state of the cell, this division may be artificial. The nucleus of astrocytes has a distinct nucleolus but no clumped chromatin.

Astrocytes often have processes (end feet) adjacent to the endothelium of capillaries (Fig. 17), and this has implicated them in a system of rapid transport of metabolites. Labeling studies show, however, that this is not the preferential path followed by some molecules. Similar studies also show that, contrary to earlier work, the barrier preventing certain molecules from passing from blood stream to brain tissue, the so-called blood-brain barrier, is a property of the endothelial cell itself rather than of the astrocytic end feet surrounding the capillary. Astrocytes often have been invoked as the skeletal element of the nervous system, and also seem to function in providing insulation between adjacent neuronal processes so preventing "cross talk." They play an important part in the removal of degenerative debris of damaged neurons. In addition, they, and perhaps also the oligodendrocytes, have been implicated in the uptake of extracellular potassium ions produced during depolarization of the neuronal membrane.

Oligodendrocytes (literally, cells with few branches) (Fig. 20B) resemble small stellate neurons and can sometimes be confused with them. They have a round nucleus with irregular chromatic clumps and nucleolus which can be seen with Nissl stains. The cytoplasm contains abundant microtubules and ribosomes. These cells are often found adjacent to neurons, where they are called satellite cells, and in bundles of myelinated axons. The myelin is, in fact, a wrapping of surface membrane of the oligodendrocyte around the axon, leaving a sheet of paired membranes, face to face, rolled around the axon, with little or no cytoplasm in between each successive roll (Fig. 21).

When viewed in longitudinal section a nerve shows discontinuities in its myelin coat. These discontinuities are called nodes of Ranvier and represent the border between two adjacent myelin-forming oligodendrocytes. The nodes usually have a small area of bare axon which allows the ion transfer necessary for saltatory conduction. A heavily myelinated axon has a larger number of membrane rings whereas a lightly myelinated axon has fewer. An unmyelinated axon lies indented in the surface of a neuroglial cell, either with several others in one indentation or singly.

In the peripheral nervous system, the Schwann cell plays an essentially similar role in relation to myelin formation and in its relationship to unmyelinated axons. Any free nerve endings of sensory neurons lying within the dermis are always surrounded by a thin sheet of Schwann cell cytoplasm.

Microglia present a great problem in interpretation, owing to the continued failure to identify clearly such types with the electron microscope. Many light microscopic studies have suggested them to be of mesodermal origin. Recent electron microscopic studies have shown a type of neuroglial cell which is neither oligodendrocyte nor astrocyte and may represent an undifferentiated state that with a suitable stimulus, such as neuronal degeneration, may divide and function as a phagocyte. This is a likely candidate for the "microglial" cell.

The reactions to damage of the nervous system involve both neurons and neuroglial cells, and may vary considerably depending, among other things, on how extensive the damage is and which part of the neuron is involved.

The simplest trauma is that of a cut dividing an axon as shown in Figure 14b. Changes occurring distal to the cut (between the cut and the axon terminal) are called *orthograde, descending,* or *Wallerian degeneration.* The degeneration breaks the axon into discontinuous beads and causes changes in the axon terminal. The terminal may shrink and the cytoplasm become densely staining as shown by electron microscopy. Such changes can be shown specifically by the Nauta techniques of light microscopy (Fig. 23). They have a time course extending from several days to several weeks (and even months). Other terminals fill up with neurofilaments and the changes can be shown with neurofibrillar methods (Figs. 22A, B). They are rather short-term and are possibly replaced in time by the dense reaction. The degeneration reaction of axon terminals is accompanied by a great increase in size of the cytoplasm of adjacent astrocytes (in the CNS) or of

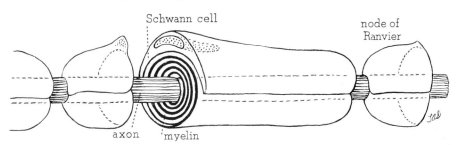

FIG. 21. Diagram of the wrapping of the Schwann cell forming a myelin sheath around a peripheral axon.

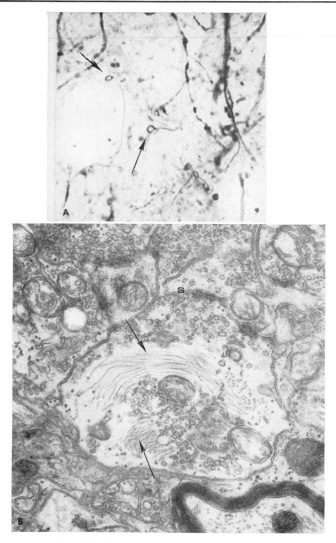

FIG. 22.   A, Degenerative terminal neurofibrillar rings (arrows). B, An electron micrograph showing neurofilaments forming part of a ring (arrows) in nerve terminal, taken from the same region as in a. There is a synaptic contact at S.

Schwann cell cytoplasm in the peripheral nervous system. The astrocytic cytoplasm more commonly contains bundles of filaments and scattered glycogen granules than does normal tissue.

In the myelinated part of the axon following trauma there is some delamination and general disruption of the ordered structure of the myelin, and this becomes broken down within the cytoplasm of the oligodendrocyte from which it was formed. In the peripheral nervous system the tube of cytoplasm is maintained for

some time so that a new axon may grow along it.

The changes in the cell body and the parts of the neuron proximal to the cut are called *retrograde degeneration*. The most obvious changes are the dispersion of Nissl substance (termed chromatolysis) and the frequent displacement of the nucleus to an eccentric position (Fig. 14b). Additional retrograde changes, stained by Nauta methods, include disintegration of the dendrites and of the axon proximal to the cut. If the neuron is able

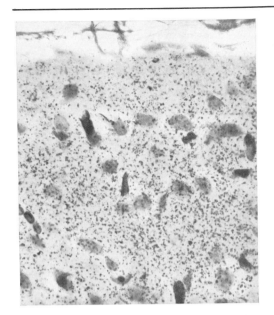

FIG. 23. Fink-Heimer modification of Nauta stain showing degeneration granules with the light microscope.

to regenerate a new axon, the Nissl substance will ultimately return to its former appearance. If regeneration is not possible, the cell body will shrink and be removed by neuroglial cells. If numbers of cell bodies are dying, there will be a massive increase in the number of neuroglia in the area termed *gliosis*. The neuroglial cells involved include astrocytes and probably oligodendrocytes already in the area as well as "microglial" cells.

Damage to a cell body and its terminals sometimes results in shrinkage of the cell onto which its terminals project. This is called *transneuronal degeneration* and can sometimes be produced by functional deafferentiation rather than a lesion. For example, transneuronal degeneration occurs in the lateral geniculate nucleus after an eye has been removed. A similar change can be induced in an experimental animal if it is kept in the dark from birth, or even if the eyelids are kept closed during a critical period of development.

The possibilities for regeneration are quite limited in the mammalian nervous system, although less so in Amphibia, for example. If a peripheral nerve is cut,

there is a good chance that a reasonable percentage of axons of motor neurons in the spinal cord and of sensory processes of cell bodies in the dorsal root ganglion will re-establish their original connections, so that, for example, stimulation of one motor neuron will result in the same movement as before the cut. Such specificity of connections, although not absolute, is, nevertheless, quite remarkable. The number of successful regenerating axons is always increased if scar tissue is removed at the cut and if the cut ends are approximated. It is even better if, rather than being cut, the nerve is only crushed.

Within the central nervous system, growth of axons across a cut is minimal, the failure being largely related to the nature of the neuroglial cells rather than the neurons themselves. There is evidence, however, that once degenerated axon terminals are removed from their synaptic site, other terminals may replace them, and this replacement could represent a structural basis for some of the return of function that is common following a neurologic lesion.

BIBLIOGRAPHY

Beresford, W. A., 1966: An evaluation of neuroanatomical methods and their relation to neurophysiology. Brain Res., *1*, 221–249.

Bodian, D., and Mellors, R. C., 1945: The regenerative cycle of motoneurons. J. Exp. Med., *81*, 469–488.

Bunge, R. P., 1968: Glial cells and the central myelin sheath. Physiol. Rev., *48*, 197–251.

Cajal, S. R., 1954: (English translation) Neurone theory or reticular theory? Consejo Superior de Investigaciones Cientificas, Instituto Ramon y Cajal, Madrid.

Galambos, R., Editor, 1964: Section on Glial Cells. Neurosciences Research Program Bulletin, *1*, 375–436. M.I.T. Press, Cambridge.

Grant, G., and Westman, J., 1968: Degenerative changes in dendrites central to axonal transection. Experientia, *24*, 169–170.

Gray, E. G., and Guillery, R. W., 1966: Synaptic morphology in normal and degenerating nervous system. Int. Rev. Cytol., *19*, 111–182.

Matthews, M. R., Powell, T. T. S., and Cowan, W. M., 1960: Transneuronal cell degeneration in the lateral geniculate nucleus of the macaque monkey. J. Anat., *94,* 145–168.

Mori, S., and Leblond, C. P., 1970: Electron microscopic identification of three classes of oligodendrocytes and a preliminary study of their proliferative activity in the corpus callosum of young rats. J. Comp. Neurol., *139,* 1–30.

Mugnaini, E., and Walberg, F., 1964: Ultrastructure of neuroglia. Ergebn. Anat. Entwickel., *137,* 193–236.

Porter, K., and Bonneville, M., 1964: *An Introduction to the Fine Structure of Cells and Tissues.* Lea & Febiger, Philadelphia.

Vaughn, J. E., and Peters, A., 1968: A third neuroglial cell type. An electron microscopic study. J. Comp. Neurol., *133,* 269–288.

Wiesel, T. N., and Hubel, D. H., 1963: Effects of visual deprivation on the morphology and physiology of cells in the cat's lateral geniculate body. J. Neurophysiol., *26,* 978–993.

Chapter 4

The Spinal Cord

GROSS TOPOGRAPHY

The spinal cord is contained within the spinal canal. The cord begins at the level of the upper border of the atlas, where it is continuous with the medulla oblongata of the brain, and extends caudally to the level of the disc between the first and second lumbar vertebrae in the adult (Fig. 24). However, its caudal extent may vary from the twelfth thoracic to the third lumbar vertebrae (Fig. 24).

The diameter of the spinal cord is small compared with the diameter of the spinal canal; this space is filled with the three meningeal coverings that surround the spinal cord. From the cord outward, the coverings are the pia mater, the arachnoid mater, and the dura mater (Fig. 25). The *pia mater* closely invests the spinal cord and is reflected into it along the courses of the blood vessels which supply it. The *arachnoid mater,* as its name implies, is spider-web-like in character; it is separated from the pia mater by the *subarachnoid space* which is normally filled with cerebrospinal fluid. The *dura mater* is the outermost covering and is separated from the arachnoid mater by the *subdural space.* It is surrounded by a thick layer of *epidural fat* containing the epidural plexus of veins. The dura mater extends caudally beyond the lower limit of the spinal cord, or to the level of the disc between the second and third sacral vertebrae, forming the *dural cul-de-sac*

(Fig. 24). The cul-de-sac is lined with arachnoid mater and contains cerebrospinal fluid. Lumbar puncture needles are usually introduced into the dural cul-de-sac for withdrawal of cerebrospinal fluid for diagnostic examination and for injection of therapeutic solutions or spinal anesthetics. This area is obviously chosen because the needle can be introduced without danger of damage to the spinal cord.

The *filum terminale* is a pia-glial process which begins at the lower end of the spinal cord and extends downward through the dural cul-de-sac and spinal canal; it is attached inferiorly to the dorsal surface of the coccyx and thus serves to anchor the spinal cord. Within the cul-de-sac the filum is surrounded by the lower lumbar and sacral nerves as they pass from the spinal cord to their foramina of exit. The lumbar and sacral nerves, surrounding the filum terminale and conus medullaris, constitute the *cauda equina.*

In **cross-section** the spinal cord is seen to have an H-shaped, centrally placed area of gray matter which is surrounded by white matter (Fig. 27). The two halves of the gray matter are connected across the midline by the *anterior* and *posterior gray commissures*—so named because of their relationships to the central canal. Posteriorly, division of the cord into right and left halves is indicated by the *posterior median septum* which is con-

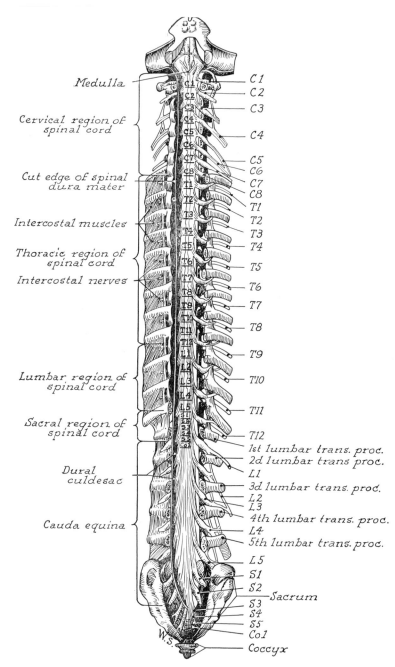

Medulla

Cervical region of
spinal cord

Cut edge of spinal
dura mater

Intercostal muscles

Thoracic region of
spinal cord

Intercostal nerves

Lumbar region of
spinal cord

Sacral region of
spinal cord

Dural
culdesac

Cauda equina

C1
C2
C3
C4
C5
C6
C7
C8
T1
T2
T3
T4
T5
T6
T7
T8
T9
T10
T11
T12

1st lumbar trans. proc.
2d lumbar trans. proc.
L1
3d lumbar trans. proc.
L2
L3
4th lumbar trans. proc.
L4
5th lumbar trans. proc.
L5
S1
S2
S3   Sacrum
S4
S5
Co1
Coccyx

W.S.

FIG. 24. Dorsal view of the spinal cord in situ with vertebral laminae removed to show the relation of the spinal cord segments to the vertebral column (after Tilney and Riley).

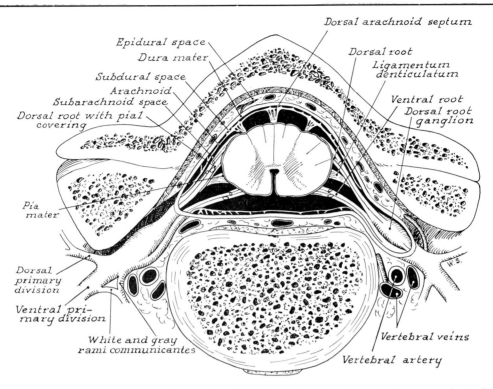

FIG. 25. Cross-section of spinal cord in the spinal canal showing meningeal coverings and the manner of exit of the spinal nerves (after Rauber).

tinuous with the pia mater. On the anterior side the two halves are separated by the *anterior median fissure*. The position of the posterior median septum is indicated on the surface of the cord by a longitudinal groove called the *posterior median sulcus*. Each lateral surface of the spinal cord presents a *posterolateral* and an *anterolateral sulcus*. The dorsal roots of the spinal nerves enter the cord in the region of the posterolateral sulcus, and the anterior roots emerge from it at the anterolateral sulcus (Figs. 25, 26).

The lateral halves of the *gray matter* present dorsal and ventral projections which are designated, respectively, *posterior* and *anterior gray columns*. The thoracic and upper lumbar levels present, in addition, a third column of gray matter, the *lateral gray column* (Fig. 29), located laterally and midway between the posterior and anterior columns; it contains the cell bodies of general visceral efferent neurons. The cell bodies of somatic efferent neurons are found in the anterior gray columns. Cervical and lumbosacral enlargements of the spinal cord appear at the levels which give origin to the brachial and lumbosacral plexuses, respectively (Figs. 28, 30, 31). The increases in size at these levels are due to the increased number of neurons required for innervation of the limbs.

GRAY AND WHITE COLUMNS

The neurons whose cell bodies are located in the posterior gray columns are of two functional types and are designated *internuncial* (or *association*) *cells* and *tract cells*. The internuncial neurons receive impulses from the dorsal root fibers; their axons are distributed to other cells in the gray matter, particularly in the anterior gray columns, and thus complete spinal reflex arcs (Fig. 32). The axons of some internuncial neurons are distributed

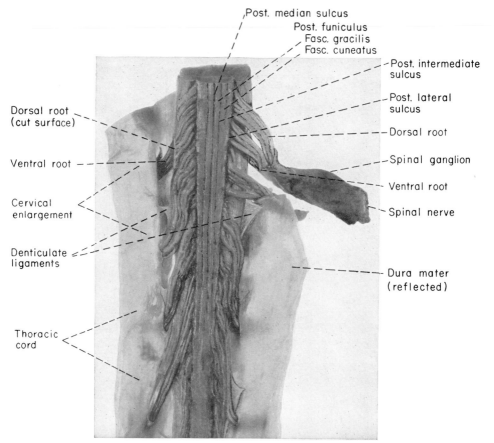

FIG. 26. Retouched photograph showing several segments of the spinal cord (posterior view) to illustrate the dorsal and ventral roots of spinal nerves in relation to the cord, dura mater, and denticulate ligaments.

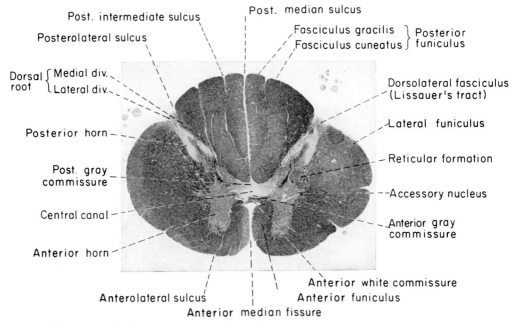

FIG. 27. Photomicrograph of a transverse section through the spinal cord at the level of C2. Weil stain.

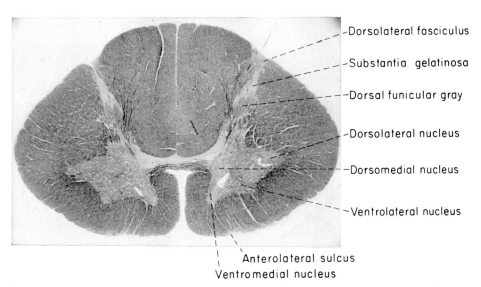

-Dorsolateral fasciculus

-Substantia gelatinosa

-Dorsal funicular gray

-Dorsolateral nucleus

-Dorsomedial nucleus

~Ventrolateral nucleus

'Anterolateral sulcus

Ventromedial nucleus

FIG. 28.   Photomicrograph of a transverse section of the spinal cord through the cervical enlargement. Weil stain.

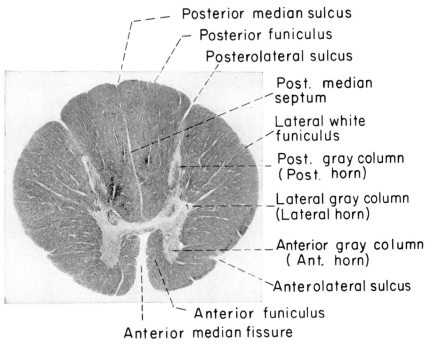

_ _ _ Posterior median sulcus

— Posterior funiculus

Posterolateral sulcus

Post. median
septum

Lateral white
funiculus

Post. gray column
(Post. horn)

Lateral gray column
(Lateral horn)

Anterior gray column
(Ant. horn)

Anterolateral sulcus

— Anterior funiculus

Anterior median fissure

FIG. 29.   Photomicrograph of a transverse section of the spinal cord through the midthoracic region. Weil stain.

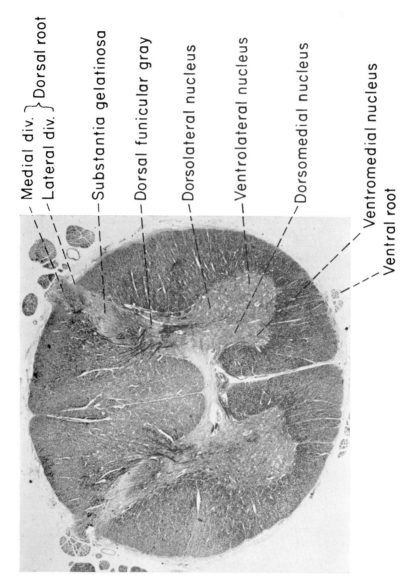

Medial div. ⎫
Lateral div. ⎭ Dorsal root

—Substantia gelatinosa

—Dorsal funicular gray

—Dorsolateral nucleus

—Ventrolateral nucleus

—Dorsomedial nucleus

Ventromedial nucleus

Ventral root

FIG. 30. Photomicrograph of a transverse section of the spinal cord through the lumbar enlargement. Weil stain.

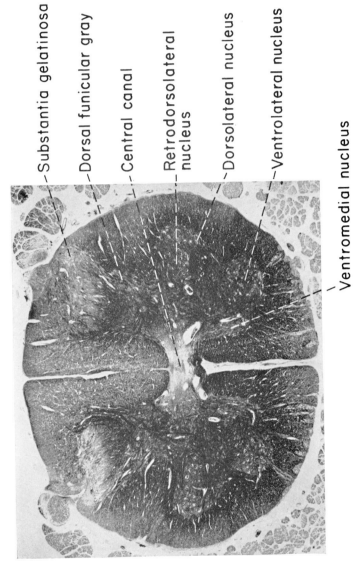

Substantia gelatinosa

Dorsal funicular gray

Central canal

Retrodorsolateral nucleus

Dorsolateral nucleus

Ventrolateral nucleus

Ventromedial nucleus

FIG. 31. Photomicrograph of a transverse section of the spinal cord through the level of S2. Weil stain.

to anterior gray column cells within their own segment of the spinal cord; others reach those of higher or lower levels; thus both intra- and intersegmental reflex arcs are made possible. They may connect with cells in the anterior gray column on the same side as that of their origin, or they may cross to those of the opposite side; through such crossed and uncrossed connections, as many muscles are brought into action on one or both sides as are necessary for a given reflex act (Fig. 32).

The tract cells also receive impulses from the periphery over the dorsal roots of the spinal nerves; their axons may course to the anterior horn cells of the same segment or to the white matter where they bifurcate and form tracts which ascend or descend for variable distances. The longest fibers eventually terminate in the brain. The ascending *fiber tracts* of the spinal cord are made up of these axons, and each tract is concerned with the conduction of relatively specific kinds of sensory information.

The *white matter* in each lateral half of the spinal cord is divided into three columns or *funiculi* (Fig. 27). The *posterior*

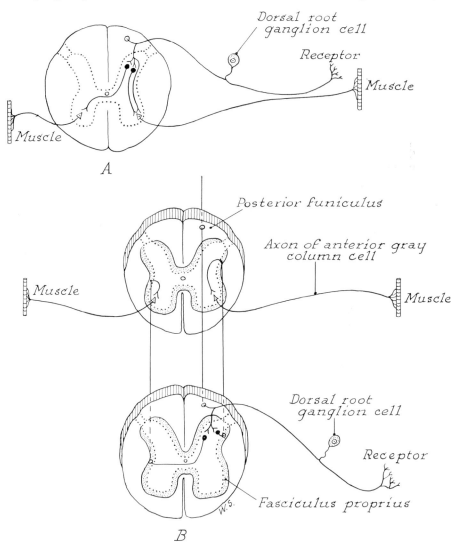

FIG. 32. Reflex arcs. A, Crossed and uncrossed intrasegmental arcs. B, Crossed and uncrossed intersegmental arcs with intersegmental connections by way of the fasciculus proprius.

funiculus is between the posterior median septum and the posterior gray column. The *lateral funiculus* occupies the area between the posterior and anterior gray columns, and the *anterior funiculus* is between the lateral funiculus and the anterior medial fissure. Each funiculus is composed of a number of fiber tracts which occupy relatively circumscribed and constant positions within it. More detailed considerations of the individual tracts are contained in following chapters.

That part of each funiculus which is in immediate relationship to the gray matter is called the fasciculus proprius (Fig. 32). There are, then, dorsal, lateral, and ventral fasciculi proprii made up of the ascending and descending processes of internuncial neurons whose cell bodies are in the gray matter. They are therefore important in intersegmental reflex arcs (Fig. 32).

Subdivisions of Gray Columns

The three major gray columns of the spinal cord, *posterior, lateral,* and *ante-rior,* are composed of more or less distinct cell groups or nuclei which may be seen in appropriately stained sections (Figs. 33–37). The various cell groups of the posterior gray column are the *substantia gelatinosa, dorsal funicular gray, thoracic nucleus* (dorsal nucleus), and the *secondary visceral gray* (Figs. 33–36).

The substantia gelatinosa primarily consists of small neurons (Golgi Type II) and extends through the length of the spinal cord. This column of cells principally receives the terminals of small dorsal root ganglion cells which mediate pain and temperature sensibilities.

The dorsal funicular gray column is composed of larger cells as well as small neurons. This column, which likewise extends through the length of the spinal cord, receives incoming tactile and proprioceptive fibers. Pain and temperature impulses also are received directly by cells in this column and after relay in the substantia gelatinosa. The larger neurons of the dorsal funicular gray column give rise to secondary ascending fibers.

The thoracic nucleus (dorsal nucleus)

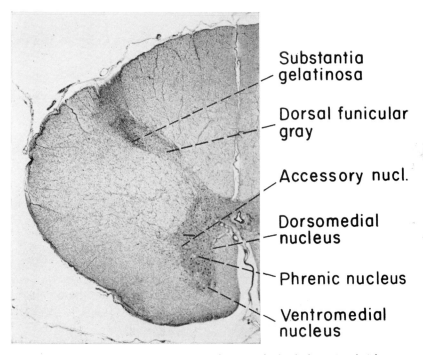

Substantia
gelatinosa

Dorsal funicular
gray

Accessory nucl.

Dorsomedial
nucleus

Phrenic nucleus

Ventromedial
nucleus

FIG. 33   Photomicrograph of a transverse section of the spinal cord at the level of C3. Cresyl violet stain.

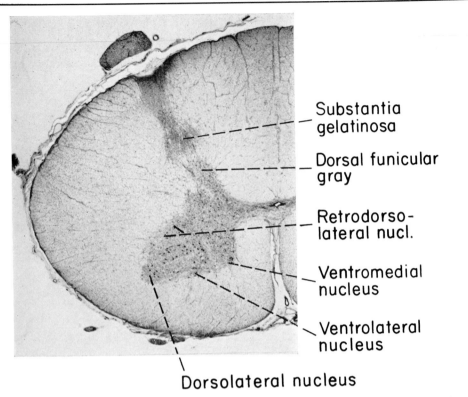

FIG. 34. Photomicrograph of a transverse section of the spinal cord through the cervical enlargement. Cresyl violet stain.

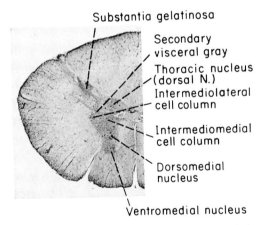

FIG. 35. Photomicrograph of a transverse section of the spinal cord at the midthoracic region. Cresyl violet stain.

(Fig. 35) is comprised of large neurons and extends approximately from cord segments C8 to L2. The posterior spinocerebellar tract (Chap. 19) originates from cells in this nucleus.

The secondary visceral gray (Fig. 35) is an indistinct column of small neurons which extends through the thoracic and upper lumbar levels. It lies at the base of the posterior horn above the cells of lateral horn gray and is believed to receive incoming visceral afferent fibers.

The lateral gray column (intermediate gray column) is composed of preganglionic neurons which are directly lateral to the central canal. From T1 to L3 levels of the cord two divisions of the lateral column are recognized, the *intermediolateral* and *intermediomedial* (Fig. 35). These columns give rise to the preganglionic sympathetic fibers (Chap. 22). At levels S2 to S4 the intermediate column is represented by the *parasympathetic* cell column. Fibers from these cells are the preganglionic efferents to the pelvic viscera (Chap. 22).

The anterior gray column is composed of relatively large multipolar neurons which give origin to somatic efferent fibers that innervate skeletal muscle fibers of somite origin. The column may be divided into three major subdivisions: the medial, lateral, and central. The medial division, represented at all levels of the cord, consists of the *ventromedial* and *dorsomedial* cell columns or nuclei which supply fibers to the axial musculature (Figs. 29, 33, 35). The lateral division is present in the

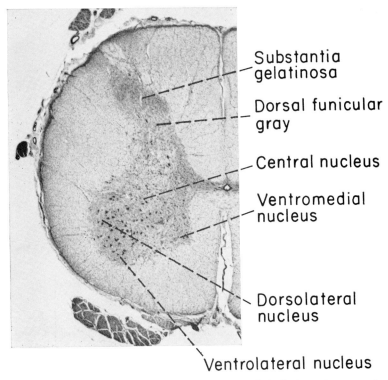

Substantia
gelatinosa

Dorsal funicular
gray

Central nucleus

Ventromedial
nucleus

Dorsolateral
nucleus

Ventrolateral nucleus

FIG. 36. Photomicrograph of a transverse section of the spinal cord through the lumbar enlargement. Cresyl violet stain.

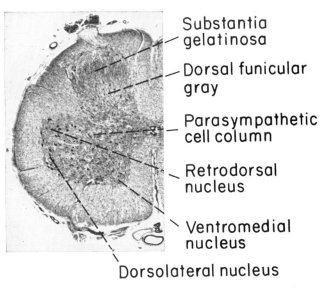

Substantia
gelatinosa

Dorsal funicular
gray

Parasympathetic
cell column

Retrodorsal
nucleus

Ventromedial
nucleus

Dorsolateral nucleus

FIG. 37. Photomicrograph of a transverse section of the spinal cord at the midsacral level. Cresyl violet stain.

cervical and lumbar enlargements and serves as the origin for fibers to muscles of the limbs. This division may be subdivided into *ventrolateral, dorsolateral,* and *retrodorsolateral* nuclei which relate to the innervation of the proximal, intermediate, and distal limb musculature, respectively (Figs. 29, 31, 34, 36, 37). It should be emphasized that there are differences in the longitudinal extent of these nuclei.

The central division of the anterior gray column includes the *phrenic, lumbosacral,* and *accessory nuclei* (Figs. 33, 36). The phrenic nucleus, which extends from about segments C3 to C6, gives origin to fibers that innervate the skeletal muscle of the diaphragm. There is no general agreement relative to the mediolateral location of this nucleus. The lumbosacral (central) nucleus extends from upper lumbar to upper sacral levels. The peripheral distribution of its axons is unknown. The accessory nucleus extends through segments C1 to C6 and gives origin to fibers that form the spinal part of the accessory nerve which innervates the trapezius and sternomastoid muscles. After emerging from the spinal cord, the fibers ascend in the spinal canal, pass through foramen magnum, and join the bulbar portion of the accessory nerve.

In recent years the cytoarchitectonic organization of cells and fibers within the gray matter of the spinal cord of experimental animals has been described which has led to definition of nine laminae of cells. The first lamina is comprised of a thin layer of small cells at the surface of the posterior horn; the ninth is composed of the large motor cells in the anterior horn. A similar lamination within the human spinal cord has been reported.

BIBLIOGRAPHY

Crosby, E. C., Humphrey, T., and Lauer, E. W., 1962: *Correlative Anatomy of the Nervous System.* Macmillan Co., New York.

Elliott, H. C., 1942: Studies on the motor cells of the spinal cord. I. Distribution in the normal human cord. Amer. J. Anat., *70,* 95–117.

Keswani, N. H., and Hollinshead, W. H., 1956: Localization of the phrenic nucleus in the spinal cord of man. Anat. Rec., *125,* 683–700.

Ralston, H. J., III, 1968: Dorsal root protections to the dorsal horn neurons in the cat spinal cord. J. Comp. Neurol., *132,* 303–330.

Rexed, B., 1952: The cytoarchitectonic organization of the spinal cord in the cat. J. Comp. Neurol., *96,* 415–495.

Rexed, B., 1954: A cytoarchitectonic atlas of the spinal cord in the cat. J. Comp. Neurol., *100,* 297–379.

Rexed, B., 1964: Some aspects of the cytoarchitectonics and synaptology of the spinal cord. In *Progress in Brain Research,* Vol. II. Organization of the Spinal Cord. J. C. Eccles and J. P. Schade, Eds. Elsevier Publishing Co., Amsterdam, pp. 58–92.

Szentágothai, J., 1964: Neuronal and synaptic arrangement in the substantia gelatinosa Rolandi. J. Comp. Neurol., *122,* 219–239.

Thomas, C. E., and Combs, G. M., 1965: Spinal cord segments. B. Gross structure in the adult monkey. Amer. J. Anat., *116,* 205–216.

Chapter 5

Somatic Tactile and Proprioceptive Pathways

TACTILE PATHWAYS

The **tactile impulses** set up by stimulation of tactile receptors are conducted to the spinal cord over the peripheral and central divisions of the processes of spinal ganglion cells. The centrally directed fibers from these ganglion cells traverse the dorsal root through its medial division and enter the posterior funiculus of the spinal cord (Figs. 38, 39) where they divide into short, descending branches and much longer, ascending ones. The descending branches aggregate into small tracts known as the *fasciculus septomarginalis* adjacent to the posterior median septum and the *fasciculus interfascicularis* between the gracile and cuneate fasciculi (Fig. 39). Both the ascending and descending branches distribute collaterals to cells in the posterior gray column and thus facilitate spinal reflexes in response to tactile stimuli (Figs. 32, 38, 39). The collaterals also terminate in relation to tract cells whose axons cross the midline through the gray or white commissure and help to form the anterior spinothalamic tract of the contralateral anterior funiculus (Fig. 38). This tract may include some uncrossed fibers which pursue an ipsilateral course.

An important major pathway in the mediation of tactile sensibility is formed by the many ascending divisions of dorsal root fibers which continue their upward course through the posterior funiculus of the same side and finally synapse on cells in the *nuclei gracilis* and *cuneatus* in the medulla (Fig. 42). Axons from cells in these nuclei cross to the opposite side and course upward to the thalamus in the fiber tract known as the *medial lemniscus* (Fig. 38). In the medulla the paired lemnisci are adjacent and appear as vertical columns of longitudinally running fibers near the midline. In the pons the lemnisci are more horizontally disposed in the ventral part of the tegmentum, and in the midbrain they migrate to a ventrolateral tegmental position. Tactile impulses reaching the thalamus by way of the medial lemnisci are relayed by thalamic neurons to the cerebral cortex. The axons of the thalamic neurons project upward through the internal capsule (Fig. 38) to the sensory receiving areas of the cortex. The internal capsule (Chap. 10) consists of nerve fibers which relay information from lower levels of the nervous system to the cerebrum and of fibers which project motor and regulatory information from the cerebrum to the lower centers.

An alternate pathway for the mediation of tactile sensibility is the anterior spinothalamic tract (Fig. 38). The fibers in this tract course upward through the

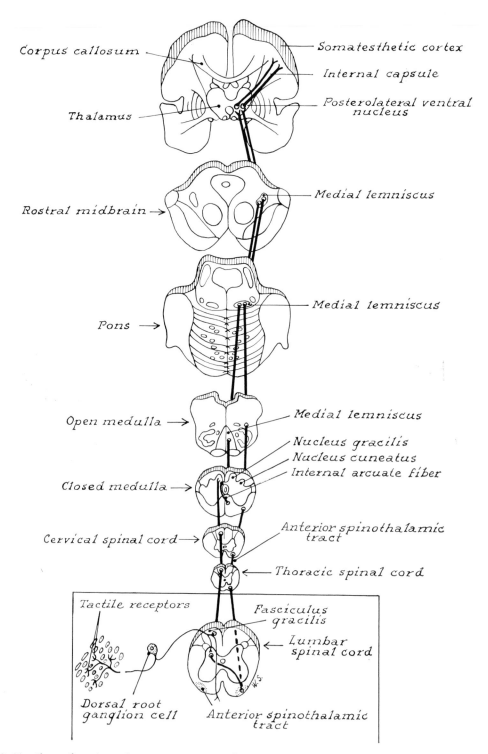

FIG. 38. The tactile pathways from receptor to somatesthetic cortex.

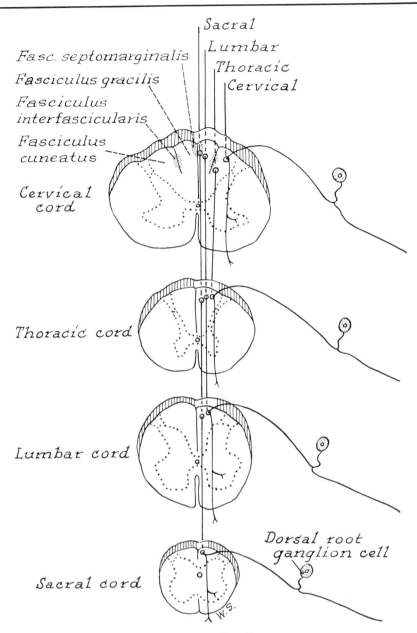

FIG. 39. Diagram illustrating the lamination of the posterior funiculi.

spinal cord and brain stem and finally terminate by synapsing on neurons in the thalamus. In its course through the medulla the anterior spinothalamic tract is generally considered to be dorsolateral to the inferior olivary nucleus in relation to the lateral spinothalamic tract. At the level of the upper pons the fibers of the anterior spinothalamic tract become incorporated in the medial lemniscus (Fig. 38) and, like other lemniscal fibers, are relayed at the thalamus to the cerebral cortex.

Hence, the pathway over the anterior spinothalamic tract and that by way of the posterior funiculus and medial lemniscus ultimately reach the cerebral cortex and the conscious level.

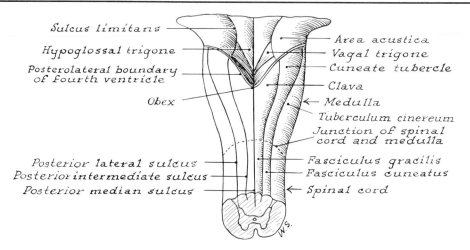

Sulcus limitans

Hypoglossal trigone

Posterolateral boundary of fourth ventricle

Obex

Area acustica

Vagal trigone

Cuneate tubercle

Clava

Medulla

Tuberculum cinereum

Junction of spinal cord and medulla

Posterior lateral sulcus

Posterior intermediate sulcus

Posterior median sulcus

Fasciculus gracilis

Fasciculus cuneatus

Spinal cord

FIG. 40. Dorsal view of medulla oblongata and cervical spinal cord showing continuity of spinal cord sulci with sulci on the dorsal aspect of the closed part of the medulla.

The fibers transmitting tactile information over the posterior funiculus and medial lemniscus are primarily concerned with the finer localizing and discriminatory aspects of tactile sensibility. The discriminatory capabilities depend on a synaptic ratio approaching 1:1 among the three levels of afferent conduction which intervene between receptor and cerebral cortex—dorsal root ganglia, nuclei gracilis and cuneatus, and thalamus. In contrast, the anterior spinothalamic pathway is concerned with less localized, more general tactile sensibility. This decreased specificity indicates that more than one primary afferent neuron synapses on a given tract cell, and several tract cells, in turn, synapse on one thalamic neuron. It is evident from this fact that some tactile sensibility will remain if either the posterior funiculi or the anterior spinothalamic tracts are not functioning, but that discrete tactile capabilities will be lost if the posterior funiculi are not operating. In addition to light touch or general tactile sensation, the anterior spinothalamic tracts are considered to subserve sexual sensations, tickle, and itch.

The **posterior funiculus** of the spinal cord is chiefly composed of the ascending rami of dorsal root fibers and is specifically laminated; fibers coming into the

funiculus at successively higher levels are more and more laterally placed. The fibers which enter below the midthoracic level constitute the *fasciculus gracilis* and those entering above that level make up the *fasciculus cuneatus* (Fig. 39). In the cervical levels of the spinal cord, the two fasciculi are separated from one another by the *posterior intermediate septum* whose position is indicated on the surface by the *posterior intermediate sulcus*. It and the other sulci on the surface of the cervical part of the cord are continued upward on to the medulla oblongata (Fig. 40).

The **medulla oblongata** consists of a caudal closed portion and of a rostral open portion. At the junction of the two portions the central canal opens out into the fourth ventricle. The open portion is so designated because of failure of approximation of the alar laminae to form a central canal in this region, such as exists in the closed portion.

Between the posterior median and posterior intermediate sulci of the medulla, and in immediate relationship to the fourth ventricle, there is a swelling referred to as the *clava* (Fig. 40). Just lateral to the posterior intermediate sulcus, and extending to a more rostral level, is a similar swelling called the *cuneate tubercle.* The clava and cuneate tubercle indicate the positions beneath the surface, of the nucleus gracilis and the nucleus cuneatus, respectively. The fasciculus gracilis terminates in the nucleus gracilis and the fasciculus cuneatus in the latter nucleus. The term "nucleus," as it is used with reference to the central nervous system, denotes a compact collection of nerve cells having more or less specific functions; the cells in a given nucleus are concerned with the reception of nervous impulses from certain neurons elsewhere in the nervous system and with the relay of those impulses to other centers or to effectors.

The **nucleus gracilis** and the **nucleus cuneatus** are clearly visible in a cross-section of the closed portion of the medulla which cuts through the clava and cuneate tubercle; they are covered on their dorsal sides by the terminal portions of the fasciculi gracilis and cuneatus (Fig. 41). In sections through this caudal level of the medulla it can be appreciated that nucleus gracilis and nucleus cuneatus are extensions of the posterior gray columns of the cervical spinal cord (Fig. 41). Fibers from the fasciculi can be traced into the nuclei where they synapse on cells whose axons course ventrally and medially to enter the contralateral medial lemniscus (Figs. 42, 43). The decussating fibers from the nuclei, because of their arched course, are called *internal arcuate fibers.* The decussation, formed by the fibers from both sides, is known as the *sensory decussation,* or, sometimes, as the *decussation of the medial lemniscus.*

The **medial lemniscus,** as was previously stated, can be traced rostrally through the medulla, pons, and mesencephalon to its termination in relation to cells in the thalamus whose axons end in the sensory area of the cerebral cortex. As will become apparent in subsequent discussions, the medial lemniscus contains some descending fibers (Chap. 14). The fact that the anterior spinothalamic tract joins the lemniscus in the pons has also been mentioned.

Pathways from receptor endings to the

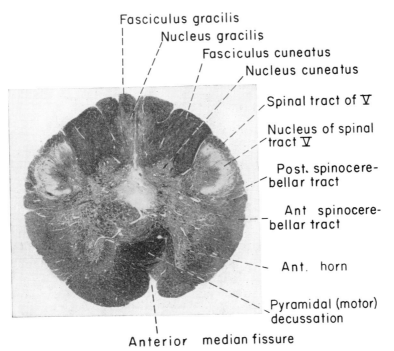

Fasciculus gracilis
Nucleus gracilis
Fasciculus cuneatus
Nucleus cuneatus
Spinal tract of Ⅴ
Nucleus of spinal tract Ⅴ
Post. spinocerebellar tract
Ant. spinocerebellar tract
Ant. horn
Pyramidal (motor) decussation
Anterior median fissure

FIG. 41. Photomicrograph of a transverse section of the neuraxis at the level of transition from spinal cord to medulla. Weil stain.

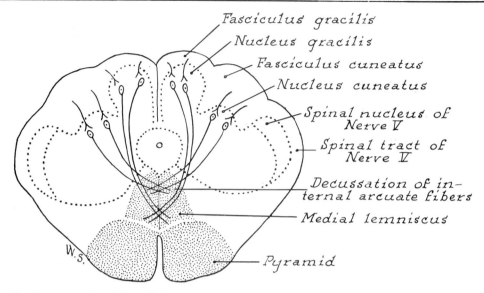

FIG. 42. Cross-section of medulla at the level of the decussation of the internal arcuate fibers.

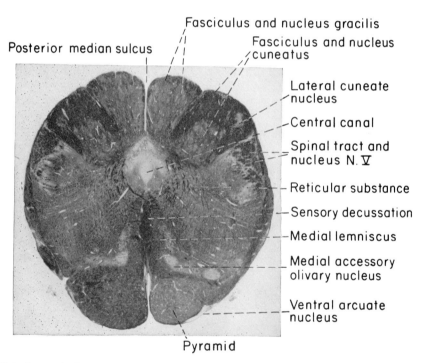

FIG. 43. Photomicrograph of a transverse section of the medulla at the level of the sensory decussation. Weil stain.

cerebral cortex require a minimum of three neurons. The first neuron (*primary* or of the *first order*) has its cell body in a peripheral ganglion (with some exceptions). The second neuron (*secondary* or of the *second order*) has its cell body in the posterior gray column of the spinal cord or in some nucleus of the brain stem and, with few exceptions, is a decussating neuron, i.e., its axon crosses to the opposite side. The cell body of the third neuron (*tertiary* or of the *third order*) is in

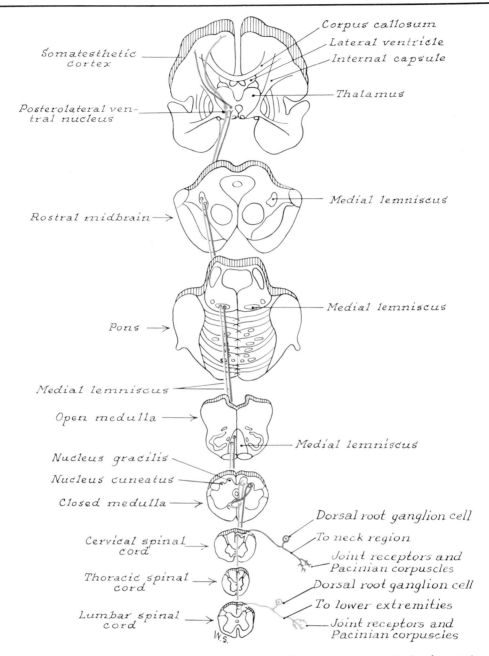

FIG. 44. The proprioceptive pathways from the receptors to somatesthetic cortex. Proprioceptive impulses entering the spinal cord below the midthoracic level are shown utilizing the fasciculus gracilis whereas those entering above that level course upward in the fasciculus cuneatus.

the thalamus and its axon courses upward to terminate in the cerebral cortex. A given sensory impulse, due to the decussation of the secondary neuron, is delivered to the side of the brain opposite that of its origin, in most instances. In addition, a topographical arrangement of fibers is usually maintained in an orderly fashion. Fibers added to a given tract at higher levels are contiguous to, but remain separate from, those already present. Similarly, when fibers cross to the contralateral side they do so, for the most part, without mixing. The exceptions to these general rules that exist in some of the pathways from the head region will be pointed out as the cranial nerves are considered. The nucleus in the thalamus, in which the medial lemniscus terminates, is situated laterally, posteriorly, and ventrally; therefore, it is designated the posterolateral ventral nucleus (Figs. 38, 78).

PROPRIOCEPTIVE PATHWAYS

Ascending fibers which carry impulses concerned with sense of **position, pressure, vibration, movement, and stereognosis** (a complex preception), like those concerned with tactile discrimination, course in the posterior funiculi. The neurons of the first order, in the dorsal root ganglia, distribute peripheral processes to proprioceptive receptors and, insofar as vibratory sense and stereognosis are concerned, to exteroceptors as well. Exteroceptors may also be concerned in pressure sense. Central processes enter the posterior funiculi over the medial divisions of the dorsal roots, and their long ascending divisions end in the nucleus gracilis or nucleus cuneatus depending on the level of the spinal cord at which they entered (Fig. 44). The further course of proprioceptive impulses over the internal arcuate fibers and medial lemniscus to the thalamus and from the thalamus to the cortex is the same as that described for tactile discriminatory impulses.

Collaterals from the central processes of primary neurons in the proprioceptive pathway terminate in relation to somatic motor neurons in the anterior gray column and thus contribute to the formation of proprioceptive spinal reflex arcs. The knee jerk is an example of a reflex that utilizes such an arc (Fig. 45). Tapping the patellar tendon effects a sudden stretch of the quadriceps muscle and stimulates the muscle spindles and musculotendinous endings therein. The impulses thus set up reach the spinal cord by way of the femoral nerve and the dorsal roots of the second, third, and fourth lumbar

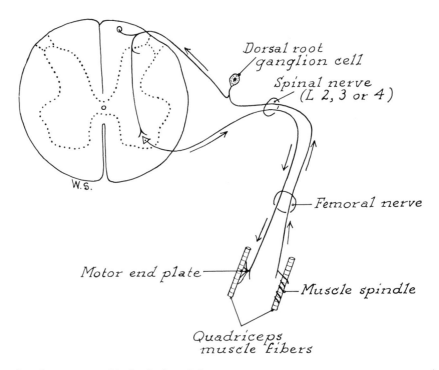

FIG. 45. The reflex arc responsible for the knee jerk.

nerves; through terminals which end directly upon motor neurons (also through internuncial cells) they activate anterior gray column cells in the corresponding lumbar segments. Through the axons of the latter cells, efferent impulses are conducted to the quadriceps muscle and account for its sudden reflex contraction. In this instance, the stimulus is an artificial one, but it illustrates the connections which facilitate proprioceptive reflexes as they normally occur in response to changes in length and tension of muscles.

Muscle spindles are complex receptor organs composed of specialized *intrafusal* muscle fibers which are separated from the regular *extrafusal* muscle fibers by a connective tissue capsule. They are arranged in parallel with the regular extrafusal fibers and, ultimately, have the same attachments on connective tissue and tendon (Fig. 46). Thus, during contraction, the tension on the muscle spindles is reduced; when the muscle is stretched, tension is increased. There are several types of receptor endings located in the noncontractile center of the extrafusal fiber. In addition, the contractile poles of the fiber are supplied by *gamma efferent* motoneurons (see Chap. 14). The gamma efferents, by causing the two polar regions to contract, increase the tension in the central region of the intrafusal fiber where the receptor endings are located. Thus, a biasing mechanism is provided by the gamma motor system which independently affects the sensitivity of the muscle spindle. It is obvious that the simple stretch reflex shown in Figure 45 is influenced by the activity of gamma motoneurons. In addition, their discharge is affected in either an excitatory or inhibitory manner by way of central nervous regulation as well as by an afferent barrage from a variety of receptors, cutaneous ones in particular (Fig. 46).

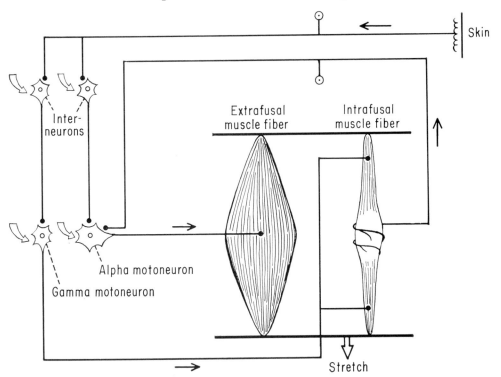

FIG. 46.   Schematic representation of intrafusal muscle fiber, its innervation, and the routes by which the stretch reflex can be influenced. Arrows pointing to the soma of interneurons and alpha and gamma motoneurons represent central nervous connections which could affect the reflex. (Modified from Fig. 115, Chap. 6, *Neurophysiology*, Ruch, Patton, Woodbury, and Towe, W. B. Saunders Co., 1962.)

FUNCTIONAL AND CLINICAL RELATIONSHIPS

It is now apparent that destruction of either posterior funiculus at any given level will result in loss of sense of position, movement, pressure, vibration, and stereognosis, as well as of tactile discrimination on the same side as the lesion and caudal to it (Figs. 38, 44). Interruption of one medial lemniscus will cause contralateral loss of all these types of sensibility. In either case some general tactile sensation remains, however, due to the representation in the anterior spinothalamic tracts. Unilateral interruption of a posterior funiculus may occur as a result of intra- or extramedullary tumor of the spinal cord and interruption of either medial lemniscus may result from thrombosis of one or more branches of the anterior spinal artery (Fig. 47).

Pernicious anemia, undiagnosed and untreated, results in degeneration of the spinal cord in the posterior and lateral funiculi—so-called *subacute combined degeneration* or sclerosis (Fig. 178). This is a bilateral condition which, so far as degeneration in the posterior funiculi is concerned, accounts for bilateral reduction and eventual loss of all types of sensibility carried by the fasciculi gracilis and cuneatus.

The posterior funiculi also exhibit degeneration with marked loss of myelin in *tabes dorsalis.* The degeneration in this condition is secondary to *radiculitis* (inflammatory involvement of the dorsal roots). The spirochete of syphilis attacks the dorsal roots whose component fibers are degenerated throughout their intramedullary course; proprioceptive sensibility is therefore diminished or completely

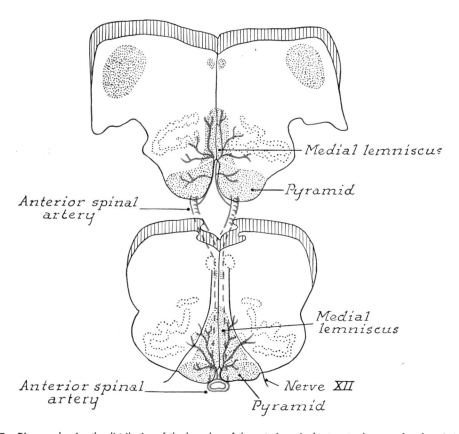

FIG. 47. Diagram showing the distribution of the branches of the anterior spinal artery to the ventral and medial areas of the medulla.

abolished. As should be expected, the radiculitis also results in some reduction of tactile, pain, and thermal sensibility. Degeneration is not found in the anterior and lateral spinothalamic tracts since they are formed by axons of secondary neurons; only the primary neurons are involved. Since the dorsal roots are the afferent limbs of proprioceptive reflex arcs, the knee jerk and other deep reflexes are diminished or absent in tabes dorsalis.

The lumbar and sacral nerves are the first to be attacked by the radiculitis of syphilis; therefore, loss of vibratory and position sense and diminution of reflexes occur in the lower extremities first. Degeneration in the posterior funiculi, if there is opportunity to examine the spinal cord from a tabetic patient in the earlier stages of the disease, will be more marked in the fasciculus gracilis than in the fasciculus cuneatus.

Sensory loss similar to that of tabes has been reported occasionally in uncontrolled diabetics. Postmortem examinations in diabetics have revealed similar changes in the spinal cord.

BIBLIOGRAPHY

Bowsher, D., 1958: Projection of the gracile and cuneate nuclei in *Macaca mulatta*: an experimental degeneration study. J. Comp. Neurol., *110,* 135–156.

Calne, D. B., and Pallis, C. A., 1966: Vibratory sense: A critical review. Brain, *89,* 723–746.

Gordon, G., and Paine, C. H., 1960: Functional organization in nucleus gracilis of the cat. J. Physiol. (London), *153,* 331–349.

Magoun, H. W., 1958: *The Waking Brain.* Charles C Thomas, Springfield, Ill.

Matzke, H. A., 1951: The course of the fibers arising from the nucleus gracilis and cuneatus of the cat. J. Comp. Neurol., *94,* 439–452.

Perl, E. R., and Whitlock, D. G., 1961: Somatic stimuli exciting spinothalamic projections to thalamic neurons in cat and monkey. Exp. Neurol., *3,* 256–296.

Rose, J. E., and Mountcastle, V. B., 1959: Touch and Kinesthesia. In *Handbook of Physiology,* Vol. I, Section I, J. Fields, Ed. American Physiological Society, Washington, D.C., pp. 387–429.

Walker, A. E., and Weaver, T. A., Jr., 1942: The topical organization and termination of the fibers of the posterior columns in *Macaca mulatta.* J. Comp. Neurol., *76,* 145–158.

Wall, P. D., 1967: The laminar organization of dorsal horn and effects of descending impulses. J. Physiol. (London), *188,* 403–423.

Chapter 6

Pain, Thermal, and Visceral Afferent Pathways

Pain and thermal sensibilities may be discussed together since they are served by the same pathway through the spinal cord and brain stem. The dorsal root ganglion cells concerned with pain and thermal sense are smaller than those which conduct tactile and proprioceptive impulses, and the processes of the cells are also of smaller caliber and are lightly myelinated. Their central divisions enter the spinal cord in the region of the posterolateral sulcus and are directed laterally as compared with the course of the tactile fibers; for this reason they have been considered to form the *lateral division of the dorsal root* in contradistinction to the *medial division* which enters the posterior funiculus (Fig. 48). It is important to understand that these are divisions of the dorsal root as a whole and not of the individual root fibers.

The **dorsolateral fasciculus** (of Lissauer) is found in the interval between the posterior and lateral funiculi (Fig. 27). It is formed in part by the short ascending and descending divisions of the pain and thermal fibers which constitute the lateral divisions of the dorsal roots. The major part of this tract is believed to be comprised of fibers which interconnect neurons at different levels of the *substantia gelatinosa* (a cap of small neurons which form the apex of the posterior gray column). Although the tract is present throughout the length of the spinal cord, the individual fibers are distributed to no more than a total of three or four segments. In the standard preparations of spinal cord sections stained with iron-hematoxylin, the dorsolateral fasciculus appears much lighter in color than the white matter of the adjacent posterior and lateral funiculi. This is due to the relative lack of myelin in this fasciculus. The intensity of the blue color produced in the white matter when such sections are stained with hematoxylin (Pal-Weigert or Weil methods) varies in proportion to the amount of myelin present.

Terminals from the ascending and descending fibers in the fasciculus and from the incoming fibers themselves terminate through synapses on neurons within the substantia gelatinosa and deeper parts of the posterior gray columns.

From these more deeply placed neurons of the posterior gray columns which comprise the dorsal funicular gray, laminae VI and VII of Rexed, fibers arise which cross to the lateral funiculus through the anterior white commissure and course upward through the spinal cord and brain stem as components of the *lateral spinothalamic tract* (Fig. 48). Although the detailed relations of the incoming pain and temperature fibers to the cells which

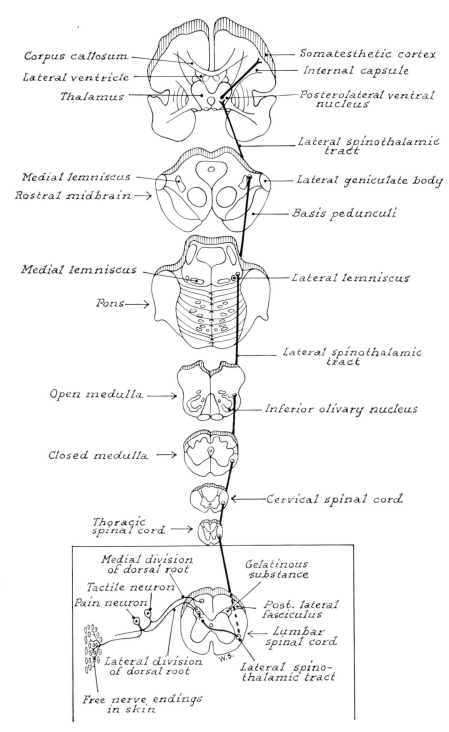

Corpus callosum

Somatesthetic cortex

Lateral ventricle

Internal capsule

Thalamus

Posterolateral ventral nucleus

Lateral spinothalamic tract

Medial lemniscus

Lateral geniculate body

Rostral midbrain →

Basis pedunculi

Medial lemniscus

Lateral lemniscus

Pons →

Lateral spinothalamic tract

Open medulla →

Inferior olivary nucleus

Closed medulla →

Cervical spinal cord

Thoracic spinal cord →

Medial division of dorsal root

Gelatinous substance

Tactile neuron

Pain neuron

Post. lateral fasciculus

Lumbar spinal cord

Lateral division of dorsal root

W.S.

Lateral spino-thalamic tract

Free nerve endings in skin

FIG. 48.   The pain and thermal pathway from receptor to somatesthetic cortex.

give rise to the lateral spinothalamic tract are not established, it appears unlikely that axons of cells in the substantia gelatinosa contribute directly to the tract. The lateral spinothalamic tract, like the medial lemniscus, terminates in the posterolateral ventral thalamic nucleus (Figs. 48, 78). It has been speculated that the termination of these two tracts in the same thalamic nucleus is significant in enhancing the localization of painful stimuli through the accompanying simultaneous tactile impulses. Pain and thermal impulses then presumably are conducted to the cerebral cortex over the axons of the thalamic neurons. Clinical observations and experimental studies indicate that conscious recognition of pain occurs at the thalamic level. This indication is supported by the failure of cortical stimulation to elicit the sensation of pain. Nevertheless, it is likely that pain has a cortical representation which is necessary for its quantitative, qualitative, and topographical assessment.

The lateral spinothalamic tract is more or less specifically laminated, like the fasciculi gracilis and cuneatus; its lamination differs from that of these fasciculi, however, in that the fibers entering at successively higher levels assume more and more medial and anterior positions in the lateral funiculus.

Investigations of the conduction of impulses resulting from stimulation of pain-sensitive receptors in tendons have led to the conclusion that the conduction of "deep pain" is exactly like that of "superficial pain." In the monkey, impulses set up by painful stimulation of exposed tendons ascend in the lateral spinothalamic tract on the side opposite their origin. No impulses from tendons, interpreted as pain by the monkey, were found to ascend in the homolateral posterior column of the spinal cord.

Spinal reflexes in response to pain and thermal stimuli are facilitated by collateral branches of the dorsal root fibers, or more likely through terminals of internuncial neurons connecting with cells of the anterior gray column. These reflexes are classified as *nociceptive*.

In **syringomyelia** there is, as the name implies, cavitation of the spinal cord. Such cavitation may result from degeneration by tumors arising in the ependymal lining of the central canal. It eventually destroys the gray and white commissures of the cord and thus interrupts the decussating axons of the second (or third) order neurons in the pain

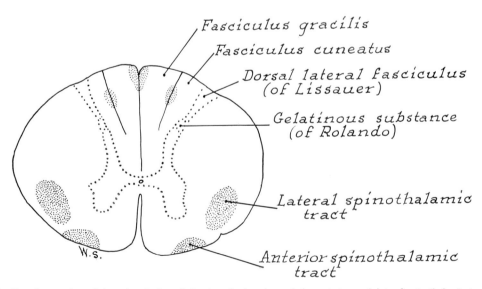

FIG. 49.   Cross-section of thoracic spinal cord showing the locations of the anterior and lateral spinothalamic tracts.

and thermal pathway. The cavity tends to extend longitudinally through several segments of the spinal cord and its presence is manifested by bilateral loss of pain and thermal sensibility, localized to those areas whose sensory innervation depends on the spinal cord segments involved. Thus, a syringomyelia of the cervical and upper thoracic segments of the cord gives rise to a "jacket" type of anesthesia (shoulder, upper extremities, and upper part of the thoracic wall). There may be preservation of all other types of sensibility, since they are conducted to the brain over spinal cord pathways which are uncrossed. It is typical of syringomyelia that the cavity expands to such an extent as to involve the anterior gray columns. This condition causes weakness localized in those muscles innervated by the same cord levels in which there is a loss of cutaneous pain and thermal sense.

The **lateral spinothalamic tract** is situated in the anterior half of the lateral funiculus of the spinal cord (Fig. 49). Damage to the tract results in loss of pain and thermal perception on the opposite side, below the level of the lesion. Practical application is made of the knowledge of the location and course of the lateral spinothalamic tract in the procedure known as cordotomy.

Cordotomy entails the surgical severance of the lateral spinothalamic tract, at an appropriate level of the spinal cord, for the relief of otherwise intractable pain. If the pain-producing disease process is unilateral the tract must, of course, be severed on the opposite side. If the pain to be relieved is from parts of the body having bilateral innervation, it becomes necessary to cut the tract on both sides.

The **dentate ligament** is an important landmark in cordotomy. It consists of eighteen to twenty-one tooth-like projections of the pia mater. The serrations arise from the lateral midline of the spinal cord (Fig. 50), pierce the arachnoid mater, and attach to the inner surface of the dura mater. If the surgeon inserts his knife into the cord ventral to the dentate ligament he can cut the lateral spinothalamic tract without danger of damage to the main motor pathway (lateral corticospinal tract) which is also in the lateral funiculus, but lies dorsal to the plane of the dentate ligaments. It has been emphasized that the lateral spinothalamic tract is not confined to a small bundle of fibers and that analgesia cannot be obtained by a "3-millimeter deep" incision between the dentate ligament and the emerging roots of spinal nerves. Instead, a ventromedial incision to include almost the entire anterior quadrant of the spinal cord is the more

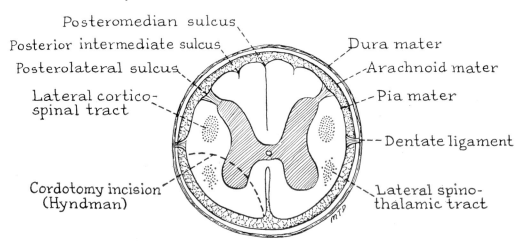

FIG. 50. Diagram showing the relationship of the dentate ligament to the spinal cord and its coverings and indicating the importance of the dentate ligament as a landmark in cordotomy.

5

generally recommended procedure (Fig. 50).

It has been noted that the ascending divisions of the dorsal root fibers carrying pain impulses course upward in the dorsolateral fasciculus for a variable number of segments, usually one to three. Therefore, it is necessary to section the lateral spinothalamic tract at a level rostral to that which represents the upper limit of the painful process.

In the medulla the lateral spinothalamic tract is situated posterolateral to the inferior olivary nucleus. The nucleus has been described as being the shape of a crumpled purse; it is located in the anterolateral area of the medulla (Figs. 51, 52). Damage to the lateral spinothalamic tract in the medulla results in complete loss of pain and thermal sense from the head down on the side opposite that of the lesion. The tract can be cut surgically in the medulla as well as at other levels in the brain stem.

The **olivary eminence** provides an important landmark for section of the lateral

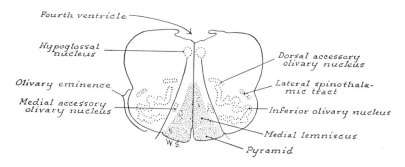

FIG. 51. Cross-section of the open part of the medulla oblongata showing the relationship of the lateral spinothalamic tract to the inferior olivary nucleus and to the olivary eminence.

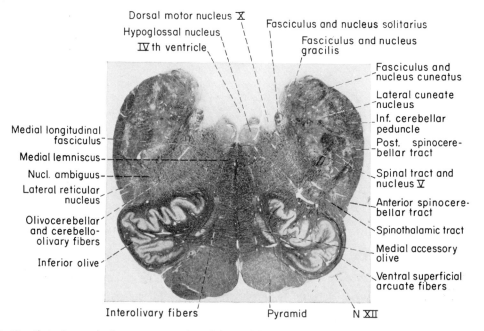

FIG. 52. Photomicrograph of a transverse section of the medulla at the caudal part of the fourth ventricle. Note the reduced pyramid on the right which is due to partial degeneration of pyramidal tract fibers resulting from hemorrhage into the internal capsule (see Chaps. 16 and 18). Weil stain.

spinothalamic tract at the level of the medulla (Fig. 51). The eminence consists of an elongated swelling on the lateral surface of the medulla which is due to the underlying olivary nucleus. If the surgeon inserts his knife immediately dorsal to the eminence and to a measured depth (about 4½ mm), he can completely sever the tract. Medullary spinothalamic tractotomies result in high cervical levels of contralateral analgesia and some sensory changes indicating injury to the trigeminal pathway (Chap. 8).

Interoceptive nervous impulses reach the conscious level, but impulses classified as *general visceral afferent* are neither accurately localized with reference to the area of stimulation nor as accurately interpreted as are exteroceptive and proprioceptive impulses. **Visceral pain** and organic sensations such as hunger, nausea, and thirst are examples of these poorly localized visceral sensations (see referred pain, page 59). The **special visceral afferent impulses** from olfactory and taste receptors are more accurately interpreted.

The cell bodies of the **primary visceral afferent neurons** are in the spinal ganglia; in the ganglia associated with the glossopharyngeal, vagus, and facial nerves; and in the olfactory mucous membrane. The peripheral processes of cell bodies in the spinal ganglia pass from the spinal nerves to the ganglia of the sympathetic chain through the *white rami communicantes* (Fig. 53). They pass through the chain ganglia without any synapse therein and may rejoin the spinal nerves by way of the *gray rami communicantes,* in which event they are distributed to vascular and glandular structures outside the body cavities. Other visceral afferent fibers are distributed from the chain ganglia to thoracic and abdominal viscera by way of the cardiac, pulmonary, and splanchnic nerves. Visceral afferent fibers to the heart and lungs arise from the upper thoracic spinal ganglia. The fibers to the digestive tract,

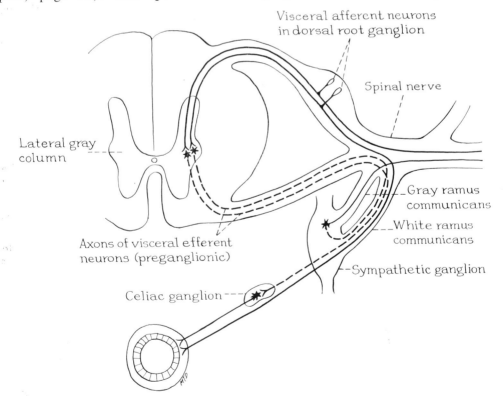

FIG. 53.   The origin and manner of distribution of visceral afferent fibers from the lower thoracic region.

liver, kidneys, ureters, bladder, gonads, and peritoneum arise from the lower thoracic ganglia and course to the celiac and other plexuses of the abdomen by way of the splanchnic nerves (Fig. 53). They eventually reach the visceral structures, in association with visceral efferent fibers, through these plexuses.

Caudal analgesia, as used in obstetrics, represents a practical application of the knowledge that the visceral afferent fibers of the eleventh and twelfth thoracic nerves, via the splanchnics, are concerned especially with the sensory innervation of the uterus. The analgesic agent is introduced into the spinal canal through the sacral hiatus in just sufficient quantity to diffuse it upward in the epidural fat to a level which includes the eleventh thoracic nerves. Thus the pain impulses from the uterus are blocked without interfering with the visceral efferent impulses to the musculature of its upper segment which come from the intermediolateral gray column in thoracic segments above the eleventh. The somatic afferent impulses from the perineum are also blocked and the pain which is otherwise associated with the marked dilatation of this region is eliminated.

General visceral afferent fibers of the vagus nerve, arising from cells in the *inferior ganglion* (Chap. 1), are also distributed to thoracic and abdominal viscera. The inferior ganglion is a sensory ganglion which is functionally and structurally analogous to spinal ganglia and whose neurons function as the afferent limbs of visceral reflex arcs; experiments have indicated, however, that these neurons are of less importance in the conscious perception of visceral sensations than neurons whose cell bodies are in the spinal ganglia.

The **interoceptive pathway** to the conscious level is not as well defined as are the exteroceptive and proprioceptive pathways. It is usually considered to consist of a series of several neurons, with cell bodies in the posterior gray columns, whose axons course upward in the fasciculi proprii through a few segments and synapse on the dendrites or cell bodies of the next higher group of neurons in the chain. If this were the only pathway for visceral impulses, section of the lateral spinothalamic tract should have no effect on visceral pain. Experiments have shown, however, that the pain pathway from the renal pelvis can be interrupted by cordotomy. Advanced neoplastic disease of the pelvic viscera is a clinical condition for which bilateral cordotomy is often employed to provide the patient relief from intractable pain. It appears, therefore, that *visceral pain impulses* are carried upward in or near the lateral spinothalamic tract. Other types of impulses arising in the viscera may be conducted by a chain of neurons with cell bodies in the posterior gray column.

It is generally believed that visceral sensations reach the conscious level in the thalamus. Somatic pain also is believed to reach consciousness in the thalamus but localization of the point of stimulation and differentiation among varying intensities of stimulation are functions of the cerebral cortex (see page 132).

Visceral reflex arcs are completed within the spinal cord. The central processes of visceral afferent neurons may synapse directly on visceral efferent neurons in the intermediolateral gray column (Fig. 54A) or on internuncial neurons in the posterior gray column (secondary visceral gray) whose axons are distributed in such a manner as to account for both intra- and intersegmental arcs.

Internuncial neurons also facilitate *viscerosomatic reflexes.* An example of such a reflex is the rigidity of the muscles of the anterior abdominal wall in the presence of acute appendicitis. Pain impulses from the regional peritoneum are conducted to the spinal cord by the splanchnic nerves and the dorsal roots of the lower thoracic nerves. Within the cord, connections are made, through internuncial cells, with the anterior gray column cells which innervate the abdominal muscles (Fig. 54B).

The existence of *somatovisceral reflexes* may be mentioned appropriately at this point although the consideration of visceral efferent impulses will be left until later (Chap. 23). The *pilomotor reflex* is an example of this type; it is manifested by the appearance of goose flesh in response to the application of cold to the skin. Thus, exteroceptors for cold and somatic afferent neurons are responsible for the afferent portion of a reflex in which the effectors are smooth muscles that are innervated by general visceral efferent fibers (Fig. 54C).

Referred pain (pain referred to the body wall or extremities) may result from visceral disease. Visceral pain may be due to over-distention of the walls of a viscus as in cases of ureteral or biliary stone, by inflammation as in appendicitis, or by impaired blood supply (ischemia). Instead of being localized in the diseased

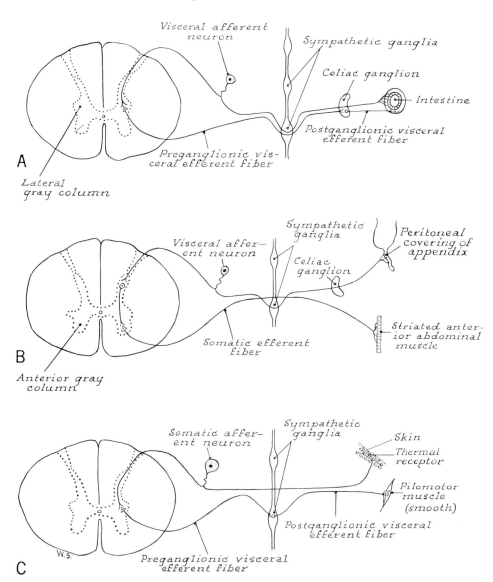

FIG. 54. Visceral reflex arcs. A, Viscerovisceral arc. B, Viscerosomatic arc responsible for abdominal rigidity in appendicitis. C, Somatovisceral arc involved in the pilomotor reflex.

viscus, the pain is referred to definite skin areas which become hyperalgesic to stimuli while the patient is experiencing the pain or in the interims between acute attacks of pain. The location of the skin areas to which visceral pain is referred is determined by the fact that the visceral afferent fibers reach the same segment of the spinal cord that innervates the particular skin zone. It has been suggested that the spinal receptive neurons within the cord segments corresponding to the dermatomes involved in the referred pain are activated (facilitated) by the stream of painful impulses from the viscus and, for this reason, have a lower threshold for impulses from the skin. An alternative explanation of referred pain is that visceral afferents converge with cutaneous afferents to end on the *same* neuron at the cord (or higher) level in the pain pathway. This neuron could then be activated by either visceral or cutaneous stimuli and presumably would relay similar information to the brain in either case. The possibility of the brain misinterpreting the source of the stimuli would be obvious. This explanation for the mechanism of referred pain is known as the convergence-projection theory.

Pain arising as the result of spasm of the coronary arteries (cardiac ischemia) is referred to the precordium and to the ulnar side of the arm, forearm, and hand. Pain from gallbladder disease is commonly referred to the region around the inferior angle of the right scapula.

Parietal pain also may be referred as in subdiaphragmatic pain which is referred to the skin of the shoulder (area supplied by the supraclavicular nerves). This referral may be explained by impulses being transmitted from the diaphragm by sensory fibers in the phrenic nerve to spinal cord segments C3 and C4. The dorsal roots of these segments are common to the phrenic and supraclavicular nerves.

Collaterals from the pain pathways which end in brain stem nuclei caudal to the classical relay nuclei in the thalamus have long been recognized. It has been shown recently that after anterolateral cordotomy in humans many degenerating fibers may be found in reticular nuclei of the medulla and pons, descending vestibular nuclei, and nuclei of the solitary and spinal trigeminal tracts. The nuclei that receive these projections form a diffuse, multisynaptic medial or extralemniscal corticipetally conducting system in the brain stem. This system has been studied in the brain stem of monkeys and has been compared with the lateral (classical lemniscal) system.

Slow conduction and prolonged response to stimulation indicates the presence of numerous relays in the medial system. Functionally, it appears that the lateral system is essential for perception, recognition, and localization of stimuli; whereas the medial system, through its slower transport of all sensory modalities, initiates and maintains the conscious state and thus provides a background of nervous activity without which integrated sensory motor and adaptive functions would be impossible. It also has been proposed that the medial system is involved in the process of concentration superimposed on inattentive wakefulness. Direct stimulation of the medial system induces alert attention whereas its depression or destruction renders the subject unconscious. The effect of anesthesia on potentials conducted in the medial and lateral systems gives support to the conclusions regarding consciousness; impulses propagated over the medial system are blocked by administration of ether or sodium pentobarbital to the animal while laterally conducted impulses reach the sensory cortex with unimpaired or augmented intensity. This evidence suggests that the multisynaptic medial system is more susceptible to anesthetic blocking than the paucisynaptic lateral pathway. Anatomically, the extralemniscal sensory system can be located only in a general manner, based on sites from which electrical activity has been recorded. These sites are found in pontile and mesencephalic tegmenti, in the reticular formation and periaqueductal gray matter, and in the subthalamus and hypothalamus, adjacent to the third ventricle. Certain thalamic nuclei are also found to be concerned in the final relay to cerebral cortex. These include the *intralaminar* and/or *reticular nuclei* (Chap. 20).

BIBLIOGRAPHY

Bonica, J. J., 1964: *An Atlas on Mechanisms and Pathways of Pain in Labor.* F. A. Davis Co., Philadelphia.

Bowsher, D., 1962: The topographical projection of fibers from the anterolateral quadrant of the spinal cord to the subdiencephalic brain stem in man. Psychiat. Neurol. (Basel), *143*, 75–99.

Crawford, A. S., and Knighton, R. S., 1953: Further observations on medullary spinothalamic tractotomy. J. Neurosurg., *10*, 113–121.

French, J. D., Verzeano, M., and Magoun, H. W., 1953a: An extralemniscal sensory system in the brain. A.M.A. Arch. Neurol. Psychiat., *69*, 505–518.

French, J. D., Verzeano, M., and Magoun, H. W., 1953b: A neural basis of the anesthetic state. A.M.A. Arch. Neurol. Psychiat., *69*, 519–529.

Fulton, J. F., 1949: *Physiology of Nervous System,* 3rd ed. Oxford University Press, New York.

Glees, P., 1953: The central pain tract (tractus spino-thalamicus). Acta Neuroveg. (Wien), *7*, 160–174.

Hingson, R. A., and Edwards, W. B., 1943: Continuous caudal analgesia in obstetrics. J.A.M.A., *121*, 225–229.

Hinsey, J. C., and Phillips, R. A., 1940: Observations upon diaphragmatic sensation. J. Neurophysiol., *3*, 175–181.

Hyndman, O. R., and Jarvis, F. J., 1940: Gastric crisis of tabes dorsalis: treatment by anterior chordotomy in eight cases. Arch. Surg., *40*, 997–1013.

Hyndman, O. R., and Wolkin, J., 1943: Anterior chordotomy: further observations on physiologic results and optimum manner of performance. A.M.A. Arch. Neurol. Psychiat., *50*, 129–148.

Magoun, H. W., 1958: *The Waking Brain.* Charles C Thomas, Springfield, Ill.

Mehler, W. R., Feferman, M. E., and Nauta, W. J. H., 1960: Ascending axon degeneration following anterolateral cordotomy. An experimental study in the monkey. Brain, *83*, 718–750.

Nathan, P. W., 1963: Results of antero-lateral cordotomy for pain in cancer. J. Neurol. Neurosurg. Psychiat., *26*, 353–362.

Nathan, P. W., and Smith, M. C., 1953: Spinal pathways subserving defaecation and sensation from the lower bowel. J. Neurol. Neurosurg. Psychiat., *16*, 245–256.

Pearson, A. A., 1952: Role of gelatinous substance of spinal cord in conduction of pain. A.M.A. Arch. Neurol. Psychiat., *68*, 515–529.

Poirier, L. J., and Bertrand, C., 1955: Experimental and anatomical investigation of the lateral spino-thalamic and spino-tectal tracts. J. Comp. Neurol., *102*, 745–757.

Ruch, T. C., 1961: Pathophysiology of pain. In *Neurophysiology,* T. C. Ruch, H. D. Patton, J. W. Woodbury, and A. L. Towe, Chapter 15. W. B. Saunders Company, Philadelphia, pp. 350–368.

Schwartz, H. G., and O'Leary, J. L., 1941: Section of the spinothalamic tract in the medulla with observations on the pathway for pain. Surgery, *9*, 183–193.

Swanson, A. G., Buchan, G. C., and Alvord, E. C., Jr., 1965: Anatomic changes in congenital insensitivity to pain. Arch. Neurol. (Chicago), *12*, 12–18.

Szentágothai, J., 1964: Neuronal and synaptic arrangement in the substantia gelatinosa Rolandi. J. Comp. Neurol., *122*, 219–239.

White, J. C., 1954: Conduction of pain in man; observations on its afferent pathways within the spinal cord and visceral nerves. A.M.A. Arch. Neurol. Psychiat., *71*, 1–23.

Yoss, R. E., 1953: Studies of the spinal cord. III. Pathways for deep pain within the spinal cord and brain. Neurology, *3*, 163–175.

Chapter 7

The Brain Stem: External and Internal Configurations

GENERAL TOPOGRAPHY

The **brain stem,** as previously stated, consists of thalamus, midbrain, pons, and medulla oblongata. It has already been observed that the medulla oblongata is a direct and expanded upward continuation of the spinal cord and that it consists of closed and open portions. The floor of the fourth ventricle, often called the *rhomboid fossa,* occupies the posterior surface of the open portion and extends rostrally to assume the same relationship to the pons (Fig. 55).

The **fourth ventricle** is bounded infero-

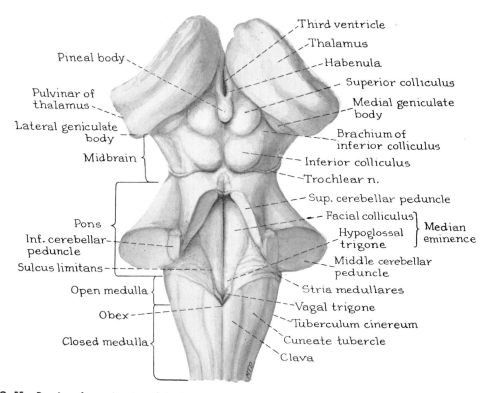

FIG. 55. Drawing of posterior view of the brain stem.

laterally, on both sides, by the inferior cerebellar peduncle, the cuneate tubercle, and the clava (Fig. 55). The rostrolateral walls of the ventricle are formed by the superior cerebellar peduncles. The inferior peduncles curve posteriorly from the medulla to enter the cerebellum. The superior peduncles course rostrally from the cerebellum to the midbrain and, as they pass forward, sink into the tegmentum (dorsal area) of the pons. The functions of the cerebellar peduncles will be considered in Chapter 19.

All of the cranial nerves except the olfactory, which terminates in the olfactory bulb (Fig. 73), and the spinal part of the accessory have a superficial origin (i.e., direct attachment) to the brain stem (Figs. 56, 57). The brain stem attachment of the optic nerve is at the optic chiasm and after partial decussation con-

tinues as the optic tract to the lateral geniculate body and to the superior colliculus of the midbrain (Fig. 57). The superficial origin of the oculomotor nerve is on the anterior aspect of the brain stem at the medial border of the cerebral peduncle just rostral to the transverse fibers of the pons (Fig. 56). The trochlear nerve arises superficially from the superior (anterior) medullary velum at the caudal margin of the inferior colliculus (Fig. 55). The trigeminal nerve arises superficially from the lateral aspect of the middle of the pons by two roots, the sensory root (portio major) and the motor root (portio minor). The superficial origin of the abducens nerve is on the anterior aspect of the brain stem at the junction of pons and medulla (Fig. 56). The facial nerve with its sensory root, the intermediate nerve, arises superficially at the anterolateral

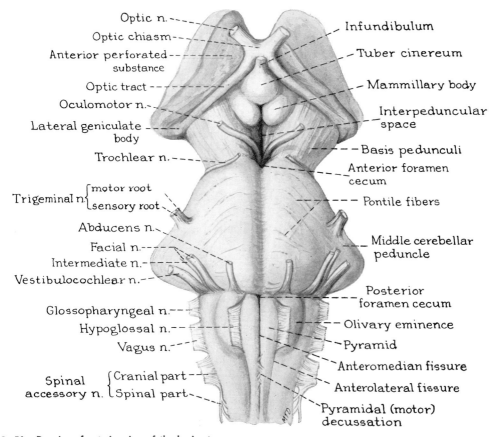

FIG. 56. Drawing of anterior view of the brain stem.

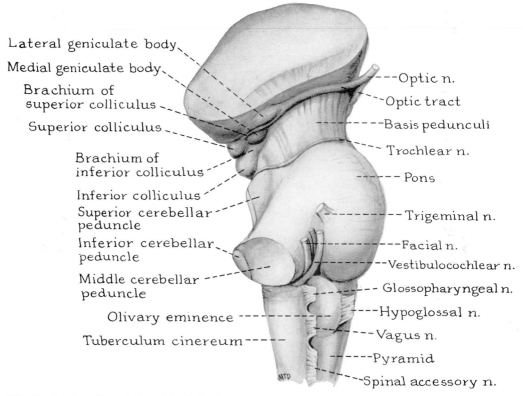

Lateral geniculate body
Medial geniculate body
Brachium of superior colliculus
Superior colliculus
Brachium of inferior colliculus
Inferior colliculus
Superior cerebellar peduncle
Inferior cerebellar peduncle
Middle cerebellar peduncle
Olivary eminence
Tuberculum cinereum

Optic n.
Optic tract
Basis pedunculi
Trochlear n.
Pons
Trigeminal n.
Facial n.
Vestibulocochlear n.
Glossopharyngeal n.
Hypoglossal n.
Vagus n.
Pyramid
Spinal accessory n.

FIG. 57.   Drawing of lateral view of the brain stem.

border of the caudal pons, and more later-alward at the caudal border of the pons is the attachment of the vestibulocochlear nerve (Figs. 56, 57). The glossopharyngeal and vagus nerves and cranial part of the accessory nerve arise as a series of rootlets from the medulla along the posterolateral sulcus in line with the dorsal roots of the spinal nerves (Figs. 56, 57). The rootlets of the spinal part of the accessory nerve arise from the first six segments of the spinal cord. These rootlets unite into a common trunk which courses cephalad and joins the cranial part of the accessory nerve (Fig. 56). The hypoglossal nerve emerges from the medulla as a series of rootlets along the anterolateral sulcus between the pyramid and olivary eminence (Figs. 56, 57).

The Medulla

On the anterior aspect of the medulla the pyramids appear as longitudinal prominences on either side of the antero-median fissure (Fig. 56). The anteromedian fissure terminates at the junction of the medulla and pons as the *posterior foramen cecum*. Its termination at this point is due to the superimposition of a broad band of transversely coursing fibers on the anterior surface of the brain stem. They are the *pontile fibers* and can be seen to become concentrated laterally and dorsally into bilateral bundles—middle cerebellar peduncles—which enter the cerebellum.

The **lateral view of the brain stem** shows to good advantage the rootlets of the spinal accessory, vagus, and glossopharyngeal nerves which emerge from the medulla through the dorsolateral sulcus (Fig. 57).

Cross-sections through the medulla at the level of the glossopharyngeal (IX) and vestibulocochlear (VIII) nerves show that these nerves traverse the widest part of the fourth ventricle (Figs. 58, 59). Note that the *lateral spinothalamic tracts* and *medial lemnisci* occupy the same relative positions as at more caudal medullary levels. In sections through the most caudal region of the pons (Fig. 60), the transversely cut bundles of fibers which comprise the medial lemnisci are oriented somewhat obliquely. This orientation reflects the rotation which the medial lemnisci undergo in passing through the transition zone from medulla to pons. This rotation, approximately 90°, brings the medial lemnisci into the transverse position at the intermediate levels of the pons (Figs. 61, 62). The rotation occurs in such a way as to bring the original posterior, or cuneate, component medially and the more anterior, or gracile, component laterally. In more rostral sections (Figs.

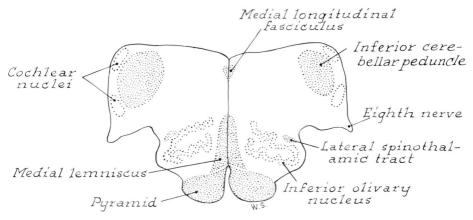

FIG. 58. Section through the open portion of the medulla oblongata.

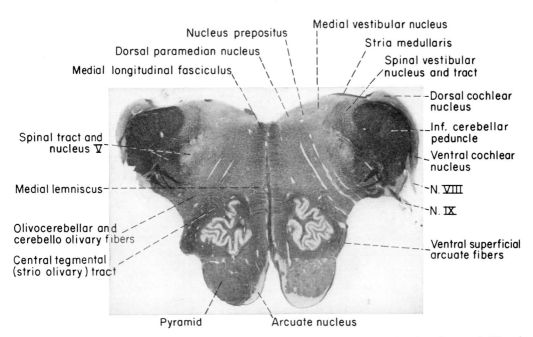

FIG. 59. Photomicrograph of a transverse section through the medulla at the level of the glossopharyngeal (IX) and cochlear division of the vestibulocochlear (VIII) nerves. Note the reduced pyramid on the right. (See explanation for Figure 52 which is a section from the same brain stem.) Weil stain.

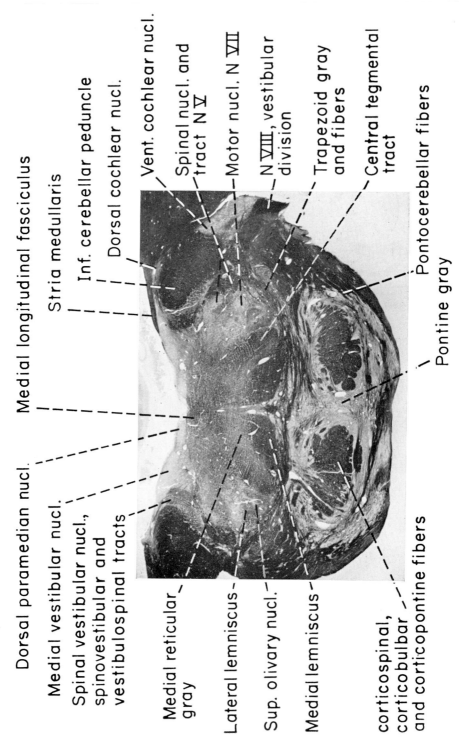

Dorsal paramedian nucl.

Medial vestibular nucl.

Spinal vestibular nucl.,
spinovestibular and
vestibulospinal tracts

Medial reticular
gray

Lateral lemniscus

Sup. olivary nucl.

Medial lemniscus

corticospinal,
corticobulbar
and corticopontine fibers

Medial longitudinal fasciculus

Stria medullaris

Inf. cerebellar peduncle

Dorsal cochlear nucl.

Vent. cochlear nucl.

Spinal nucl. and
tract N V

Motor nucl. N VII

N VIII, vestibular
division

Trapezoid gray
and fibers

Central tegmental
tract

Pontocerebellar fibers

Pontine gray

FIG. 60. Photomicrograph of a transverse section through the caudal pons at the level of the nuclei of the facial (VII) and vestibulocochlear (VIII) nerves.

63, 64) the medial lemnisci are seen to have migrated laterally from the median raphé and are in relation to the spinothalamic tracts.

The Pons

Transverse sections of the pons (sections cut at right angles to its rostrocaudal axis) reveal that it consists of posterior and anterior portions which are quite different from one another in appearance (Figs. 61, 62). The *tegmentum,* or posterior part, is continuous with that portion of the medulla dorsal to the pyramids (Fig. 58). The *basis pontis,* or anterior part, is composed, in great part, of the transversely coursing *pontile fibers* already referred to. Intermingled with the pontile fibers are bundles of longitudinally coursing fibers and numerous nuclear masses. The corticospinal fibers which are included in the longitudinal group continue caudally into the pyramids of the medulla (Figs. 56, 58); they will be discussed later. The cells of the *pontile nuclei,* or nuclear masses, give origin to the pontile or pontocerebellar fibers (Figs. 60, 61, 63).

The **lateral lemniscus**—another smaller bundle of longitudinally coursing fibers—lies posterolateral to the medial lemniscus in the tegmentum of the pons (Figs. 61, 62). It is an important link in the central auditory pathway and is readily identified in Weil-stained sections of the pons; it becomes important at this point in the discussion because the *lateral spinothalamic tract* is located just posterolateral to it.

The *lateral lemniscus,* at the extreme rostral limit of the pons (Figs. 65, 66), moves to a more dorsal position; it lies immediately lateral to the lower half of the superior cerebellar peduncle which here is completely submerged in the tegmentum of the pons. The *lateral spinothalamic tract* at this level lies posterolateral to the medial lemniscus near the surface of the pons.

The Midbrain

The posterior surface of the midbrain presents four rounded eminences or *colliculi* (Fig. 55). The two rostral eminences usually are termed the *superior colliculi* and the two caudal ones the *inferior colliculi.* The colliculi are also called *quadrigeminal bodies.* The two *bases pedunculi,* separated from one another by the *interpeduncular space* are seen on the anterior aspect of the midbrain (Fig. 56). The interpeduncular space terminates

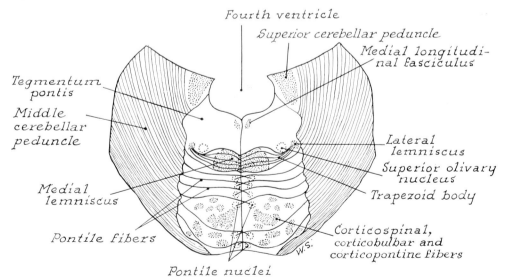

FIG. 61. A transverse section through the caudal third of the pons.

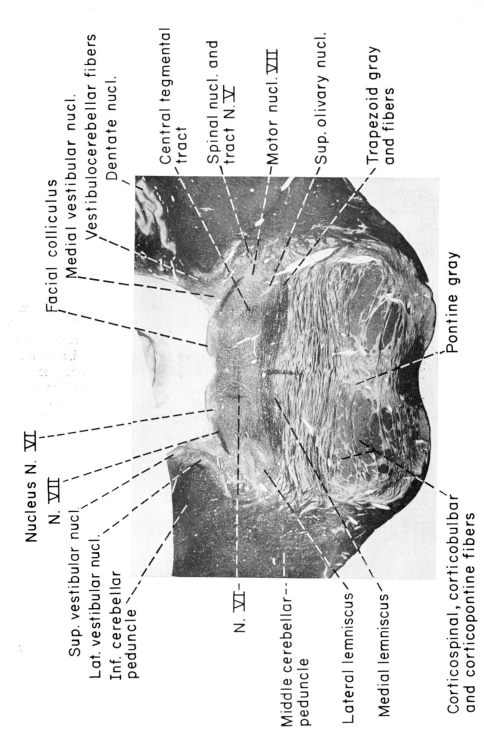

Nucleus N. VI
N. VII

Facial colliculus
Medial vestibular nucl.
Vestibulocerebellar fibers
Dentate nucl.

Central tegmental tract
Spinal nucl. and tract N. V
Motor nucl. VII
Sup. olivary nucl.
Trapezoid gray and fibers

Sup. vestibular nucl.
Lat. vestibular nucl.
Inf. cerebellar peduncle

N. VI

Middle cerebellar peduncle
Lateral lemniscus
Medial lemniscus

Corticospinal, corticobulbar and corticopontine fibers

Pontine gray

FIG. 62.   Photomicrograph of a transverse section through the caudal pons at the level of the motor nuclei of the abducens (VI), and facial (VII) nerves. Weil stain.

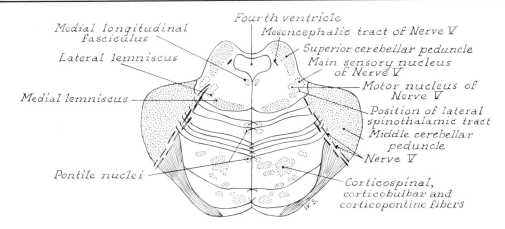

FIG. 63. Section through the pons at the level of the trigeminal nerve.

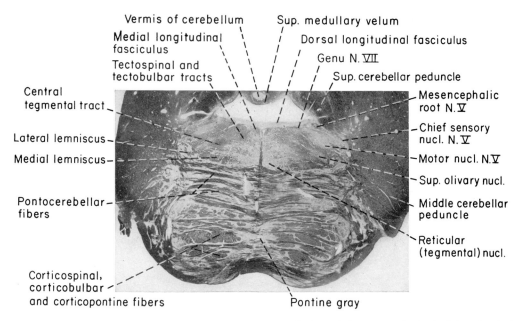

FIG. 64. Photomicrograph of a transverse section through the middle third of the pons at the level of the trigeminal (V) nerve. Weil stain.

caudally as the *anterior foramen cecum* at the point where the bases pedunculi disappear under cover of the pontile fibers (Fig. 56).

In transverse sections through the midbrain (Figs. 67–70) the original cavity of the embryonic neural tube is represented by the *cerebral aqueduct (aqueduct of Sylvius)* which connects the third and fourth ventricles (Fig. 74). The *central gray matter,* within the ventral area

of which the oculomotor and trochlear nuclei are found, surrounds the cerebral aqueduct. The part of the midbrain that lies posterior to the level of the aqueduct, including the quadrigeminal bodies, is called the *quadrigeminal lamina,* or *tectum.* The *tegmentum* of the midbrain lies between the quadrigeminal lamina and the *bases pedunculi.* Its contact with the bases pedunculi, on both sides, is marked by a pigmented layer of gray matter called

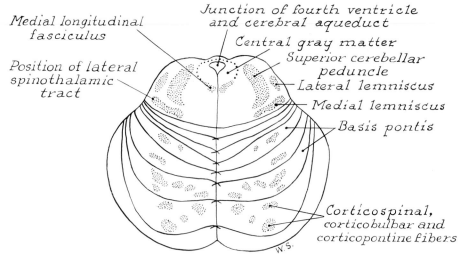

FIG. 65.   Section through the rostral part of the pons.

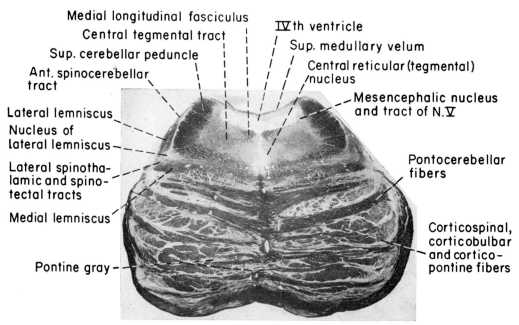

FIG. 66.   Photomicrograph of a transverse section through the rostral third of the pons (Isthmus region). Weil stain.

the *substantia nigra.* The tegmentum is continuous with the correspondingly named area of the pons, and the bases pedunculi continue caudally into the basis pontis. The corticospinal, corticobulbar, and corticopontile fibers that constitute the bases pedunculi account for the longitudinally coursing bundles of fibers previously noted in the basilar part of the pons.

In the midbrain, the *medial lemniscus* is forced into a more lateral and posterior position by the *decussation of the superior cerebellar peduncles* and by the *red nucleus;* the former are seen at the level of the interior colliculi and the latter at the level of the superior colliculi (Figs. 67–70). The peduncles cross the midline and distribute large proportions of their component fibers to the red nuclei. The

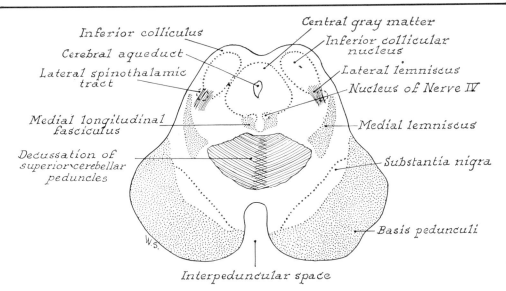

Inferior colliculus
Cerebral aqueduct
Lateral spinothalamic tract
Medial longitudinal fasciculus
Decussation of superior cerebellar peduncles
Central gray matter
Inferior collicular nucleus
Lateral lemniscus
Nucleus of Nerve IV
Medial lemniscus
Substantia nigra
Basis pedunculi
Interpeduncular space
W. S.

FIG. 67.   Section through the midbrain at the level of the inferior colliculi.

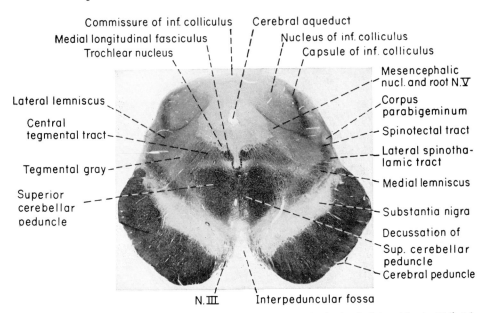

Commissure of inf. colliculus
Medial longitudinal fasciculus
Trochlear nucleus
Cerebral aqueduct
Nucleus of inf. colliculus
Capsule of inf. colliculus
Lateral lemniscus
Central tegmental tract
Tegmental gray
Superior cerebellar peduncle
Mesencephalic nucl. and root N.V
Corpus parabigeminum
Spinotectal tract
Lateral spinothalamic tract
Medial lemniscus
Substantia nigra
Decussation of Sup. cerebellar peduncle
Cerebral peduncle
N. III
Interpeduncular fossa

FIG. 68.   Photomicrograph of a transverse section through the inferior collicular level of the midbrain. Weil stain.

red nuclei are so-called because they are pinkish in appearance in freshly cut sections.

The *lateral lemniscus,* at the level of the inferior colliculi, is actually posteromedial to the medial lemniscus. Most of its fibers terminate in the *nucleus of the inferior colliculus* (Figs. 67, 68). At the level of the superior colliculi the *inferior quadrigeminal brachium* (peduncle of the inferior colliculus), composed of axons originating in the inferior collicular nucleus, occupies a superficial position, dorsolateral to the medial lemniscus (Figs. 69, 70). The *lateral spinothalamic tract* intermingles with the terminal fibers of the lateral lemniscus at the level of the inferior colliculi and lies medial to the inferior quadrigeminal brachium at the superior collicular level.

6

It should be noted that the lateral spino-thalamic tract is superficial in the tegmentum at midbrain levels and is thus accessible to the surgical procedure known as mesencephalic tractotomy. This procedure has been used effectively for treatment of intractable pain without surgical complications. Incisions at this level also sever the secondary trigeminal pathway and serve to relieve pain originating in the head region. The course of the trigeminothalamic fibers from the spinal nucleus of the trigeminal nerve will be described in Chapter 8.

The Diencephalon

The diencephalon is so completely and intimately surrounded by the cerebral hemispheres as to appear to be a part of them (Fig. 71). Only its anterior surface can be observed in the intact brain (Fig. 73). Two rounded prominences at the caudal limit of its anterior surface are known as *mammillary bodies.* The *tuber cinereum,* from which the hypophysis is suspended, is immediately rostral to the mammillary bodies; the *optic chiasm* is rostral to it.

The **third ventricle** appears as a slit-like cavity in sections of the diencephalon (Figs. 71, 72). It communicates with the fourth ventricle by way of the cerebral aqueduct. Rostrally, it communicates, through the paired *interventricular fora-mina,* with the right and left lateral ventricles in the cerebral hemispheres (Fig. 74). The floor of the third ventricle is formed by the *hypothalamus,* which includes the structures previously mentioned as being visible on the inferior surface of the diencephalon as well as several nuclei and fiber tracts which will be discussed later (Chap. 21). The lateral walls of the ventricle are formed by the medial surfaces of the right and left *thalami.* The *interthalamic adhesion (massa intermedia),* which is not always present, bridges the ventricle and connects the two thalami with each other (Fig. 75). The roof of the third ventricle is formed by a thin layer of ependyma which stretches between the superior and medial borders of the two thalami and by the pia mater overlying the ependyma. The pia mater, which is rich in blood vessels, constitutes the tela choroidea of the third ventricle (Figs. 71, 72). From this vascular layer tufts of blood vessels, covered by epithelium, invaginate into the ventricle and form the choroid plexus (Fig. 239).

When observed from above following removal of the cerebral hemispheres and corpus callosum, the **thalami** are seen to consist of ovoid masses of gray matter on both sides of the third ventricle (Fig. 55). Each side is considerably expanded at its caudal limit; the expansion is termed the *pulvinar.* The superior and lateral sur-

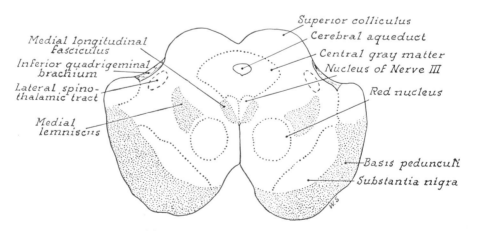

FIG. 69.   Section through the midbrain at the level of the superior colliculi.

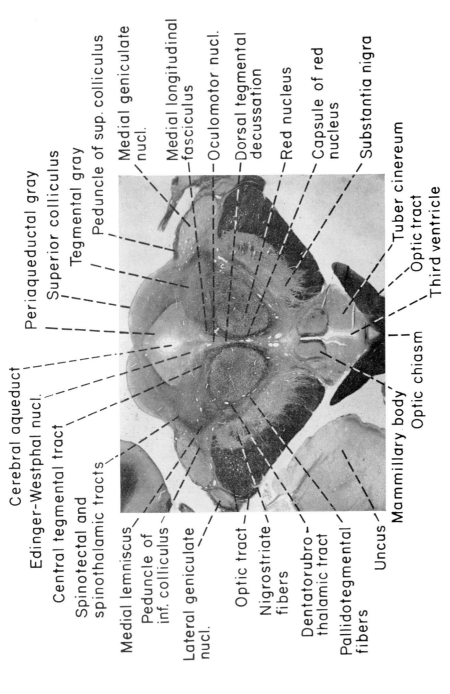

FIG. 70. Photomicrograph of a transverse section through the superior collicular level of the midbrain. Weil stain.

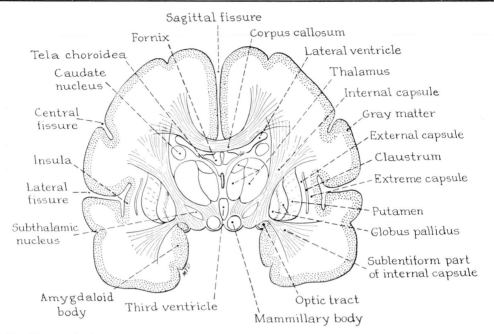

FIG. 71. Diagram of a frontal section through the brain at the diencephalic level.

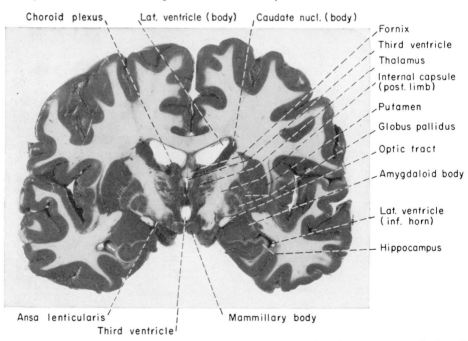

FIG. 72. Anterior view of a coronal section of brain at the level of the mammillary bodies stained by the ferric ferrocyanide method of Tompsett.

faces of the thalamus are covered by thin layers of white matter (Fig. 75). The layer on the superior surface is called the *stratum zonale;* that on the lateral surface, the *external medullary lamina.* A Y-shaped reflection from the stratum zonale into the substance of the thalamus, as seen in sections, is termed the *internal medullary lamina* (Fig. 75). It divides the thalamus into *medial, lateral,* and

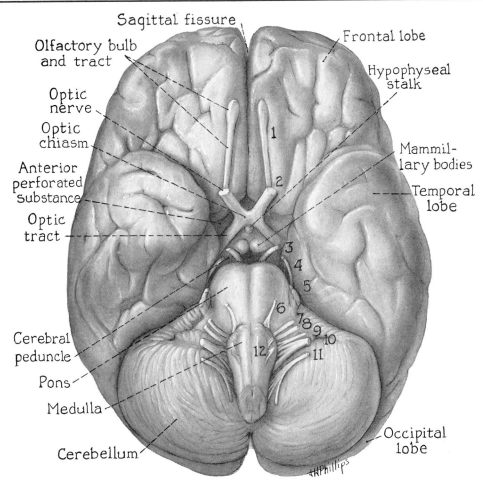

FIG. 73. Drawing of inferior surface of the brain.

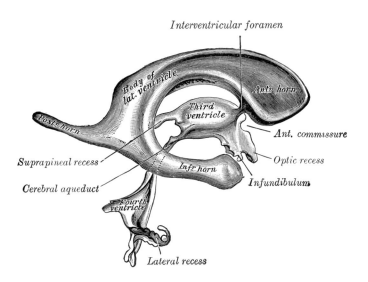

FIG. 74. Drawing of a cast of the ventricular system of the brain as seen from the side. (Retzius in Gray's Anatomy.)

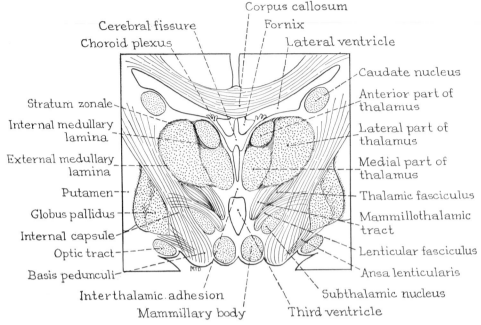

Corpus callosum
Cerebral fissure
Fornix
Choroid plexus
Lateral ventricle
Caudate nucleus
Stratum zonale
Anterior part of thalamus
Internal medullary lamina
Lateral part of thalamus
External medullary lamina
Medial part of thalamus
Putamen
Thalamic fasciculus
Globus pallidus
Mammillothalamic tract
Internal capsule
Lenticular fasciculus
Optic tract
Basis pedunculi
Ansa lenticularis
Interthalamic adhesion
Subthalamic nucleus
Mammillary body
Third ventricle

FIG. 75. Diagram of a frontal section through the diencephalon.

anterior parts. The anterior part, in frontal sections through the middle third of the thalamus, is superiorly placed; the reason for its being called anterior is quite obvious in horizontal sections, however (Figs. 76, 77).

Each of the three parts of the thalamus contains a number of nuclei which have more or less specific functions. The nucleus in which the medial lemniscus and lateral spinothalamic tract terminate is ventrally and caudally placed in the lateral part (Fig. 78) and is designated the *posterolateral ventral nucleus.* Medial to it is the posteromedial ventral nucleus in which impulses from the head region are received. The two nuclei have been described as a "ventrobasal complex." Within the posterolateral portion the body segments are represented in an orderly fashion with cervical segments most medial and sacral segments most lateral. The posteromedial portion contains representation of contralateral head, face, and intraoral structures with mouth and face most medially located.

The regions of the external and internal medullary laminæ (Figs. 75–77) contain the reticular and/or intralaminar nuclei which play an important role in the conduction of nonspecific sensory impulses to the cerebral cortex. These impulses reach the intralaminar nuclei by way of the extralemniscal sensory system (Chap. 6) and, through this thalamic relay, contribute to the "arousal" of the cerebrum, making it receptive to visual, auditory, and general sensory impulses.

The **internal capsule**—so-called because it appears to form the inner part of a capsule of white matter surrounding the lentiform nucleus—lies immediately lateral to the external medullary lamina of the thalamus (Figs. 71, 72, 75). It is composed of axons of cells in the thalamus which are proceeding to the cerebral cortex and of axons of cells in the cortex which are distributed to lower levels of the central nervous system. The *thalamocortical fibers* include fibers which carry general sensory impulses from the posterolateral ventral nucleus to the sensory area of the cortex (Fig. 78).

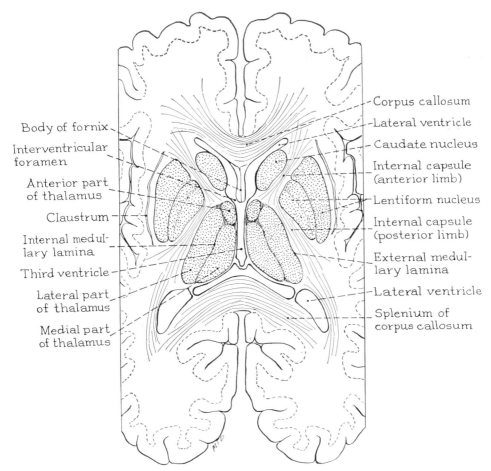

Corpus callosum

Lateral ventricle

Caudate nucleus

Internal capsule
(anterior limb)

Lentiform nucleus

Internal capsule
(posterior limb)

External medul-
lary lamina

Lateral ventricle

Splenium of
corpus callosum

Body of fornix

Interventricular
foramen

Anterior part
of thalamus

Claustrum

Internal medul-
lary lamina

Third ventricle

Lateral part
of thalamus

Medial part
of thalamus

FIG. 76. Diagram of a horizontal section through the diencephalon.

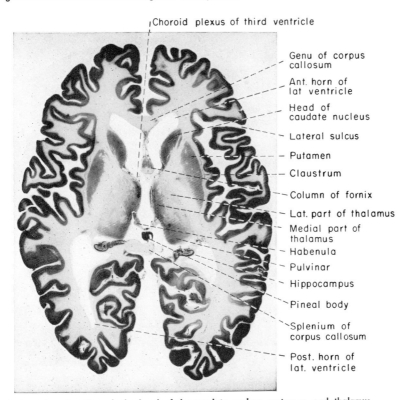

Choroid plexus of third ventricle

Genu of corpus
callosum

Ant. horn of
lat ventricle

Head of
caudate nucleus

Lateral sulcus

Putamen

Claustrum

Column of fornix

Lat. part of thalamus

Medial part of
thalamus

Habenula

Pulvinar

Hippocampus

Pineal body

Splenium of
corpus callosum

Post. horn of
lat. ventricle

FIG. 77. A horizontal section through the head of the caudate nucleus, putamen, and thalamus.

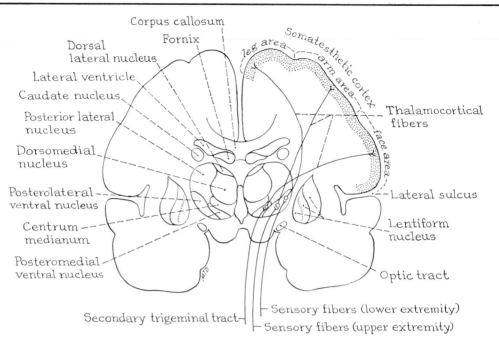

FIG. 78. Diagram showing the termination of sensory tracts in the nuclei of the lateral part of the thalamus, and the projection of these nuclei on the somatesthetic cortex by way of the internal capsule (modified from Ranson).

BIBLIOGRAPHY

Carpenter, M. B., Stein, B. M., and Shriver, J. E., 1968: Central projections of spinal dorsal roots in the monkey. II. Lower thoracic, lumbosacral and coccygeal dorsal roots. Amer. J. Anat., *123,* 75–118.

Cohen, S. M., and Grundfest, H., 1954: Thalamic loci of electrical activity initiated by afferent impulses in cat. J. Neurophysiol., *17,* 193–297.

Fisher, C. M., 1965: Pure sensory stroke involving face, arm and leg. Neurology (Minneap.), *15,* 76–80.

Glees, P., 1953: The central pain tract (tractus spino-thalamicus). Acta Neuroveg. (Wein), *7,* 160–174.

Morin, F., Schwartz, H. G., and O'Leary, J. L., 1951: Experimental study of the spinothalamic and related tracts. Acta Psychiat. Neurol. Scand., *26,* 371–396.

Mountcastle, V. B., and Henneman, E., 1952: The representation of tactile sensibility in the thalamus of the monkey. J. Comp. Neurol., *97,* 409–439.

Poirier, L. J., and Bertrand, C., 1955: Experimental and anatomical investigation of the lateral spino-thalamic and spino-tectal tracts. J. Comp. Neurol., *102,* 745–757.

Rasmussen, A. T., and Peyton, W. T., 1941: The location of the lateral spinothalamic tract in the brain stem of man. Surgery, *10,* 699–710.

Soffin, G., Feldman, M., and Bender, M. B., 1968: Alterations of sensory levels in vascular lesions of lateral medulla. Arch. Neurol. (Chicago), *18,* 178–190.

Walker, A. E., 1942: Relief of pain by mesencephalic tractotomy, A.M.A. Arch. Neurol. Psychiat., *48,* 865–883.

Whitlock, D. G., and Perl, E. R., 1961: Thalamic projections of spinothalamic pathways in monkey. Exp. Neurol., *3,* 240–255.

Chapter 8

General Afferent Pathways from the Head

The pathways to the thalamus traversed by afferent impulses originating in the trunk and extremities have now been described in considerable detail. Before discussing their further course through the internal capsule and their manner of termination in the cerebral cortex, we shall trace the pathways concerned in the conduction of afferent impulses from the head region to the thalamus. A diagrammatic representation of major brain stem nuclei which receive afferent fibers from the head is shown in Fig. 79.

General somatic afferent fibers are contained in the *trigeminal, facial, glossopharyngeal, vagus, oculomotor, trochlear,* and *abducens nerves.* Since the great majority of these fibers are in the trigeminal nerve, it will be considered first.

The *trigeminal ganglion,* like the spinal ganglia, is developed from the neural crest. Like the spinal ganglia, it contains unipolar neurons. It is located between the two layers of the cranial dura mater, on the anterior surface of the petrosa of the temporal bone (Meckel's cave). The peripheral processes of the ganglion cells are distributed to exteroceptive endings throughout the head region by way of the *ophthalmic, maxillary,* and *mandibular divisions* of the trigeminal nerve. The central processes form the *sensory root* of the nerve which crosses the superior border of the petrosa and enters the pons at a point approximately midway between its rostral and caudal borders and in the region where the pontile fibers enter into, and form, the middle cerebellar peduncle (Figs. 56, 57).

The *motor root* of the trigeminal nerve emerges from the pons immediately anterior (rostral) to the entering fibers of the sensory root; it is chiefly motor in function but also contains proprioceptive fibers which are distributed to the muscles of mastication.

Some of the **fibers of the sensory root** terminate in the *main sensory nucleus* of the trigeminal nerve which, in transverse sections through the middle third of the pons, is seen in the posterolateral area of the pontile tegmentum (Figs. 64, 80). The nucleus is anterior to the superior cerebellar peduncle, medial to the middle cerebellar peduncle, and posterolateral to the motor nucleus of the trigeminal. The motor and sensory nuclei are separated from one another by a layer of trigeminal nerve fibers. The fibers that terminate in the main sensory nucleus are concerned only with tactile sensibility.

Other central fibers of the trigeminal nerve turn caudally to form its *descending* or *spinal tract;* this tract continues downward through the caudal third of the pons and through the entire length of the me-

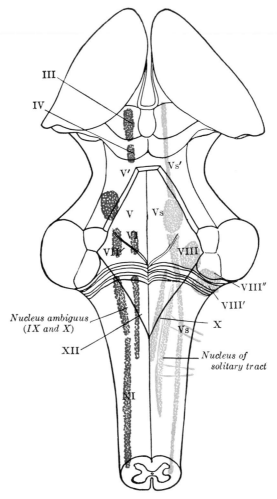

FIG. 79. The cranial nerve nuclei schematically represented; posterior view. Motor nuclei in sensory in blue. (The olfactory and optic centers are not represented.) (From Gray's Anatomy, 28th ed. Charles Mayo Goss, Ed., Lea & Febiger, Philadelphia.)

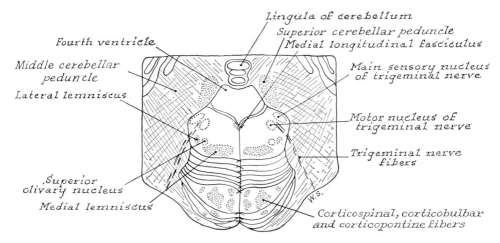

FIG. 80. Section through the pons at the level of the main sensory and motor nuclei of the trigeminal nerve.

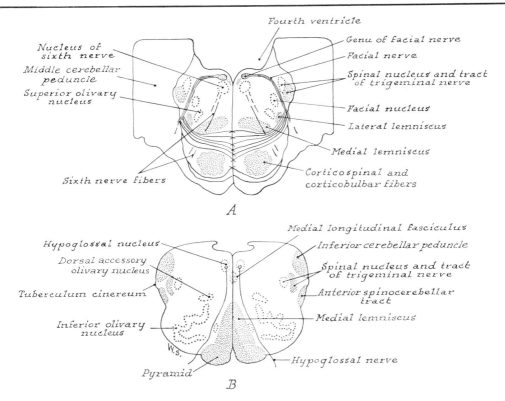

FIG. 81. A, Section through the pons at the level of the abducens nucleus. B, Section through the medulla near the caudal end of the fourth ventricle.

dulla (Fig. 81). In the pons it lies in the lateral part of the tegmentum and in intimate relation to the middle cerebellar peduncle (Fig. 81A).

In the medulla the tract is relatively superficial and, with its nucleus, accounts for a narrow longitudinal prominence observable on the surface and known as the *tuberculum cinereum;* it lies considerably dorsal to the inferior olivary nucleus and immediately anterior to the inferior cerebellar peduncle (Figs. 43, 81B). Throughout its course the tract distributes fibers to the *spinal nucleus* of the trigeminal; the spinal nucleus extends caudally from the main sensory nucleus in the pons to the level of the junction of medulla and spinal cord and lies just medial to the tract (Fig. 82). The spinal tract and nucleus are chiefly concerned with pain and thermal impulses. Following medullary spinothalamic tractotomy

(Chap. 6), ipsilateral analgesia of the face has been observed which may be attributed to destruction of, or injury to, the spinal tract and nucleus of the trigeminal nerve. On the basis of the order in which recovery of pain sense has been observed to occur following this surgical procedure, it appears that the fibers in the spinal tract are arranged from posterior to anterior in the following order: mandibular, maxillary, and ophthalmic. This arrangement of fibers in the spinal tract has also been described from experiments with cats. In addition to the posterior-anterior arrangement, there is a cephalo-caudal pattern within the spinal tract which reflects the differences in caudal extent of pain and temperature fibers from the three main divisions of the fifth nerve. The ophthalmic fibers terminate on cells in the most caudal part of the spinal nucleus; some reach the level of the sec-

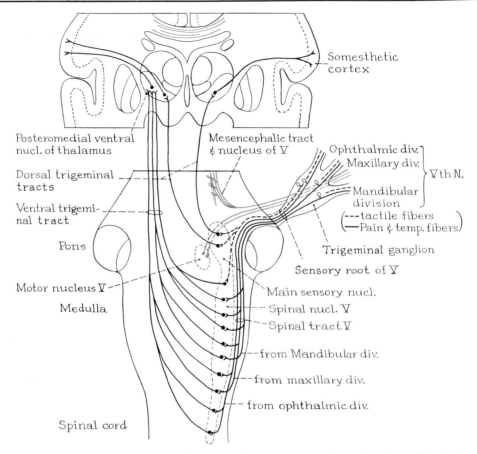

Posteromedial ventral nucl. of thalamus

Mesencephalic tract & nucleus of V

Ophthalmic div.
Maxillary div. } V th N.
Mandibular division

Somesthetic cortex

Dorsal trigeminal tracts

Ventral trigeminal tract

(---tactile fibers
—Pain & temp. fibers)

Pons

Trigeminal ganglion

Sensory root of V

Motor nucleus V

Main sensory nucl.

Medulla

Spinal nucl. V

Spinal tract V

from Mandibular div.

from maxillary div.

from ophthalmic div.

Spinal cord

FIG. 82.   Diagram of the central connections of the trigeminal nerve superimposed on a dorsal view of the brain stem.

ond or third cervical segment. The mandibular fibers end on cells in the more cephalic part of the nucleus and fibers of the maxillary nerve synapse with cells in the intermediate region (Fig. 82). There is some overlap in the termination of descending spinal tract fibers as well as variation in caudal extent. Significantly, complete facial analgesia may be obtained by section of the spinal tract at the level of the obex.

Some tactile impulses are conducted through the spinal tract to its nucleus. A considerable number of the central processes of trigeminal ganglion cells concerned with the transmission of tactile impulses divide into ascending branches which terminate in the main sensory nucleus and descending branches which end in the spinal nucleus.

It should be noted that the spinal tract and nucleus are, in effect, upward extensions into the brain stem of the posterior-lateral fasciculus of Lissauer and the gelatinous substance of the posterior gray column (Figs. 41, 83). Moreover, the spinal nucleus has a gelatinous appearance similar to that of its counterpart in the spinal cord. The fact that the nucleus and tract are primarily concerned with pain and thermal sensibilities is also of interest in view of the pain and thermal functions of the analogous spinal cord structures.

Cell bodies of secondary neurons in sensory pathways to the cerebral cortex from levels served by the spinal nerves are found in the posterior gray columns—so-called tract cells. Cells similar in function are found in the sensory nuclei of

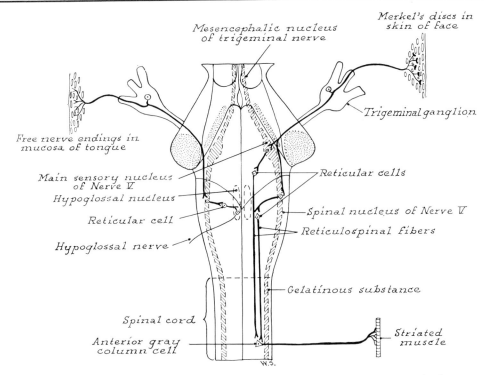

FIG. 83. Diagram showing a reflex arc through the spinal nucleus of the trigeminal nerve, reticular formation, and hypoglossal nucleus (left side) and trigeminoreticulospinal arcs (right side).

cranial nerves and are responsible for transmission of sensory impulses upward to the thalamus (Fig. 82). There are also association or internuncial cells in the sensory nuclei; they connect, through the reticular formation, with efferent neurons in the brain stem and thus enter into reflex arcs (Fig. 83). The efferent neurons may have their cell bodies in motor nuclei of cranial nerves or in the reticular formation.

The term, **reticular formation,** is applied to the network of gray and white matter in the medulla (Fig. 91) and in the tegmental areas of the pons and midbrain. The rather large cells scattered through the formation contribute to numerous reflex arcs within the brain stem and give rise to *reticulospinal fibers.* As their name implies, the reticulospinal fibers descend into the spinal cord where they come into direct or indirect relationship with anterior gray column cells to complete reflex arcs (Fig. 83) whose

effectors are striated muscles of the trunk and extremities.

A third sensory nucleus is associated with the trigeminal nerve. It is concerned with proprioceptive impulses from the muscles of mastication and, because it extends rostrally into the midbrain, it is called the *mesencephalic nucleus* (Figs. 68, 84). Proprioceptive impulses from the extrinsic muscles of the eye may also enter this nucleus. The *mesencephalic root* (or tract) of the trigeminal is associated with the nucleus and both are found at the periphery of the central gray matter surrounding the cerebral aqueduct and in the anterolateral angle of the rostral part of the fourth ventricle (Figs. 64, 84*B, C*).

Whereas the cells in the main sensory and spinal nuclei of the trigeminal, like those in the posterior gray columns of the spinal cord, are multipolar in type. cells in the mesencephalic nucleus are unipolar with axons that divide into peripheral and central processes. The peripheral processes are distributed to proprioceptive endings in the muscles of mastication by way of the mesencephalic root and motor root of the trigeminal nerves (Fig. 82); others may course to the eye muscles with the oculomotor, trochlear, and abducens nerves. The central processes may enter the trigeminal tracts and,

through them, may proceed upward to the thalamus. The fact that the cells in the mesencephalic nucleus are of the unipolar variety leads to the assumption that this nucleus is developed from the rostral limit of the neural crest and that it failed to separate from the neural tube as did those portions which developed into true sensory ganglia.

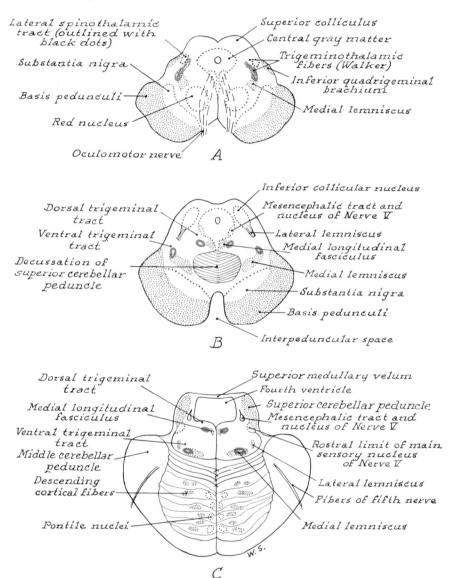

FIG. 84. A, Section through the midbrain at the level of the superior colliculi showing intermingling of trigeminothalamic fibers with fibers of the medial lemniscus and lateral spinothalamic tract (Walker). B, Section through the midbrain at the inferior collicular level showing the locations of the trigeminal tracts and of the mesencephalic tract and nucleus of the trigeminal nerve. C, Section through the rostral part of the pons with the locations of trigeminal tracts and mesencephalic tract and nucleus indicated.

The **secondary afferent pathways of the trigeminal** are usually designated as *ventral* and *dorsal trigeminal tracts (lemnisci)* (Fig. 84). The *ventral tract* is composed chiefly of crossed fibers arising in the opposite spinal and main sensory nuclei (Fig. 82). It terminates in the *posteromedial ventral thalamic nucleus* (Fig. 78). In the medulla the ventral trigeminal tract is closely associated with the lateral spinothalamic tract; this relationship has been thought to account for contralateral analgesia, limited to the ophthalmic distribution of the fifth nerve, subsequent to medullary spinothalamic tractotomy. The ventral tract in the pons forms a flattened bundle on the dorsal aspect of the medial lemniscus.

Experimental studies in monkeys have shown that at the level of the superior colliculi trigeminothalamic fibers are intermingled with the posterolateral fibers of the medial lemniscus and with those of the lateral spinothalamic tract (Fig. 84*A*).

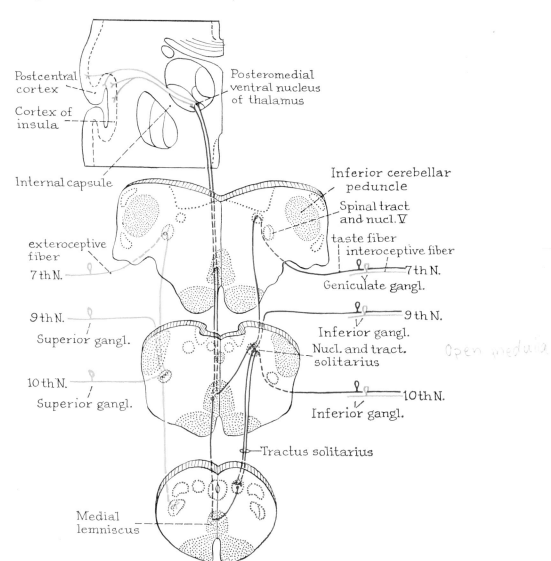

FIG. 85. Diagram showing the central connections of the sensory fibers in the facial, glossopharyngeal, and vagus nerves. The general and special visceral afferent components are shown in blue and red respectively on the right. The general somatic afferent components are shown in green on the left.

The fact that *mesencephalic tractotomy* accomplishes interruption of both the lateral spinothalamic tract and the ventral trigeminal tract has already been mentioned (Chap. 7).

The *dorsal trigeminal tract* is generally considered to be situated anterolateral to the central gray matter surrounding the cerebral aqueduct in the mesencephalon and just ventral to the floor of the fourth ventricle in the pons (Fig. 84*B, C*). Its fibers terminate in the posteromedial ventral nucleus of the thalamus.

GENERAL SOMATIC AFFERENT FIBERS

The general somatic afferent fibers of the *vagus, glossopharyngeal,* and *facial nerves* are distributed to skin in the region of the external ear. These cutaneous fibers of the vagus, auricular branch (Arnold's nerve), arise from cells in the superior ganglion (jugular). Fibers of the glossopharyngeal nerve arise from cells in the superior ganglion (petrosal) of this nerve and are distributed peripherally through the auricular branch of the vagus. The fibers of the facial nerve originate from cell bodies in the geniculate ganglion and their distribution to the ear is through the auricular branch of the facial. The central processes of these fibers enter the medulla and pons, join the spinal tract of the trigeminal, and terminate in the spinal nucleus (Fig. 85).

The general somatic afferent fibers of the *oculomotor, trochlear,* and *abducens nerves,* as was implied in the discussion of the mesencephalic nucleus of the trigeminal, may arise from unipolar cells located in that nucleus and may be distributed to proprioceptive endings in the extrinsic eye muscles. Another view, supported by neurophysiological evidence, is that the afferent fibers to the proprioceptive endings in the extraocular muscles arise from neurons within the oculomotor and trochlear nuclei. Despite the fact that complete information as to the origin of these fibers is still lacking, it is obvious that they have a very important function in coordination of the extraocular muscles. A very delicate balance among all the extrinsic muscles of both eyes is essential to accurate binocular vision.

GENERAL VISCERAL AFFERENT FIBERS

These fibers are present in the *glossopharyngeal* and *vagus nerves.* The fibers of the glossopharyngeal have their cell bodies in the *inferior ganglion* (petrosal). Peripheral processes are distributed to the pharynx, to the posterior third of the tongue, and to the carotid sinus. Central processes enter the medulla in the region of the posterolateral sulcus and through the tractus solitarius synapse on cells in the nucleus solitarius (Figs. 52, 85). The tract is surrounded by the nucleus and, in the open part of the medulla, both are located somewhat medial to the inferior cerebellar peduncle in the reticular formation. They extend throughout almost the entire length of the medulla and at their caudal limit are in the gray matter surrounding the central canal.

The general visceral afferent fibers of the vagus nerve arise from cells in the *inferior ganglion* (nodose) of this nerve. Peripheral processes are distributed to the pharynx, larynx, trachea, esophagus, and thoracic and abdominal viscera. The central processes, like those from the inferior ganglion of the glossopharyngeal and the superior ganglion of the vagus, enter the medulla through the posterolateral sulcus. They are then distributed to cells in the *nucleus solitarius* in the same manner as those from the inferior ganglion of the glossopharyngeal (Fig. 85).

The facial nerve contains some afferent fibers classified as *general visceral afferent.* They arise from cells in the *geniculate ganglion* and are distributed to the posterior part of the nasal cavity and soft palate by way of the *greater (superficial) petrosal* branch of the intermediate nerve. The central processes of these fibers end in the nucleus solitarius.

The **axons of cells in the nucleus soli-**

tarius, on which the general visceral afferent fibers of the glossopharyngeal and vagus nerves synapse, make numerous indirect and direct connections with efferent neurons in visceral and somatic motor nuclei and with neurons in the reticular formation and so complete important visceral and viscerosomatic reflex arcs. The carotid sinus reflex (reflex for control of blood pressure), the respiratory reflexes, the cough reflex, and the vomiting reflex are dependent on such intramedullary connections (Chap. 23). The secondary pathway to the thalamus, for general visceral afferent impulses conducted to the nucleus solitarius by the vagus and glossopharyngeal nerves, is incorporated into the medial lemniscus of the opposite side (Fig. 85).

BIBLIOGRAPHY

Brodal, A., 1947: Central course of afferent fibers for pain in facial glossopharyngeal and vagus nerves. A.M.A. Arch. Neurol. Psychiat., *57*, 292–306.

Carpenter, M. B., and Hanna, G. R., 1961: Fiber projections from the spinal trigeminal nucleus in the cat. J. Comp. Neurol., *117*, 117–132.

Corbin, K. B., 1940: Observations on the peripheral distribution of fibers arising in the mesencephalic nucleus of the fifth cranial nerve. J. Comp. Neurol., *73*, 153–177.

Corbin, K. B., and Harrison, F., 1942: Further attempts to trace the origin of afferent nerves to the extrinsic eye muscles. J. Comp. Neurol., *77*, 187–190.

Corbin, K. B., and Oliver, R. K., 1942: The origin of fibers to the grape-like endings in the insertion third of the extra-ocular muscles. J. Comp. Neurol., *77*, 171–186.

Crawford, A. S., and Knighton, R. S., 1953: Further observations on medullary spinothalamic tractotomy. J. Neurosurg., *10*, 113–121.

Foley, J. O., and DuBois, F. S., 1943: An experimental study of the facial nerve. J. Comp. Neurol., *79*, 79–105.

Kerr, F. W. L., 1963: The divisional organization of afferent fibers of the trigeminal nerve. Brain, *86*, 721–732.

Kimmel, D. L., Kimmel, C. B., and Zarkin, A., 1961: The central distribution of afferent nerve fibers of the facial and vagus nerves in the guinea pig. Anat. Rec., *139*, 245.

Morest, D. K., 1967: Experimental study of the projections of the nucleus of the tractus solitarius and the area postrema in the cat. J. Comp. Neurol., *130*, 277–299.

Papez, J. W., and Rundles, W., 1937: The dorsal trigeminal tract and the centre median nucleus of Luys. J. Nerv. Ment. Dis., *85*, 509–519.

Pearson, A. A., 1949: The development and connections of the mesencephalic root of the trigeminal nerve in man. J. Comp. Neurol., *90*, 1–46.

Ranson, S. W., and Clark, S. L., 1959: *The Anatomy of the Nervous System,* 10th Ed. W. B. Saunders Co., Philadelphia.

Rhoton, A. L., O'Leary, J. L., and Ferguson, J. P., 1966: The trigeminal, facial, vagal and glossopharyngeal nerves in the monkey. Arch. Neurol., *14*, 530–540.

Russell, G. V., 1954: The dorsal trigeminothalamic tract in the cat reconsidered as a lateral reticulo-thalamic system of connections. J. Comp. Neurol., *101*, 237–263.

Sjöqvist, O., 1938: Eine neue Operationsmethode bei Trigeminusneuralgie: Durchschneidung des Tractus spinalis trigemini. Zbl. Neurochir., *2*, 274–281.

Szentagothai, J., and Kiss, T., 1949: Projection of dermatomes on the substantia gelatinosa. A.M.A. Arch. Neurol. Psychiat., *62*, 734–744.

Walker, A. E., 1942: Somatotopic localization of spinothalamic and secondary trigeminal tracts in mesencephalon. A.M.A. Arch. Neurol. Psychiat., *48*, 884–889.

Woodburne, R. T., 1936: A phylogenetic consideration of the primary and secondary centers and connections of the trigeminal complex in a series of vertebrates. J. Comp. Neurol., *65*, 403–501,

Chapter 9

The Special Senses of Taste, Hearing, Equilibrium, Sight, and Smell

TASTE

Taste is classified as a *special visceral afferent* sense. The receptors are the *taste buds* that develop during fetal life from local thickenings of the lingual epithelium. The cells in these thickenings elongate and reach the surface; the epithelial mass thus produced differentiates into taste cells and columnar supporting cells and eventually assumes its characteristic flask shape (Fig. 86). Recent evidence

indicates that cells of the taste buds undergo renewal and that the so-called supporting cells are precursors of the more differentiated neuroepithelial taste cells. The taste cells end at the surface in hair-like receptive tips. The *taste fibers* of the *facial, glossopharyngeal,* and *vagus nerves* ramify on the surfaces of the cells. In the adult, taste buds persist on the surfaces of the vallate and foliate papillae and on a few fungiform papillae of the

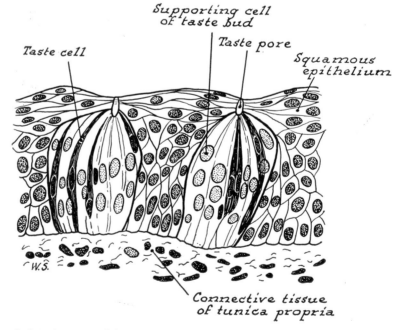

FIG. 86.   Taste buds in the mucosa of the tongue (after Schaffer).

tongue, on the soft palate, and on the laryngeal surface of the epiglottis.

Taste fibers to the anterior two-thirds of the tongue are components of the facial nerve and arise from unipolar cells in the *geniculate ganglion* (Fig. 85). The peripheral processes reach the tongue by way of the *chorda tympani nerve*. The nerve leaves the facial canal through an opening in its anterior wall, traverses the tympanic cavity and the petrotympanic fissure, and joins the lingual nerve with which it proceeds to the tongue. The central processes course inward through the facial and internal auditory canals and enter the brain stem at the junction of the pons and medulla. Within the me-

dulla the fibers enter the *tractus (fasciculus) solitarius* (Figs. 52, 85) through which the taste impulses are conducted to the *nucleus solitarius*.

Taste fibers to the posterior one-third of the tongue are from the *glossopharyngeal nerve*. The fibers originate as the peripheral processes of cells in the *inferior ganglion*. The central processes of these cells enter the medulla and terminate in the *nucleus solitarius*. If there are taste buds in the epithelium of the soft palate, as has been reported, they may receive special visceral afferent fibers from the inferior ganglion of the vagus by way of the pharyngeal plexus or from the geniculate ganglion by way of the major

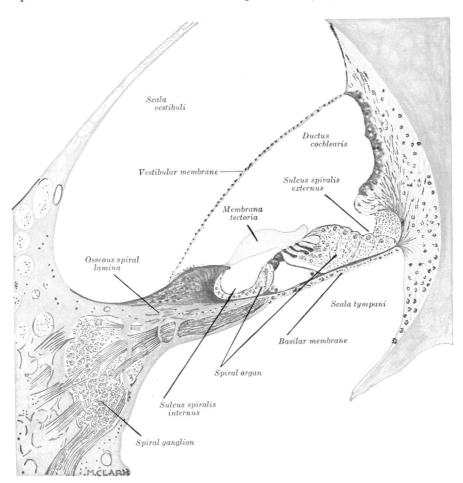

FIG. 87.   Drawing of a section through the second turn of the human cochlea. Mallory's stain. (From Gray's Anatomy, 28th ed., Charles Mayo Goss, Ed., Lea & Febiger, Philadelphia.)

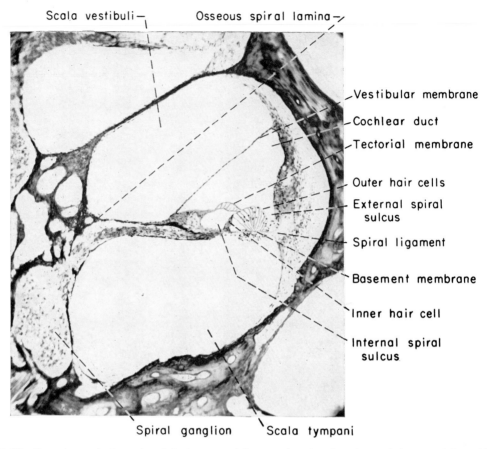

Scala vestibuli—   Osseous spiral lamina—

Vestibular membrane

Cochlear duct

Tectorial membrane

Outer hair cells

External spiral sulcus

Spiral ligament

Basement membrane

Inner hair cell

Internal spiral sulcus

Spiral ganglion   Scala tympani

FIG. 88. Photomicrograph of a section of the inner ear of the squirrel monkey through one of the turns of the cochlea. (Section of specimen provided by Dr. Catherine A. Smith.)

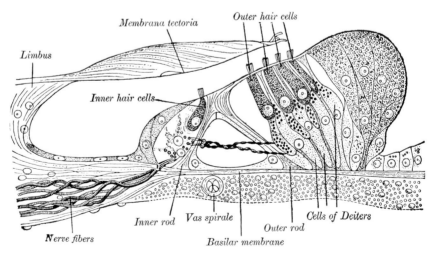

Membrana tectoria   Outer hair cells

Limbus

Inner hair cells

Inner rod   Vas spirale   Cells of Deiters

Outer rod

Nerve fibers   Basilar membrane

FIG. 89. Section through the spiral organ of Corti. Magnified. (G. Retzius from Gray's Anatomy, 28th ed., Charles Mayo Goss, Ed., Lea & Febiger, Philadelphia.)

petrosal nerve. In either case, taste impulses from the soft palate would be conducted to the nucleus solitarius.

The *secondary afferent pathway for taste* (from nucleus solitarius to thalamus) apparently is incorporated into the contralateral *medial lemniscus* (Fig. 85). On reaching the thalamic level such secondary fibers terminate in the *posteromedial ventral nucleus* (Figs. 78, 85) with the other secondary afferent fibers from the head region. From this nucleus, tertiary taste fibers apparently project to the inferior part of the postcentral gyrus and adjacent insular cortex.

As is true of the general visceral afferent fibers that terminate in the nucleus solitarius, the taste fibers also serve as the afferent limbs of numerous visceral and viscerosomatic reflex arcs.

Before proceeding to the description of the other special visceral afferent pathway—that for the special sense of smell—the special somatic senses of hearing, equilibrium, and vision are considered. This procedure is used in order that those sensory pathways which utilize the brain stem in their course to the cerebral cortex may be studied consecutively. The olfactory pathway to the cortex does not traverse the brain stem.

HEARING

The auditory portion of the eighth nerve is made up of the central processes of axons of bipolar cells in the *spiral ganglion* (Figs. 87, 88). The peripheral processes, or dendrites, of these cells are distributed to the *spiral organ of Corti* in the cochlea. (Figs. 87, 88, 89.)

The **cochlea** consists of a bony canal which spirals forward around a central core; the core is termed the *modiolus* and the canal completes approximately two and one-half turns around it. The *cochlear duct,* often referred to as the *scala media,* occupies a median position in the bony canal; it is separated from the *scala vestibuli* on the one side by the *vestibular* (Reissner's) *membrane* and from the

scala tympani on the other side by the bony *spiral lamina, spiral ligament,* and *basilar membrane;* the last-named structure stretches between the spiral ligament and lamina. The scala tympani ends at the *round window (fenestra rotunda)* in the base of the cochlea (Fig. 90*A*). The round window is a deficiency in the bony wall between the tympanic cavity and the internal ear which is normally closed by the *secondary tympanic membrane.* The scala vestibuli and the scala tympani, which are normally filled with perilymph, communicate with one another at the apex of the cochlea (helicotrema).

The cochlear duct, saccule, utricle, and membranous semicircular canals are developed from the otic vesicle. The vesicle (see Chapter 2) comes from a thickened ectodermal plate known as the *auditory placode* which develops alongside the rhombencephalon. Invagination of the placode creates the *auditory pit;* this pit closes to form the vesicle which then migrates inward and occupies a position in the mesenchyme between the ectoderm and the hind-brain. The cochlear duct, as finally developed, ends blindly at the apex of the cochlea; it contains the spiral organ of Corti and is filled with endolymph. At its basal limit it communicates with the saccule through the *ductus reuniens* (Fig. 90*B*).

The **spiral organ of Corti**—the end organ for auditory stimuli—extends throughout the length of the cochlear duct where it rests upon the basilar membrane. In cross-section it is seen to have a triangular tunnel running through it, known as the tunnel of Corti (Figs. 87–89). On both sides of the tunnel, and contributing to its formation, are the inner and outer rods or pillars of Corti. A single row of hair cells lies on the inner side of the inner rod; on the outer side of the outer rod there are three or four rows of similar cells. Each hair cell is surmounted by about twenty hair-like processes. Both the inner and outer hair cells are supported by rows of columnar cells. A space

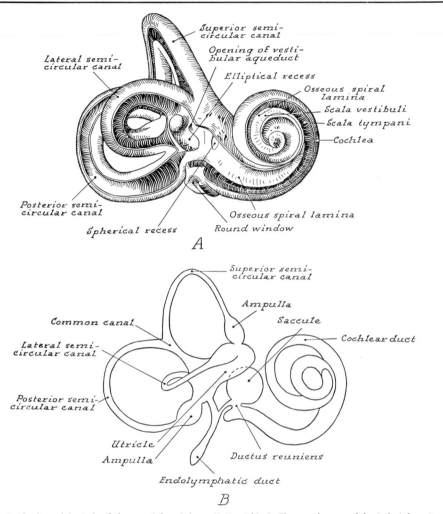

FIG. 90. A, The bony labyrinth of the ear (after Sobotta-McMurrich). B, The membranous labyrinth (after Gray).

medial to the organ of Corti is known as the internal spiral sulcus. The tectorial membrane overhangs the sulcus and the organ of Corti.

Sound waves strike the tympanic membrane and cause it to vibrate; the vibrations are transmitted to the perilymph of the vestibule by the ossicular chain whose final component is the stapes with its footplate in the oval window. The waves set up in the perilymph cause the basilar membrane to vibrate; since the organ of Corti rests upon the membrane it, too, vibrates and the processes of the hair cells are moved about in the endolymph or against the undersurface of the tectorial membrane. The nerve impulses thus set up in the hair cells are transferred to the dendrites of the spiral ganglion cells. Although not usually demonstrable in fixed sections of the cochlea, it is frequently stated that the processes of the hair cells are actually embedded in the undersurface of the tectorial membrane. A dampening effect on the hair cells is ascribed to the tectorial membrane by some investigators.

The basilar membrane appears to be specifically segmented as to the frequencies to which it will respond maximally. That this situation is true appears to have been proved in animal experiments in which certain segments of the membrane and organ of Corti have been removed. Animals thus treated are found to be deaf to certain frequency ranges. These observations support the "place theory" of hearing, and in fact, there is good evidence that the part of the basilar membrane evidencing the most pronounced response to stimulation, changes with changes of frequency. The response of the basilar membrane to different sound frequencies has been explained by the traveling wave theory.

The **spiral ganglion** is situated within the bony spiral lamina (Figs. 87, 89). The dendrites of its bipolar cells course outward through the spiral lamina and basilar membrane and terminate in relation to the hair cells of the organ of Corti. The central processes, or axons, enter the modiolus and emerge through the lamina cribrosa at its base to form the auditory portion of the eighth nerve which then traverses the internal auditory canal and terminates in the *dorsal* and *ventral cochlear nuclei* at the junction of the medulla and pons (Figs. 59, 91). Experiments have indicated that the various levels of the cochlear spiral are topically represented in the cochlear nuclei.

The **cochlear nuclei** are attached to the external surface of the inferior cerebellar peduncle. They contain the cell bodies of the *secondary neurons* in the *auditory pathway*. Axons of these cells enter the tegmentum of the pons where they either

decussate in and form a transverse band of fibers known as the *trapezoid body* (Figs. 60, 92) or end in the homolateral superior olivary nucleus. The *superior olivary nucleus* is dorsal to the trapezoid body and in the angle formed between the medial and lateral lemnisci (Figs. 60, 92). As components of the trapezoid body, the secondary auditory fibers are intermingled with the longitudinally coursing fibers of the medial lemnisci. In their course to the trapezoid body they form *dorsal* and *ventral striae* (Fig. 92); the former originate in the dorsal cochlear nucleus and pass dorsal to the inferior cerebellar peduncle whereas the latter originate in both dorsal and ventral nuclei and pass ventral to the inferior cerebellar peduncle. After decussating in the trapezoid body some of the fibers turn rostrally in the *lateral lemniscus,* whose course through the pons was observed in the study of the lateral spinothalamic tract (Figs. 63, 65, 66). Other fibers, after traversing the dorsal stria and trapezoid body, end in the contralateral superior olivary nucleus.

The **lateral lemniscus,** as shown by degeneration experiments, terminates in the nucleus of the inferior colliculus. The **brachium of the inferior colliculus** is formed by axons of cells in this nucleus (Figs. 68, 92) and courses rostrally and anteriorly across the lateral aspect of the mesencephalon and terminates in the *medial geniculate body* (Fig. 94). The

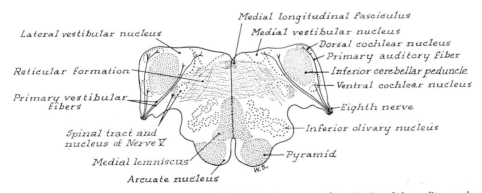

FIG. 91. Section through the rostral limit of the medulla showing the manner of termination of the auditory and vestibular fibers of the eighth nerve.

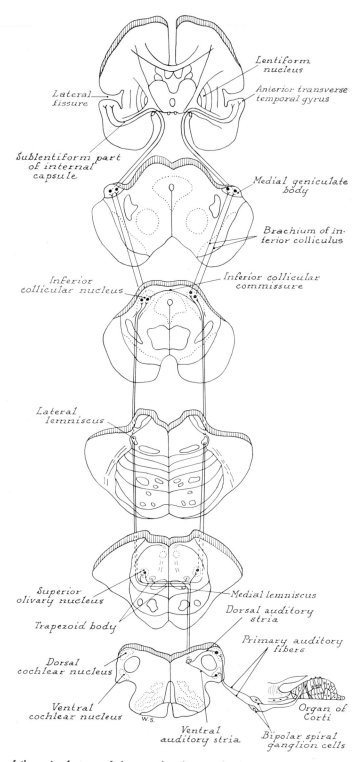

FIG. 92. Diagram of the major features of the central auditory pathway.

latter structure is a posterior thalamic nucleus located just posterior to the lateral limit of the basis pedunculi at the level of the superior colliculi. Axons from cell bodies therein course through the sublentiform portion of the internal capsule and terminate in the auditory area (anterior transverse temporal gyrus) of the cerebral cortex (Figs. 92, 93).

It appears, therefore, that the *auditory pathway* to the cortex consists of a series of at least *four neurons* instead of the usual three. The first neuron has its cell body in the *spiral ganglion,* the second in one of the *cochlear nuclei,* the third in the *inferior collicular nucleus,* and the fourth in the *medial geniculate body* (Fig. 92).

The **conduction of auditory impulses** is further complicated by the existence of other relay stations along the pathway; they include the superior olivary nucleus (Figs. 60, 92) and the nucleus of the lateral lemniscus (Fig. 66). The *nucleus of the lateral lemniscus* consists of numerous cells scattered among the fibers of the lemniscus in its pontile portion. Secondary auditory fibers from the cochlear nuclei end in the superior olivary nuclei of the same side and of the opposite side as noted above; other fibers terminate in,

or send collaterals to, the nucleus of the lateral lemniscus. The axons of the cells in these nuclear structures, in turn, course rostrally in the lateral lemniscus and, for the most part, terminate in the nucleus of the inferior colliculus; those from the superior olivary nucleus may enter the lemniscus of the same side or they may decussate through the trapezoid body and enter the contralateral one. Some fibers of the lateral lemniscus cross to the inferior collicular nucleus of the opposite side through the *commissure of the inferior colliculi* (Figs. 68, 92). The nucleus of the lateral lemniscus projects to some extent to adjacent reticular formation. This suggests a mechanism for cerebral arousal through the extralemniscal system, resulting in "attention" to auditory impulses (Chap. 6).

It is evident that there are a number of possibilities for auditory impulses arising in either ear to be projected on the auditory areas of both cerebral hemispheres. The possibilities include the termination in the superior olivary nuclei of both sides of axons of cells in the cochlear nuclei, the contribution of fibers to the lateral lemnisci of both sides by either superior olivary nucleus, and the decussation of some of the fibers of the lateral

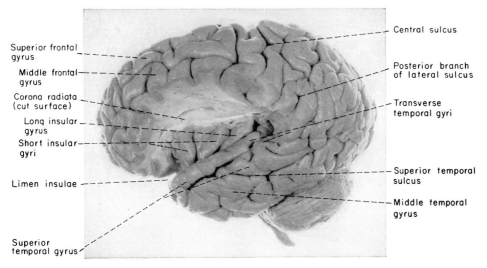

FIG. 93. Photograph of the lateral surface of the adult brain, partially dissected to illustrate the insular and the transverse temporal gyri.

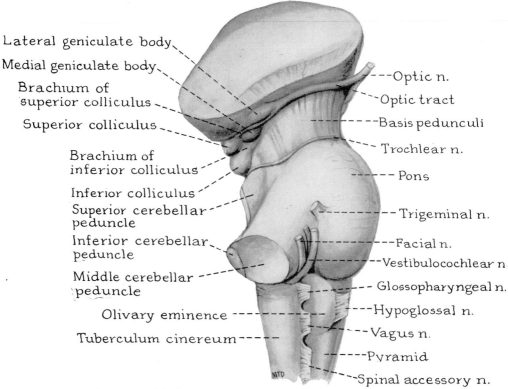

Lateral geniculate body
Medial geniculate body
Brachium of superior colliculus
Superior colliculus
Brachium of inferior colliculus
Inferior colliculus
Superior cerebellar peduncle
Inferior cerebellar peduncle
Middle cerebellar peduncle
Olivary eminence
Tuberculum cinereum

Optic n.
Optic tract
Basis pedunculi
Trochlear n.
Pons
Trigeminal n.
Facial n.
Vestibulocochlear n.
Glossopharyngeal n.
Hypoglossal n.
Vagus n.
Pyramid
Spinal accessory n.

MTD

FIG. 94. Drawing of lateral view of the brain stem.

lemniscus at the level of the inferior colliculi (Fig. 92). That the ear is bilaterally represented in the cortex is indicated by the clinical observation that unilateral destruction of the lateral lemniscus, medial geniculate body, internal capsule, or auditory area of the cortex may exist without detectable deafness in either ear.

Auditory reflexes are effected through connections in the inferior and superior colliculi (Fig. 95). The *nucleus* of the inferior colliculus, in which the lateral lemniscus terminates, has already been referred to. The area dorsomedial to the nucleus presents a laminated appearance and contains several large cells that give origin to some of the fibers of the *tectobulbar* and *tectospinal tracts*. It is probable, however, that the majority of fibers in these tracts arise from the deeper layers of the superior colliculus which receive input from the inferior colliculus through internuncial connections. *Tecto-*

bulbar and *tectospinal fibers* cross to the opposite side through the *dorsal tegmental decussation* (Fig. 95) and course downward through the brain stem and cervical portion of the spinal cord; the former terminate in relation to cells of the brain stem reticular formation and the latter in relation to anterior gray column cells of the cervical cord. Uncrossed tectospinal fibers also have been described. At medullary levels the tectospinal fibers become incorporated in the *medial longitudinal fasciculus* which, in large part, is composed of *reticulospinal fibers*. Although there are apparently no direct connections of the tectobulbar and tectospinal fibers respectively to the motor nuclei of the brain stem and to the anterior horn cells of the cervical cord segments, it may be assumed that connections are made via internuncial neurons since these tracts function in mediating reflex movements of the eyes, head, and

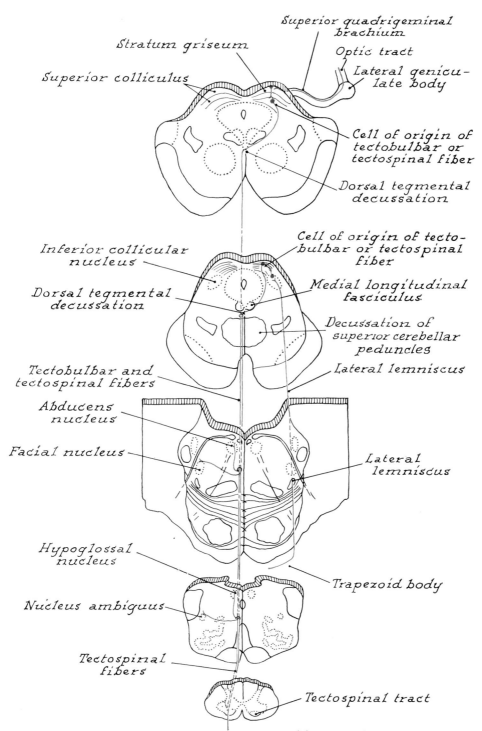

FIG. 95.   Diagram illustrating the function of tectobulbar and tectospinal fibers in visual and auditory reflexes.

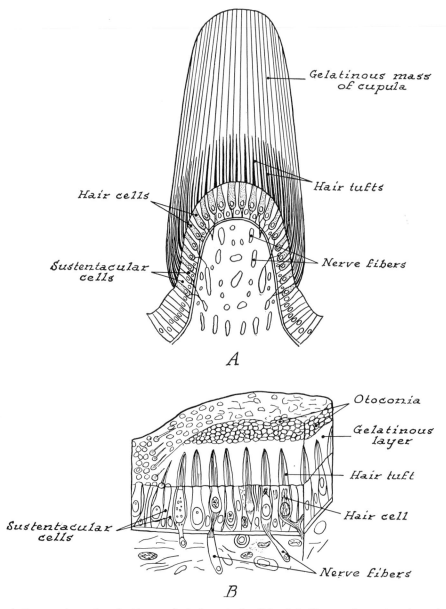

FIG. 96.   A, Diagram of a section of crista ampullaris (in part after Kolmer). B, Diagram of a section of macula (after Kolmer).

neck in response to auditory and visual stimuli. In addition, reflexes involving movement of the eyes and head are facilitated by direct projections from the superior olivary nuclei to the abducens nuclei and the medial longitudinal fasciculi. Such reflexes include turning the head and eyes toward a sudden noise or elevating the hands before the face as protection against injury which is likely to be a concomitant of a blast or explosion.

EQUILIBRIUM

The **special somatic sense of equilibrium** involves the vestibular portion of the eighth nerve. The cells of origin of the *vestibular nerve* are in the *vestibular ganglion* that is found in the internal auditory canal. Like those in the spiral ganglion of the cochlea, these neurons are of the bipolar type. Their peripheral processes pierce the lamina cribrosa at the outer limit of the internal auditory canal and are distributed to the *cristae ampullares* of the membranous semicircular canals and to the maculae of the utricle and saccule.

The **membranous semicircular canals** are located within the bony canals and are completely surrounded by perilymph. The **utricle and saccule,** within the bony vestibule of the internal ear, are also surrounded by perilymph. The perilymph spaces of the semicircular canals and vestibule are continuous with the scala vestibuli of the cochlea (Fig. 90).

The **cristae** develop from the epithelium lining the ampullae of the membranous semicircular canals. A curved ridge transverse to the long axis of the canal appears in each ampulla; within it two types of cells are differentiated—sensory and supporting (Fig. 96A). The sensory cells have bristle-like hairs at their free surfaces. It has been suggested that the supporting cells secrete the jelly-like substance which is seen on the sur-

face of the crista and which forms its so-called cupula. The **maculae** (Figs. 96B, 97) develop within the utricle and saccule in the same manner as described for the development of the cristae and are considerably larger. Their surfaces are covered by a gelatinous membrane within which are calcareous bodies called *otoconia* or *otoliths.*

The hair cells of the cristae are stimulated by currents set up in the endolymph which fills the membranous canals, utricle, and saccule. The currents result from movements of the head in the planes of the respective canals. The hair cells of the maculae are stimulated by the effect of gravity on the otoliths embedded in the gelatinous masses surmounting them. The hair cells of the cristae are concerned with dynamic equilibrium; the hair cells of the maculae with static equilibrium.

The **axons of the vestibular ganglion cells** accompany the auditory portion of the eighth nerve through the internal auditory canal and enter the brain stem at the junction of the pons and medulla. They pass ventral to the inferior cerebellar peduncle and for the most part terminate in the vestibular nuclei; some

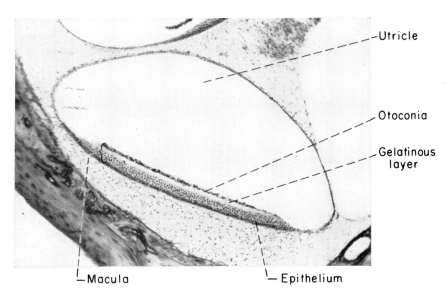

FIG. 97. Photomicrograph of a section of the utricle of the squirrel monkey showing the macula. (Specimen provided by Dr. Catherine A. Smith.)

vestibular fibers, however, continue past the nuclei and enter the cerebellum by way of the inferior cerebellar peduncle.

Four pairs of vestibular nuclei are found in the medullary and pontile portions of the brain stem (Figs. 59, 62, 99). The *inferior* or *spinal vestibular nucleus* is limited to the medulla where it lies just medial to the inferior cerebellar peduncle. This nucleus is continuous rostrally with the *lateral vestibular nucleus* (*Deiters*) which extends through the rostral part of the medulla and into the caudal part of the pons. The most rostrally placed of the nuclei is the *superior vestibular nucleus* which is located entirely within the pons. The *medial vestibular nucleus* is bounded laterally and rostrally by the other three. It extends forward into the pons and its caudal extremity is near the

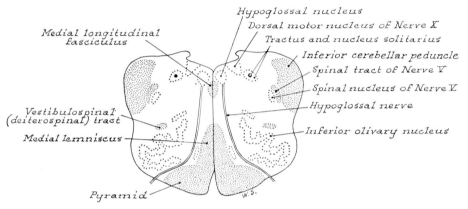

FIG. 98. Section through medulla showing the positions of the medial longitudinal fasciculi and vestibulospinal tracts.

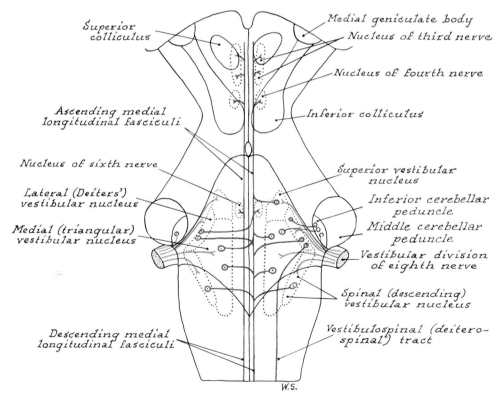

FIG. 99. Diagram of the central connections of the vestibular nerve superimposed on a dorsal view of the brain stem.

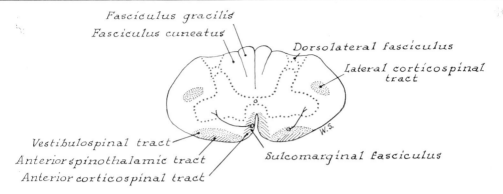

FIG. 100. Section through cervical spinal cord showing the locations of the sulcomarginal and vestibulospinal tracts in the anterior funiculi.

caudal limit of the fourth ventricle. Its medial border is near the midline of the brain stem. All the vestibular nuclei are immediately beneath the floor of the fourth ventricle, and they account for a prominence in the floor that is called the *area vestibularis.*

The vestibular nuclei are concerned mainly with the completion of vestibular reflex arcs. All the nuclei give origin to *vestibulospinal fibers* which course caudally into the spinal cord in the *medial longitudinal fasciculi* (Figs. 60, 98, 99); in the cord they enter the *sulcomarginal fasciculi* (Fig. 100). The medial longitudinal fasciculi are situated on both sides of the median raphé of the brain stem close to the floor of the fourth ventricle. The lateral vestibular nucleus also gives origin to the *vestibulospinal tract* which courses caudally in the reticular formation of the medulla just dorsal to the inferior olivary nucleus (Fig. 98) and enters the anterior funiculus of the spinal cord (Fig. 100). Although there are probably no direct connections to the large motor cells, all of the vestibulospinal fibers eventually terminate through synapses on neurons in the anterior gray columns of the spinal cord. Through these connections the musculature of the neck, trunk, and extremities is reflexly affected by vestibular impulses arising in the internal ear. The effects of the vestibular mechanism on postural muscles have been dem-

onstrated by stimulation or destruction, unilaterally, of the lateral vestibular nucleus. Stimulation is responsible for postural asymmetry of the entire body consisting of ipsilateral extension, contralateral flexion, deviation of the head toward the opposite side and, in cats, a tendency to fall toward the contralateral side; destruction of the lateral vestibular nucleus results in postural asymmetry that is the exact reciprocal of that produced by stimulation. Cutting the vestibular nerve unilaterally gives rise to similar but more pronounced and more lasting postural asymmetry than destruction of the vestibular nucleus. The close functional relationship of the vestibular and cerebellar mechanisms is indicated by the fact that stimulation or destruction of the medial cerebellar nuclei (*tectal* or *fastigial*), unilaterally, produces postural effects exactly like those resulting from stimulation or destruction of the lateral vestibular nucleus.

Direct vestibulocerebellar connections (from the vestibular ganglion to the cerebellum) have been mentioned. These fibers are joined by others from the vestibular nuclei which also reach the cerebellum by way of the inferior cerebellar peduncle (Fig. 99). Thus connections are made between the semicircular canals and the cerebellum in two ways—one of which involves a single neuron with its cell body in the vestibular ganglion and the other of which is a two-neuron pathway with the cell body of the second neuron in one of the vestibular nuclei. The cerebellar influence on postural reflexes is mediated by fastigiobulbar fibers (from the fastigial nucleus of cerebellum to the brain stem) which traverse the inferior cerebellar peduncle and end in vestibular nuclei and in the reticular formation of the medulla and pons. The significance of the vestibulocerebellar connections will become more apparent when the structure and function of the cerebellum are considered (Chaps. 19, 20).

A pathway from the vestibular nuclei to the cerebral cortex has not been defi-

nitely established although it is recognized that the special sense mediated by the vestibular nerve does reach the conscious level. In the cat the vestibular area is adjacent to and overlaps the posterior margin of the general sensory area of the arm and face and the anterior margin of the auditory cortex. There is good evidence that axons of second order neurons in the vestibular nuclei decussate in the region of the trapezoid body and then ascend between the lateral and medial lemnisci to the levels of the medial geniculate body and posterolateral ventral thalamic nucleus, one or both of which may project to the cortical vestibular area.

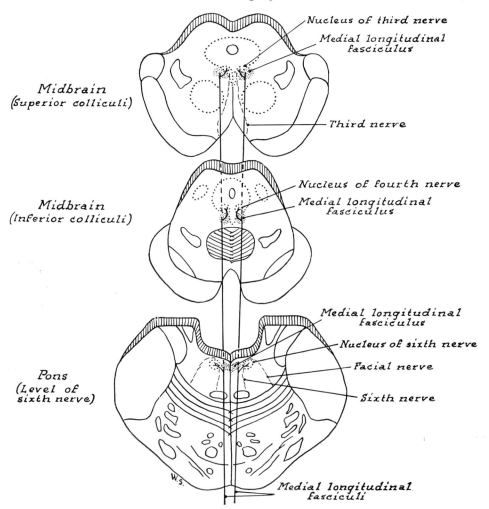

FIG. 101. Diagram illustrating the close relationships of the medial longitudinal fasciculi to the motor ocular nuclei in the pons and midbrain and the connections with the nuclei.

Evidence that vestibular impulses are projected to the cerebrum in man includes the observation that there is an area of the cortex close to that on which auditory impulses are known to be projected which, when stimulated electrically, gives rise to a feeling of vertigo in the conscious subject.

Other axons from cells in the vestibular nuclei course rostrally in the *medial longitudinal fasciculi* and terminate on motor neurons in the *abducens, trochlear,* and *oculomotor nuclei* (Figs. 100, 101). In the mesencephalon the medial longitudinal fasciculi are ventrolateral to the central gray matter surrounding the cerebral aqueduct and therefore are in close relationship to the trochlear and oculomotor nuclei (Fig. 101). *Vestibulo-ocular reflex arcs* are responsible for movements of the eyes in response to changes in the position of the head. They also appear to be concerned in the maintenance of

balanced tonicity in the eye muscles. If the semicircular canals, eighth nerve, or vestibular nuclei are injured the eyes are usually deviated to one side or the other; horizontal, vertical, or rotary nystagmus also appears in most cases of injury to the vestibular system.

Nystagmus is a term applied to a more or less rhythmic oscillation of the eyes. One phase of the oscillation is more prolonged than the other and is referred to as the slow component. The shorter phase is spoken of as the quick component. Clinically, nystagmus usually is described as being in the direction of its quick component.

Tumor of the eighth nerve (acoustic neurinoma) occurs not uncommonly; it gives rise to the so-called *cerebellopontile angle syndrome.* The *cerebellopontile angle* is located on the lateral aspect of the brain stem at the junction of the pons and medulla; it is bounded superiorly by

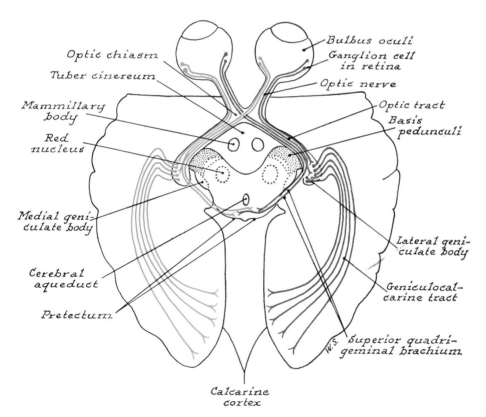

FIG. 102. Diagram of the visual pathway. Reflex connections between the retinae and the pretectum are indicated also.

8

the biventral lobule of the cerebellum. The eighth, ninth, tenth, seventh, sixth, and fifth cranial nerves are closely related to one another and to the cerebellopontile angle (Fig. 56). A tumor of the eighth nerve is responsible, during its early stages, for deafness in the corresponding ear and symptoms of vestibular dysfunction (nystagmus). As it increases in size it presses on the other nerves in the region and interferes with their function. Thus, the symptoms of such a tumor, in addition to eighth nerve symptoms, may include partial or complete ipsilateral paralysis of the soft palate (tenth nerve), paralysis of the face on the side of the lesion (seventh nerve), diminished sensibility (hypesthesia) over the distribution of the ipsilateral fifth nerve, double vision due to internal strabismus in the ipsilateral eye (sixth nerve), and ipsilateral loss of the sense of taste (ninth, tenth, and seventh nerves).

SIGHT

Vision is a special somatic afferent sense. The visual pathways are more complex than most others for the reason that impulses arising in the temporal half of the retina are conducted to the cerebral cortex of the same side while those from the nasal half are projected on the visual cortex of the contralateral hemisphere. The crossing of the fibers from the nasal halves of the two retinae occurs in the optic chiasm (Fig. 102).

The **optic vesicle** appears as a spherical evagination from the prosencephalon in embryos 3 to 4 millimeters in length. The outer or distal half of the vesicle invaginates into the inner half to form the *optic cup* that develops into the retina. As the

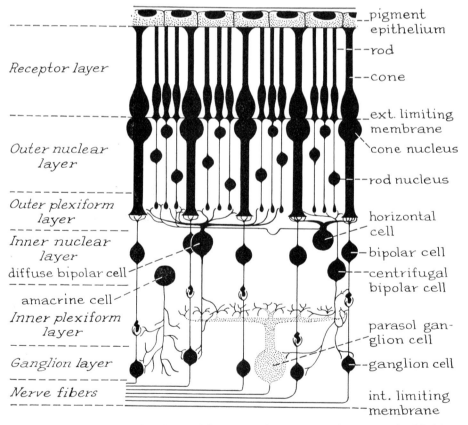

FIG. 103. Diagram showing the histologic layers of the retina and its interneuronal connections (modified from Walls, 1942).

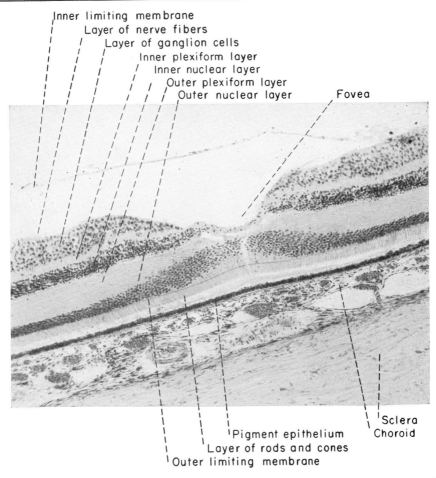

Inner limiting membrane
Layer of nerve fibers
Layer of ganglion cells
Inner plexiform layer
Inner nuclear layer
Outer plexiform layer
Outer nuclear layer   Fovea

Sclera
Choroid
Pigment epithelium
Layer of rods and cones
Outer limiting membrane

FIG. 104. Photomicrograph of a section through the retina, choroid, and sclera of the human eye. (Section of specimen provided by Dr. Carl Kupfer.)

optic cup migrates forward it maintains its attachment to the brain through the *optic stalk* that becomes the optic nerve when it is invaded by the axons of the ganglion cells in the developing retina. The *optic nerves,* since they develop as outgrowths from the brain, are not strictly peripheral in type; they are nevertheless commonly included in that category. That they are processes of the brain is manifested by the presence in them of all three types of glia cells (astrocytes, oligodendrocytes, and microgliacytes). *Glioma,* a tumor that develops from glia cells, not infrequently occurs in the optic nerve. It will be recalled that true peripheral nerve fibers have neurilemmal sheaths; these are not present in optic nerves which fail to regenerate when severed.

The **retina** contains three layers of cells: an outer layer of *rod and cone cells,* a middle layer of *bipolar cells,* and an inner layer of *ganglion cells* (Figs. 103, 104). The rods and cones are the peripheral processes of the rod and cone cells; they extend outward through the external limiting membrane and constitute the receptor organs for vision. In adequate light, cones are much more discriminating receptors, but in dim light, rods are much more efficient. The cones alone are found in the fovea centralis where vision and sensibility to color are at their maximum. The term, *fovea centralis,* applies to a depression in the macula lutea of the retina (Fig. 104).

The **macula lutea** is located directly posterior to the pupil, or in the visual axis of the eye; in this position it is approximately 3 mm temporal to the optic disc where the optic nerve fibers leave the eye (Figs. 105, 106). As regards the absence of rods in the fovea, it is of interest that sailors are trained, when on watch at night, to direct their eyes upward or downward in relation to their visual objectives; thus, these objectives are focused on the areas of the retina where rods are present; if they looked directly at the object it would be focused on the fovea and might not be seen at all.

The axons of the rod and cone cells synapse on the dendrites of the bipolar cells (Fig. 103). The area at which these synapses occur has been termed the *outer plexiform layer*. The axons of the bipolar cells, in turn, synapse on the dendrites of the ganglion cells; these synapses occur in the *inner plexiform layer*. The axons of the ganglion cells converge on the region of the optic disc and emerge from

the eye as the components of the optic nerve.

The **optic nerve** (Figs. 105, 106) enters the cranial cavity through the optic foramen. The fibers that originate in the temporal half of the retina continue past the optic chiasm into the optic tract of the same side; those from the nasal half decussate through the chiasm and enter the contralateral tract (Fig. 102).

The **optic tract** courses posteriorly around the cerebral peduncle and ends at the lateral geniculate body. Most of its fibers terminate by synapsing on cells in that body, but some continue past it and form the *brachium of the superior colliculus* (superior quadrigeminal brachium) which connects the lateral geniculate body with the superior collicular region. The latter fibers synapse on cells in the superior colliculus and in the area just rostral to the colliculus, or pretectum (Fig. 102).

The **lateral geniculate body,** like the medial one, is a posterior thalamic nucleus. It is located just lateral to the medial geniculate body under cover of

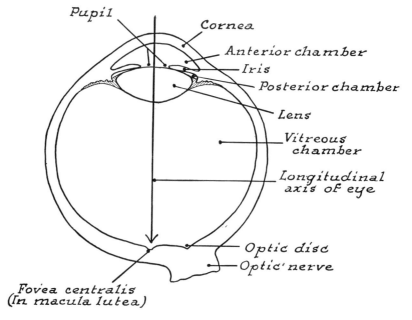

FIG. 105. Coronal section of the bulbus oculi showing the relation of the macula lutea to the optic disc and to the longitudinal axis of the eye.

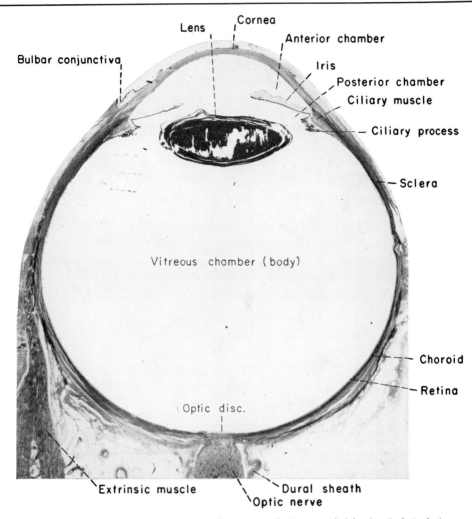

FIG. 106. Photomicrograph of a section through the human eye. (Section provided by Dr. Carl Kupfer.)

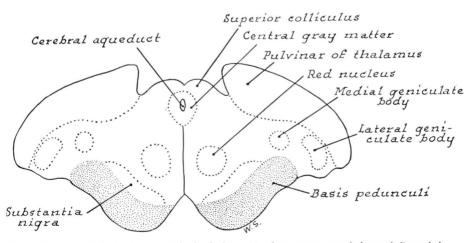

FIG. 107. Section through the brain stem at the level of transition between mesencephalon and diencephalon.

the pulvinar of the thalamus (Figs. 107, 108, 110). Axons of its cells traverse the sublenticular and, in part, the retrolenticular portions of the internal capsule. All terminate in the visual area of the cerebral cortex which is located in and around the calcarine fissure, and this group of fibers is, therefore, frequently referred to as the *geniculocalcarine tract* (Fig. 102). The fibers from the part of the lateral geniculate which receive impulses from the superior retinal quadrants course directly posteriorly to the superior lip of the calcarine fissure. Those from the part of the lateral geniculate related to the inferior retinal quadrants loop for-

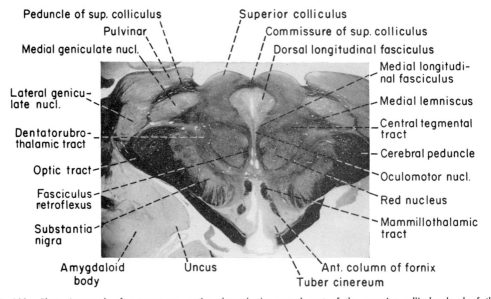

FIG. 108. Photomicrograph of a transverse section through the rostral part of the superior collicular level of the midbrain which passes through the posterior thalamic nuclei. Weil stain.

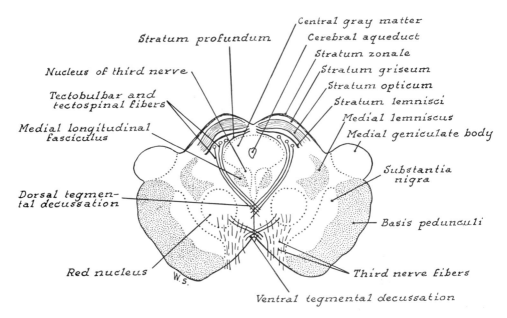

FIG. 109. Section through the mesencephalon at the level of the superior colliculi.

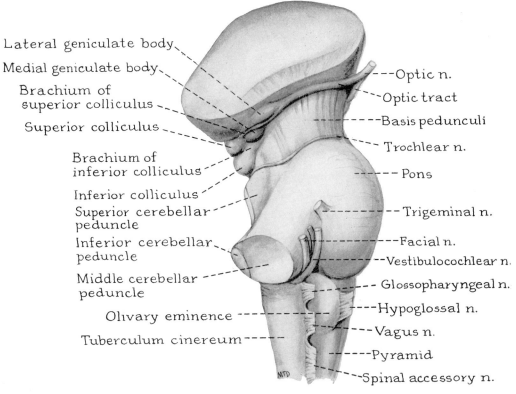

Lateral geniculate body

Medial geniculate body

Brachium of superior colliculus

Superior colliculus

Brachium of inferior colliculus

Inferior colliculus

Superior cerebellar peduncle

Inferior cerebellar peduncle

Middle cerebellar peduncle

Olivary eminence

Tuberculum cinereum

Optic n.

Optic tract

Basis pedunculi

Trochlear n.

Pons

Trigeminal n.

Facial n.

Vestibulocochlear n.

Glossopharyngeal n.

Hypoglossal n.

Vagus n.

Pyramid

Spinal accessory n.

FIG. 110.   Drawing of lateral view of the brain stem.

ward into the rostral temporal region before coursing posteriorly to the inferior lip of the calcarine fissure (Fig. 111).

The **superior colliculi** are laminated structures whose layers, from superficially inward, are designated: stratum zonale, stratum griseum, stratum opticum, stratum lemnisci, and stratum profundum (Fig. 109). The colliculi function as reflex centers and are particularly concerned with *visual reflexes*. The optic nerve fibers that reach the superior colliculus by way of its brachium (Figs. 102, 110) enter the stratum opticum; they terminate chiefly in relation to cells in the stratum griseum. These fibers, in turn, connect with large cells in the superior colliculus that give origin to many of the fibers of the *tectobulbar* and *tectospinal* *tracts* (Fig. 109) whose termination (directly or indirectly) in relation to motor neurons in the nuclei of cranial nerves and in the anterior gray columns

of the cervical segments of the spinal cord has been described (Fig. 95). *Reflex reactions* to *visual stimuli* are facilitated by these connections. Through direct or indirect connections of tectobulbar fibers with cells in the nucleus of the facial nerve the eyes are closed when there is danger of flying objects entering them. Through synapses of tectospinal fibers on anterior gray column cells in the lower cervical segments, the arms and hands are raised to further protect the eyes.

The fibers in the brachium of the superior colliculus that terminate in the *pretectum* (Fig. 102) synapse on cells whose axons enter the *Edinger-Westphal nuclei* (Chap. 23). Visceral efferent fibers from these nuclei leave the mesencephalon and enter the orbits as components of the oculomotor nerves where they end in the *ciliary ganglia*. Axons of cells in the ciliary ganglia supply the *constrictor pupillae muscles* (Fig. 218). This reflex arc, beginning in the retina and ending in the constrictor muscles, is responsible for constriction of the pupils in response to strong light. Loss of the light reflex without loss of vision often indicates some type of pathologic process in the rostro-dorsal area of the mesencephalon (pretectum). A more detailed description of the light reflex and its pathway is presented in Chapter 23.

Lesions of the Central Visual Pathways

Blindness is routinely described with reference to the fields of vision rather than with reference to the part of the retina involved. Since light rays enter the eye only through the pupil and since they travel in straight lines, it is obvious that the nasal half of the retina functions in the perception of objects in the temporal field of vision whereas the temporal half is responsible for the nasal field.

It is readily apparent that destruction of one optic nerve will produce total blindness in the eye on that side (Fig. 111,1). Destruction of the optic chiasm, such as may occur with pituitary tumor, results in blindness that is limited to those parts of the fields of vision that are projected on the nasal halves of both retinae. This is designated as *bitemporal hemianopia* since the patient fails to see objects in either temporal field (Fig. 111,2). Destruction of the fibers from the temporal hemiretina produces a unilateral nasal hemianopia (Fig. 111,3). This may result from enlargement of the internal carotid artery at the site were it lies in the angle formed by the optic nerve and optic tract.

Any lesion which destroys the optic tract on one side will result in blindness in the contralateral fields of vision (the nasal field of the ipsilateral eye and the

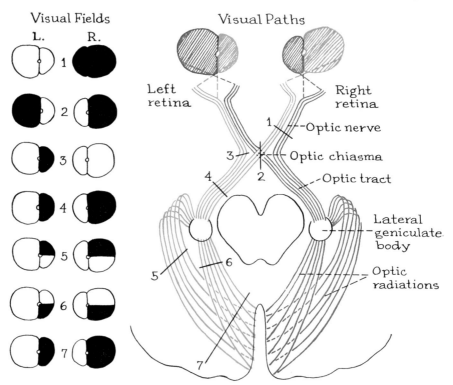

FIG. 111. Diagram of the central visual pathways and the effects of various lesions of the visual pathway. The black areas of the inserts indicate the visual field defects resulting from the lesions indicated by the corresponding numbers on the figure at the right. 1, Complete blindness of right eye; 2, bitemporal hemianopia; 3, left nasal hemianopia; 4, right homonymous hemianopia; 5, right upper quadrant hemianopia; 6, right lower quadrant hemianopia; 7, right homonymous hemianopia. (In part after Homans.)

temporal field of the contralateral eye). This type of visual defect is referred to as right or left *homonymous hemianopia* (Fig. 111,4). The same type of blindness results from complete unilateral destruction of the geniculocalcarine tract or of the visual cortex (Fig. 111,7). Destruction of the upper lip of the calcarine cortex on one side produces a visual loss in the lower quadrant of the contralateral visual field (contralateral inferior quadrantic anopia). A contralateral superior quadrantic anopia would result from destroying the lower lip of the calcarine cortex. The geniculocalcarine fibers, as they approach the visual cortex, are so arranged that lesions in the upper or lower parts of the tract would result in quadrantic field defects comparable to those described for destruction of the respective calcarine lips (Fig. 111,5 and 6 respectively). It is important to note that the quadrantopia frequently found in individuals with tumors in the temporal

lobe of the cerebrum most commonly involves the upper fields of vision. This may be explained by the concept of separate courses for the geniculocalcarine fibers at their origin from the lateral geniculate body, which are activated respectively by visual stimuli in the upper and lower quadrants of the visual fields. According to this concept, those fibers representing the upper visual fields course forward and then laterally along the outer boundary of the inferior horn of the lateral ventricle (Meyer's loop) whereas those of the lower visual fields course directly backward beneath the floor of the ventricle (Fig. 111). Thus the fibers in the more exposed position (Meyer's loop) would be interrupted without injury to the more direct (medio-inferior) fibers.

SMELL

The **special visceral sense of smell** is mediated by the olfactory cells found in the olfactory mucous membrane. The

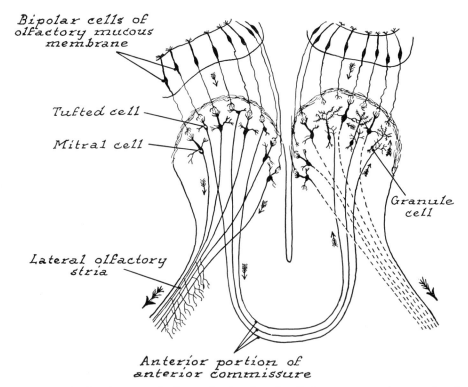

FIG. 112. Diagram showing the course of olfactory impulses from the olfactory mucous membrane to the olfactory bulbs and from the bulbs to the olfactory cortex (after Cajal).

peripheral processes, or *dendrites,* of the *olfactory cells* reach the surface of the mucous membrane by traversing the spaces between the supporting cells. The central processes, or *axons,* form the unmyelinated *olfactory nerves* which enter the cranial cavity through the openings in the cribriform plates of the ethmoid. Within the anterior cranial fossa they end in the olfactory bulbs which rest upon the cribriform plates (Fig. 112).

The **olfactory bulb** (Figs. 114, 115) is a laminated structure whose superficial

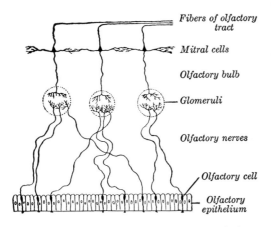

FIG. 113. Plan of olfactory neurons. (From Gray's Anatomy, 28th ed., Charles Mayo Goss, Ed., Lea & Febiger, Philadelphia.)

layer consists of unmyelinated nerve fibers from the olfactory nerves. Under this superficial layer there are several layers of gray matter and, finally, a layer of myelinated nerve fibers passing to and from the olfactory tract. A central core of neuroglia replaces the cavity which is present in some of the lower animals (Fig. 114).

Three types of cells—mitral, granule, and tufted—are found in the gray matter of the olfactory bulb. The dendrites of the *mitral* and *tufted cells* receive olfactory impulses from the olfactory nerves (Figs. 112, 113); their axons enter the layer of myelinated fibers and are thus directed into the *olfactory tract;* the tract connects the bulb with the ventral aspect of the cerebrum (Fig. 115). The thicker axons of the mitral cells mainly enter the olfactory areas of the brain by way of the *lateral olfactory stria;* the finer axons of the tufted cells pass through the *anterior commissure* to the opposite olfactory bulb (Fig. 112). The *granule cells* probably function as internuncial neurons.

The **secondary olfactory fibers** terminate in the olfactory cortex by way of the

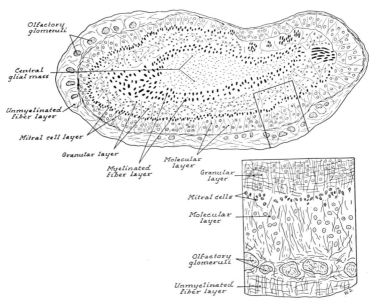

FIG. 114. Cross-section of the olfactory bulb (after Koelliker).

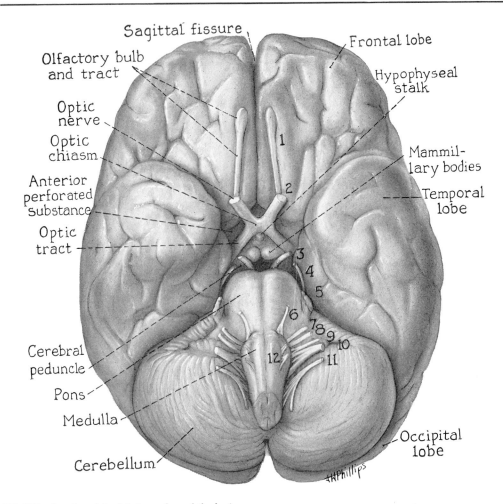

Sagittal fissure

Olfactory bulb and tract

Optic nerve

Optic chiasm

Anterior perforated substance

Optic tract

Cerebral peduncle

Pons

Medulla

Cerebellum

Frontal lobe

Hypophyseal stalk

Mammillary bodies

Temporal lobe

Occipital lobe

FIG. 115.   Drawing of the inferior surface of the brain.

olfactory tract and its two main divisions —the *lateral* and *medial olfactory striae*. It thus appears that the olfactory pathway may include only two neurons—the first in the olfactory mucous membrane and the second in the olfactory bulb. At least one more neuron must be involved when the impulse is shunted to the opposite olfactory bulb through the anterior commissure and then relayed to the cortex from there (Fig. 112).

The **nervus terminalis** is closely associated with the olfactory nerve, but whether it is olfactory in function has not been determined. The peripheral fibers of the nerve originate from ganglion cells in the *ganglion terminalis* and are distributed chiefly to the nasal septum and its epithelium. In the human embryo, the ganglion consists of groups of cells along the medial border of the olfactory bulb. The central processes of the sensory cells in the ganglion have been traced into the forebrains of embryos. Multipolar cells, associated with the unipolar and bipolar sensory cells in the ganglion terminalis, are thought to have an autonomic function.

The smell brain, or *rhinencephalon*, has lost much of its importance as such in man and, for that reason, it will not be considered in all its manifold and complex details. In some of the lower animals the rhinencephalon is extremely important—so important that the very existence of the animal may depend on it. Perhaps the greatest significance of the rhinencephalon in man is in the regulation of visceral functions and its involvement in emotional expression. The major aspects of its anatomy are described in Chapter 24.

BIBLIOGRAPHY

Allen, W. F., 1923a: Origin and distribution of the tractus solitarius in the guinea pig. J. Comp. Neurol., 35, 171–204.

Allen, W. F., 1923b: Origin and destination of the secondary visceral fibers in the guinea pig. J. Comp. Neurol., 35, 275–311.

Altman, J., and Carpenter, M. B., 1961: Fiber projections of the superior colliculus in the cat. J. Comp. Neurol., 116, 157–158.

Bagshaw, M. H., and Pribram, K. N., 1953: Cortical organization in gustation (Macaca mulatta). J. Neurophysiol., 16, 499–508.

Barnes, W. T., Magoun, H. W., and Ranson, S. W., 1943: The ascending auditory pathway in the brain stem of the monkey. J. Comp. Neurol., 79, 129–152.

Békésey, G., and Rosenblith, W. A., 1951: Handbook of Experimental Psychology, S. S. Stevens, Ed. John Wiley & Sons, New York, Chap. 27.

Benjamin, R. M., 1963: Some thalamic and cortical mechanisms of taste. In Olfaction and Taste, Y. Zotterman, Ed. The Macmillan Company, New York, pp. 309–329.

Börnstein, W. S., 1940–1941: Cortical representation of taste in man and monkey. II. The localization of the cortical taste area in man and a method of measuring impairment of taste in man. Yale J. Biol. Med., 13, 133–156.

Bucher, V. M., and Burgi, S. M., 1953: Some observations on the fiber connections of the di- and mesencephalon in the cat. Part III. The supraoptic decussations. J. Comp. Neurol., 98, 355–379.

Chambers, W. W., and Sprague, J. M., 1955: Functional localization in the cerebellum. I. Organization in longitudinal cortico-nuclear zones and their contribution to the control of posture, both extrapyramidal and pyramidal. J. Comp. Neurol., 103, 105–129.

Crosby, E. C., Humphrey, T., and Lauer, E. W., 1962: Correlative Anatomy of the Nervous System. The Macmillan Co., New York.

Emmers, R., 1966: Separate relays of tactile, thermal and gustatory modalities in the cat

thalamus. Proc. Soc. Exp. Biol. Med., 121, 527–531.

Eyster, J. A. E., Bast, T. H., and Krasno, M. R., 1935: Studies on the electrical response of the cochlea. Amer. J. Physiol., 113, 40.

Fitzgerald, G., and Hallpike, C. S., 1942: Studies in human vestibular function: I. Observations on the directional preponderance ("Nystagmusbereitschaft") of caloric nystagmus resulting from cerebral lesions. Brain, 65, 115–137.

Fredrickson, J. M., Figge, U., Scheid, P., and Kornhuber, H. H., 1966: Vestibular nerve projection to the cerebral cortex of the Rhesus monkey. Exp. Brain Res., 2, 318–327.

Hubel, D. H., and Wiesel, T. N., 1962: Receptive fields, binocular interaction and functional architecture in the cat's visual cortex. J. Physiol., 160, 106–154.

Kempinsky, W. H., 1951: Cortical projection of vestibular and facial nerves in cat. J. Neurophysiol., 14, 203–210.

Lewy, F. H., and Kobrak, H., 1936: The neural projection of the cochlear spirals on the primary acoustic centers. A.M.A. Arch. Neurol. Psychiat., 35, 839–852.

Magoun, H. W., and Ranson, S. W., 1935: The central path of the light reflex. A.M.A. Arch. Ophthal., 13, 791–811.

Mickle, W. A., and Ades, H. W., 1954: Rostral projection pathway of the vestibular system. Amer. J. Physiol., 176, 243–246.

Moulton, D. G., and Beidler, L. M., 1967: Structure and function in the peripheral olfactory system. Physiol. Rev., 47, 1–52.

Nauta, W. J. H., 1961: Fibre degeneration following lesions of the amygdaloid complex in the monkey. J. Anat., 95 515–531.

Nyberg-Hansen, R., 1966: Functional organization of descending supraspinal fibre systems to the spinal cord. Anatomical observations and physiological correlations. Ergebn. Anat. Entwicklungsgesch., 39, 1–48.

Nyberg-Hansen, R., and Mascitti, T. A., 1964: Sites and mode of termination of fibers of the vestibulospinal tract in the cat. An experimental study with silver impregnation methods. J. Comp. Neurol., 122, 369–387.

Patton, H. D., Ruch, T. C., and Walker, A. E., 1944: Experimental hypogeusia from Horsley-Clarke lesions of the thalamus in Macaca mulatta. J. Neurophysiol., 7, 171–184.

Patton, H. D., and Ruch, T. C., 1946: The relation of the foot of the pre- and postcentral gyrus to taste in the monkey and chimpanzee. Fed. Proc., 5, 79.

Pearce, G. W., and Glees, P., 1953: Experimental studies on the descending tectal pathways of the cat. J. Anat., *87,* 443.

Pearson, A. A., 1941: The development of the nervus terminalis in man. J. Comp. Neurol., *75,* 39–66.

Penfield, W., and Rasmussen, T., 1950: *The Cerebral Cortex of Man,* The Macmillan Co., New York.

Purves-Stewart, J., and Worster-Drought, C., 1952: *The Diagnosis of Nervous Diseases,* 10th ed., Edward Arnold Co., London.

Rasmussen, G. L., 1964: Anatomical relationships of the ascending and descending auditory systems. In *Neurological Aspects of Auditory and Vestibular Disorders,* W. S. Fields and B. R. Alford, Eds., Charles C Thomas, Springfield, Ill., Chap. 1, pp. 1–14.

Rhoton, A. L., O'Leary, J. L., and Ferguson, J. P., 1966: The trigeminal, facial, vagal and glossopharyngeal nerves in the monkey. Arch. Neurol., *14,* 530–540.

Rose, J. E., Galambos, R., and Hughes, J. R., 1957: Tonotopic organization of frequency sensitive units in the cochlear nuclei of the cat. Anat. Rec., *127,* 358.

Rose, J. E., and Woolsey, C. N., 1958: Cortical connections and functional organization of the thalamic auditory system of the cat. In *Biological and Biochemical Bases of Behavior,* H. F. Harlow and C. N. Woolsey, Eds. Univ. of Wisconsin Press, Madison, pp. 127–150.

Snyder, M., Hall, W. C., and Diamond, I. T., 1966: Vision in tree shrews after removal of striate cortex. Psychoneurol. Sci., *6,* 243–244.

Stevens, S. S., Davis, H., and Lurie, M. H., 1935: The localization of pitch perception on the basilar membrane. J. Genet. Psychol., *13,* 297–315.

Stotler, W. A., 1953: An experimental study of the cells and connections of the superior olivary complex of the cat. J. Comp. Neurol., *98,* 401–431.

Walberg, F., and Jansen, J., 1961: Cerebellar corticovestibular fibers in the cat. Exp. Neurol., *3,* 32–52.

Walls, G. L., 1942: *The Vertebrate Eye and Its Adaptive Radiation.* Hafner Publishing Co., New York.

Whitfield, I. C., 1967: *The Auditory Pathway,* Edward Arnold, Ltd., London.

Chapter 10

The Internal Capsule

All the pathways to the cerebral cortex, with the single exception of that for smell, have relay stations in the thalamus; in the case of each pathway it has been shown that the axon of the final neuron reaches the cortex by way of the internal capsule (Fig. 116).

The position of the internal capsule in frontal sections of the brain at the thalamic level has been noted. Its posterior limb is placed between the thalamus and the lentiform nucleus and some of its fibers course laterally beneath the lentiform nucleus (Fig. 117). Also, recall that the internal capsule is continuous with the cerebral peduncle (Figs. 117, 118).

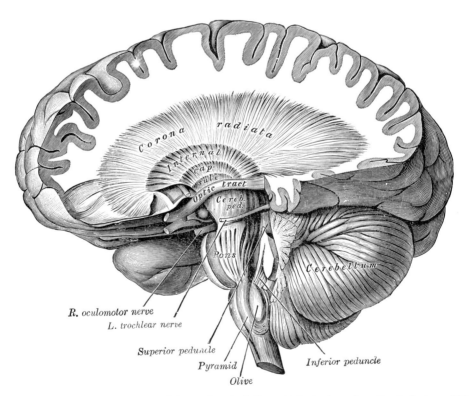

FIG. 116. Dissection showing the course of the cerebrospinal fibers. (E. B. Jamieson from Gray's Anatomy, 28th ed., Charles Mayo Goss, Ed. Lea & Febiger, Philadelphia.)

Visual fibers from the lateral geniculate body and auditory fibers from the medial geniculate body to the cortex traverse the retrolenticular and the sublentiform parts of the internal capsule respectively.

In horizontal sections of the brain which pass through the thalamus and lentiform nucleus, the **internal capsule** is seen to have the conformation of a widely opened "V" (Fig. 119). The point at which the anterior and posterior limbs of the capsule meet is termed the *genu*. The *posterior*

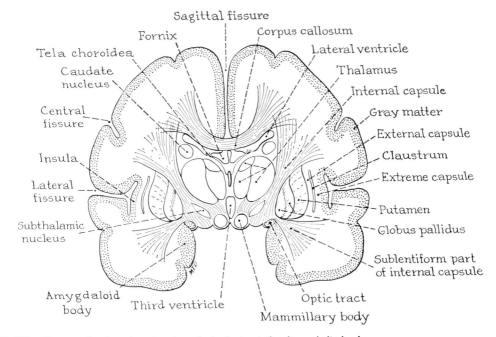

FIG. 117.   Diagram of a frontal section through the brain at the diencephalic level.

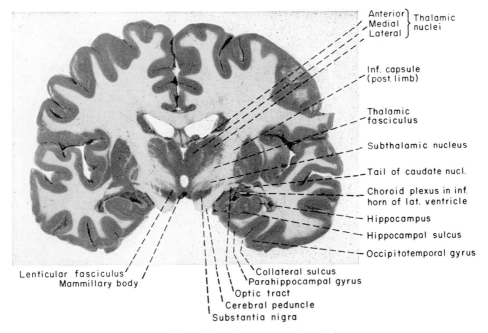

FIG. 118.   Coronal section at the level of the subthalamic area (posterior view).

limb, because of its position between the thalamus and lentiform nucleus, is often called the *thalamolentiform* or *lenticulo-thalamic* portion; the *anterior limb,* which lies between the lentiform and caudate nuclei, is designated *lenticulocaudate.* The V shape of the internal capsule is due to the conformation of the lentiform nucleus and to the positions of the thalamus and the caudate nucleus.

The **lentiform and caudate nuclei** with the **amygdaloid body** and **claustrum** constitute the **basal ganglia** whose structure (and function so far as it has been established) will be discussed later (Chap. 17), The caudate nucleus is continuous with the lower part of the rostral end of the lentiform nucleus (Fig. 121). From this

origin it arches superiorly around the thalamus and terminates in relation to the amygdaloid body in the roof of the temporal horn of the lateral ventricle. The claustrum is a narrow strip of gray matter lateral to the lentiform nucleus from which it is separated by the external capsule (Figs. 117–119).

The **anterior limb of the internal capsule** courses forward, upward, and laterally through the space developed between the lentiform and caudate nuclei (Figs. 119, 120). Numerous strands of gray matter connect the two nuclei and pass through the internal capsule (Fig. 119). They are responsible for the striated appearance of this part of the internal capsule and for the name—*corpus striatum*

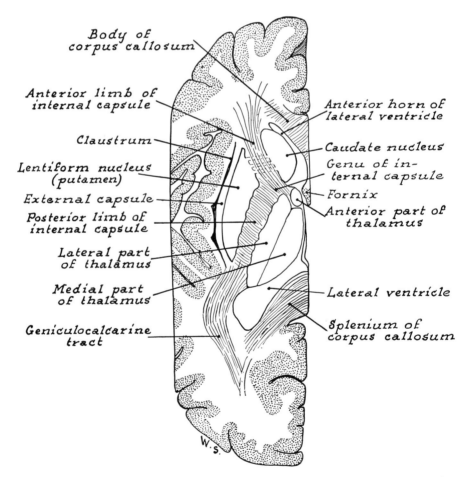

FIG. 119. Horizontal section of the left half of the brain showing the configuration of the internal capsule (modified from Toldt).

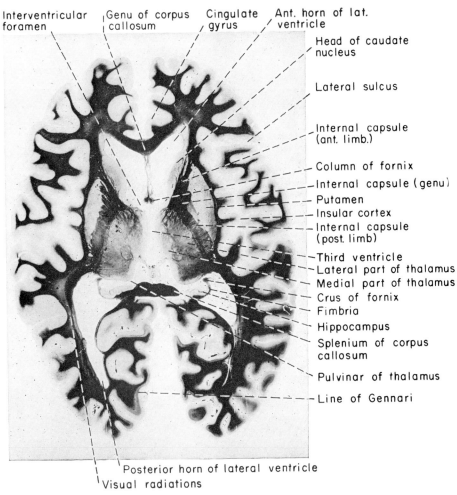

Interventricular foramen | Genu of corpus callosum | Cingulate gyrus | Ant. horn of lat. ventricle

Head of caudate nucleus

Lateral sulcus

Internal capsule (ant. limb.)

Column of fornix
Internal capsule (genu)
Putamen
Insular cortex
Internal capsule (post. limb)
Third ventricle
Lateral part of thalamus
Medial part of thalamus
Crus of fornix
Fimbria
Hippocampus
Splenium of corpus callosum
Pulvinar of thalamus
Line of Gennari

Posterior horn of lateral ventricle
Visual radiations

FIG. 120. Horizontal section through the anterior limb, genu, and posterior limb of the internal capsule.

—that has been applied to the area composed of the two nuclei and the intervening limb of the internal capsule.

The internal capsule contains *corticipetal* and *corticifugal fibers*. The former are processes of neurons in the thalamus; the latter are processes of cortical neurons.

Corticobulbar fibers course downward through the genu of the internal capsule (Fig. 122). Component fibers of the anterior limb (Figs. 120, 122) include the *frontopontine* (of cortical origin), *anterior thalamic radiations* (thalamocortical), and *corticothalamic fibers*. The posterior limb (Figs. 120, 122) contains *thalamocortical, corticospinal, corticothalamic,*

and *corticorubral fibers*. Other fibers in the posterior limb which are not indicated in the diagram are *corticotectal, corticonigral,* and *corticotegmental fibers*. Thalamocortical fibers include those which branch from the posterior limb to course through the sub- and retrolentiform parts of the capsule (auditory and visual radiations).

Corticobulbar fibers originate mainly in the motor and premotor areas of the cerebral cortex and terminate in relation to cells in the motor nuclei of cranial nerves. **Corticopontile fibers** arise in the frontal, temporal, parietal, and occipital areas of the cerebral cortex and terminate by synapsing on neurons whose cell

9

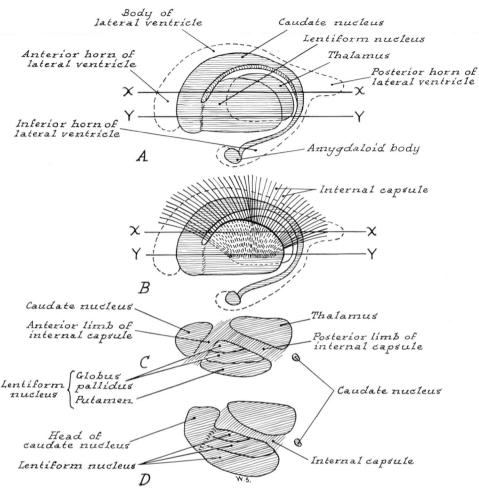

FIG. 121. *A*, Diagram of basal ganglia (not including the claustrum) as seen from the lateral side. The relationship of the lateral ventricle to the nuclei is indicated. *B*, Diagram of the basal ganglia showing the relationship of the internal capsule to its component nuclei. *C*, Horizontal section through the basal ganglia and thalamus at the level designated "X" in *A* and *B*. *D*, Horizontal section at the level "Y" in *A* and *B* (modified from Jackson-Morris).

bodies are in the pontile nuclei in the basilar part of the pons (Fig. 61). The corticobulbar fibers are concerned with the voluntary activity of muscles in the head region while the corticopontile fibers function in the coordination of voluntary muscles of the head, neck, trunk, and extremities.

Corticothalamic fibers in the anterior limb of the internal capsule originate in the frontal lobe cortex and terminate principally in the medial and anterior parts of the thalamus. Fibers in the posterior limb originate from parietal, temporal, and occipital cortices and end in the lateral part of the thalamus and in the geniculate bodies.

Thalamocortical fibers in the anterior limb of the internal capsule arise from nuclei in all three parts of the thalamus and are concerned with visceral and somatic reflexes. Those concerned with visceral reflexes terminate in the more anterior areas of the frontal lobe where frontal corticothalamic fibers have their origin. Those having to do with somatic reflexes connect the lateral part of the thalamus with the cortical areas in the posterior part of the frontal lobe from which large numbers of corticopontile fibers originate.

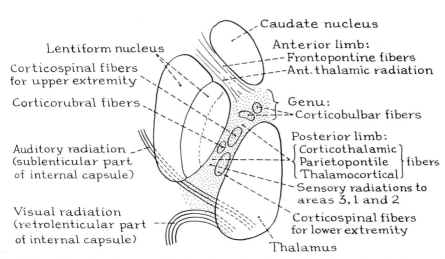

FIG. 122. Diagram illustrating the parts of the internal capsule and the various fiber systems in the respective parts as seen in horizontal section.

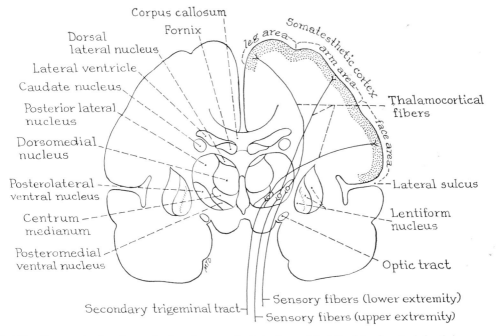

FIG. 123. Diagram showing the termination of sensory tracts in the nuclei of the lateral part of the thalamus, and the projection of these nuclei on the somatesthetic cortex by way of the internal capsule (modified from Ranson).

The relation of the latter to cerebellar reflex arcs will be considered in Chapter 19.

The **posterior half of the posterior limb of the internal capsule** contains those *thalamocortical fibers* that reach the *general sensory* or *somatesthetic area* of the cortex. Therefore, they arise from the *posterolateral* and *posteromedial ventral nuclei* in the lateral part of the thalamus (Fig. 123). *General sensory impulses* from the head, neck, trunk, and extremities reach the cortex by way of these fibers. Such impulses have previously been traced from the receptors to the thalamic nuclei by way of the ventral and lateral spinothalamic tracts, the fasciculi gracilis and cuneatus and medial lemniscus, and the ventral trigeminal tract.

A **nonspecific thalamocortical projection system** originates in the thalamus and is discussed in Chapter 21.

BIBLIOGRAPHY

Brion, S., and Guist, G., 1964: Topographie des faisceaux de projection du cortex dans la capsule interne et dans pédoncle cérébral. Étude des dégénérescences secondaires dans la sclérose latérale amyotrophique et la maladie de Pick. Rev. Neurol. (Paris), *110,* 123–144.

Kuypers, H. G. J. M., 1958: Corticobulbar connexions to the pons and lower brainstem in man. An anatomical study. Brain, *81,* 364–388.

Rosett, J., 1933: *Intercortical Systems of the Human Cerebrum, Mapped by Means of New Anatomic Methods.* Columbia University Press, New York.

Truex, R. C., and Kellner, C. E., 1948: *Detailed Atlas of the Head and Neck.* Oxford University Press, New York.

Chapter 11

The Cerebral Hemispheres

The **cerebrum** contains the highest centers of the nervous system and is the most massive portion of the brain; it occupies the greater part of the cranial cavity and covers the brain stem and cerebellum (Fig. 124). It is divided into two lateral *hemispheres* by the *sagittal fissure* into which dips the double fold of dura mater known as the falx cerebri (Fig. 125). The *frontal poles* of the hemispheres project forward into the anterior cranial fossa and rest on the orbital plates of the frontal bone. The *occipital poles* project posteriorly into the posterior cranial fossa where they rest on the tentorium cerebelli (Fig. 125). The tentorium, which is a double fold of dura mater, separates the occipital poles from the superior surface of the cerebellum. The *temporal poles* project forward and downward into the middle cranial fossa on both sides of the body of the sphenoid bone; they rest on the horizontal portions of the temporal squamae and the greater wings of the

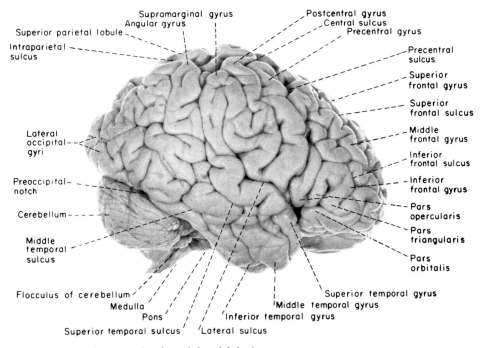

FIG. 124. Photograph of the lateral surface of the adult brain.

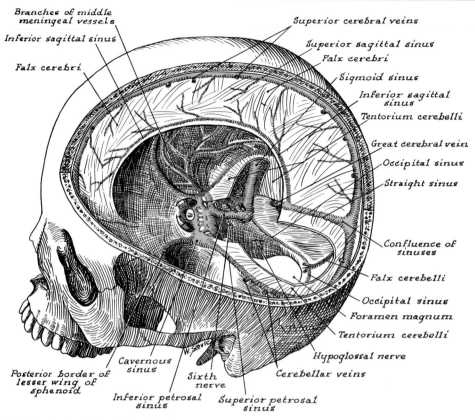

FIG. 125. The interior of the skull with the brain removed to show the dural reflections (after Sobotta-McMurrich).

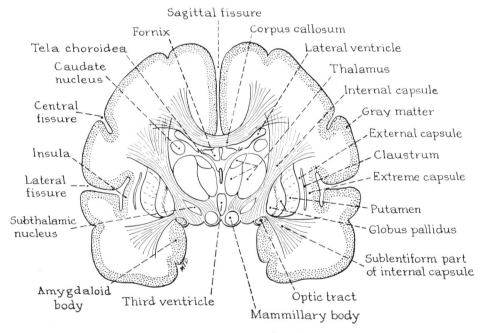

FIG. 126. Diagram of a frontal section through the brain at the diencephalic level.

sphenoid. Each cerebral hemisphere consists of a central core of white matter completely surrounded by gray matter. The gray masses (caudate and lentiform nuclei, amygdaloid body, and claustrum), which constitute the basal ganglia, are buried in the white matter (Fig. 126).

The **white matter** consists of *corticipetal (afferent) and corticifugal (efferent) projection fibers, association fibers* that connect the neurons of one cortical area with those of another, and *commissural fibers* that cross from one hemisphere to the other in the massive *corpus callosum* and in the lesser commissure of the fornix and *anterior commissure.* The corpus callosum is found at the inferior limit of the sagittal fissure.

The **gray matter,** or **cortex,** contains the cell bodies of neurons on which the various sensory impulses are projected, those of neurons giving rise to corticospinal, corticobulbar, corticopontile, and other fibers destined for lower levels of the central nervous system and those of association and commissural neurons.

Each cerebral hemisphere has three surfaces—superolateral, medial, and in-

ferior. The superolateral surface is in relation to the calvarium, the medial surface is in relation to the falx cerebri, and the inferior surface rests on the floor of the cranial cavity anteriorly and on the tentorium cerebelli posteriorly. All the surfaces are highly convoluted, thus increasing the cortical surface area. The convolutions, or gyri, are separated from one another by intervening sulci.

The **superolateral surface** is the most extensive and is markedly convex (Figs. 125, 127). It presents a deep fissure and a number of sulci which divide it into numerous lobes and gyri. The *lateral,* or *Sylvian, fissure* begins on the inferior surface of the hemisphere, on a line with the optic chiasm; it courses laterally between the temporal and frontal lobes and, on reaching the dorsolateral surface, lies between these two lobes. It divides into *anterior horizontal, anterior ascending,* and *posterior rami;* the two anterior rami project forward and upward, respectively, on the frontal lobe; the posterior ramus continues posteriorly, at first between the frontal and temporal lobes, and then between the temporal and parietal lobes

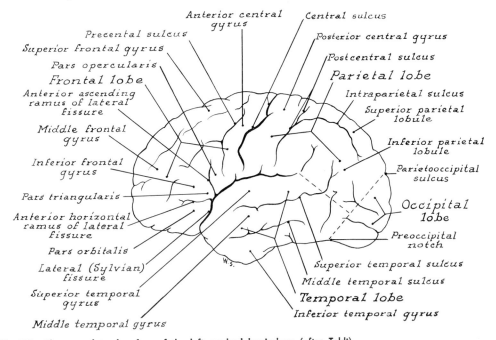

FIG. 127. The superolateral surface of the left cerebral hemisphere (after Toldt).

(Figs. 124, 127). The *central sulcus* begins about 1 centimeter posterior to the midpoint of the superior border of the hemisphere and extends downward and forward (Figs. 125, 127). It forms an angle of about 70 degrees with the superior border and terminates at or near the posterior ramus of the lateral fissure. The central sulcus separates the frontal and parietal lobes. The lateral fissure and central sulcus are constant in position, although the latter is sometimes interrupted at one or more points. Other sulci on the dorsolateral surface are subject to considerable variation.

The **occipital lobe** is more or less arbitrarily delimited anteriorly by a line drawn from the preoccipital notch on the inferior border, to the parietooccipital sulcus on the dorsal border of the hemisphere. It is a triangular lobe with its apex at the occipital pole (Fig. 127). A second line drawn from the posterior limit of the posterior ramus of the lateral fissure to the midpoint of the first line completes the boundary between the parietal and temporal lobes.

The **frontal lobe** usually presents certain well-marked sulci which divide it into relatively well-demarcated gyri (Fig. 127). The *precentral sulcus* parallels the central fissure and forms the anterior boundary of the *anterior central gyrus*. The *superior* and *inferior frontal sulci*, which more or less parallel the superior border, divide the area anterior to the precentral sulcus into *superior, middle,* and *inferior frontal gyri*. The inferior frontal gyrus is divided by the anterior horizontal and the anterior ascending rami of the lateral fissure into *pars orbitalis, pars triangularis,* and *pars opercularis*.

The **parietal lobe** is crossed by the *postcentral sulcus* which parallels the central fissure and forms the posterior boundary of the *posterior central gyrus* (Fig. 127). The *intraparietal sulcus* begins a little above the midpoint of the postcentral sulcus and extends backward and downward to terminate near the anterior boundary of the occipital lobe. It divides that part of the parietal lobe posterior to the postcentral sulcus into *superior* and *inferior parietal lobules*.

The **temporal lobe** is divided into *superior, middle,* and *inferior temporal gyri* by the *superior, middle,* and *inferior tem-*

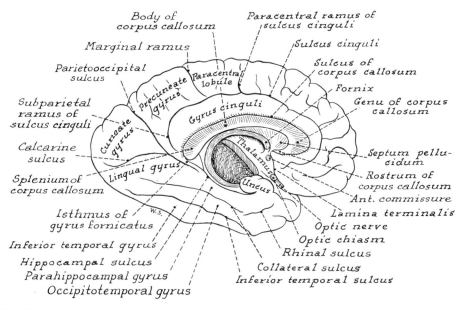

FIG. 128. The medial surface of the left cerebral hemisphere (after Toldt).

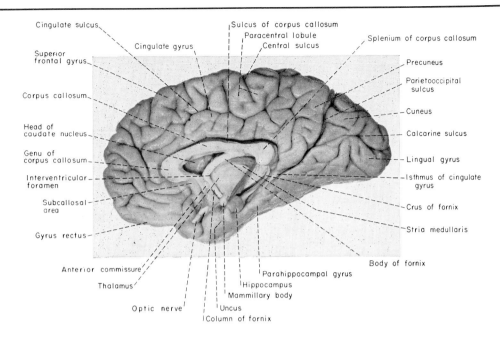

FIG. 129.   Photograph of the medial surface of the adult brain cut in sagittal section and partially dissected to show the hippocampus and fornix.

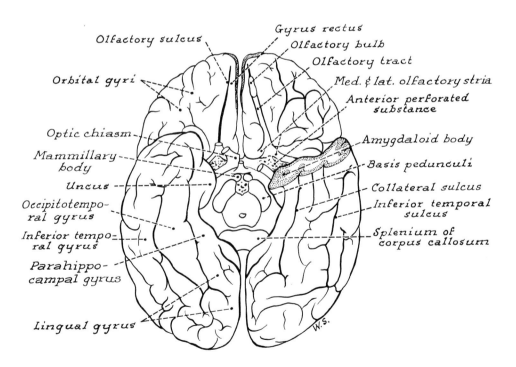

FIG. 130.   The inferior surface of the cerebrum (after Toldt). The anterior part of the left temporal lobe, the brain stem caudal to the mesencephalic level, the right olfactory tract and bulb, and the left half of the optic chiasm have been removed.

poral sulci. The inferior temporal sulcus is on the inferior surface of the temporal lobe (Fig. 130), but the three gyri are all visible on the lateral surface (Fig. 127).

The **medial surface of the cerebral hemisphere** can be examined in its entirety only if the brain is sectioned in the median sagittal plane and the brain stem is then removed by cutting through the thalamus (Figs. 128, 129). In such a preparation the remaining portion of the thalamus is partially surrounded by the *fornix* which, in turn, is partially surrounded by the *corpus callosum.* The corpus callosum, which constitutes the great commissure connecting the two hemispheres, is seen in cut section. It consists of an inferiorly placed *rostrum,* attached to the lamina terminalis, a *genu,* a *body,* and a posterior expanded *splenium.* Anteriorly the fornix is attached to the corpus callosum by the *septum pellucidum.* The fornix is a projection pathway from the hippocampi (within the temporal lobes) to the mammillary bodies. The thalamus, fornix, and corpus callosum, as seen in a median sagittal section of the brain (Figs. 128, 129), are completely surrounded by the convoluted medial surface of the hemisphere.

The *sulcus of the corpus callosum* is in immediate relationship to that structure (Figs. 128, 129) and is continuous around the splenium with the *hippocampal sulcus.* The *sulcus cinguli* parallels the callosal sulcus and forms the peripheral boundary of the *gyrus cinguli.* It gives off a *paracentral ramus* which reaches the superior border a few centimeters anterior to the notch formed by the central fissure. The sulcus cinguli terminates by dividing into *marginal* and *subparietal rami.*

The quadrilateral gyrus between the paracentral and marginal rami of the sulcus cinguli is called the *paracentral lobule.* The anterior and posterior central gyri extend over the superior border into

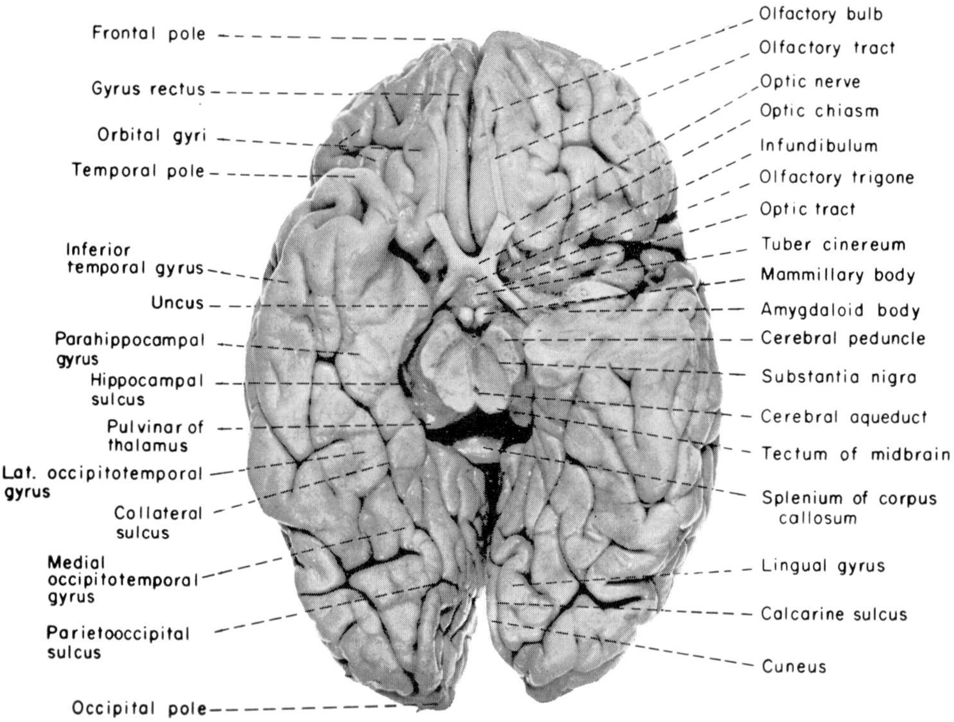
Frontal pole
Gyrus rectus
Orbital gyri
Temporal pole
Inferior temporal gyrus
Uncus
Parahippocampal gyrus
Hippocampal sulcus
Pulvinar of thalamus
Lat. occipitotemporal gyrus
Collateral sulcus
Medial occipitotemporal gyrus
Parietooccipital sulcus
Occipital pole
Olfactory bulb
Olfactory tract
Optic nerve
Optic chiasm
Infundibulum
Olfactory trigone
Optic tract
Tuber cinereum
Mammillary body
Amygdaloid body
Cerebral peduncle
Substantia nigra
Cerebral aqueduct
Tectum of midbrain
Splenium of corpus callosum
Lingual gyrus
Calcarine sulcus
Cuneus

FIG. 131. Photograph of the inferior surface of the adult brain. The rostral portion of the left temporal lobe and the brain stem caudal to the midbrain have been removed.

this lobule. The area peripheral to the sulcus cinguli and anterior to the paracentral sulcus is a medial extension of the superior frontal gyrus.

The *calcarine sulcus* begins slightly inferior to the splenium of the corpus callosum (Figs. 128, 129); from there it extends posteriorly and upward and then posteriorly and downward to terminate a short distance above the occipital pole of the hemisphere. At about its midpoint, it gives origin to the *parietooccipital sulcus* which courses upward and slightly backward to end at the superior border. Remember that the termination of the parietooccipital sulcus at the superior border, apparent on the dorsolateral surface, indicates the boundary between parietal and occipital lobes. On the medial surface the sulcus itself serves to separate these two lobes.

The *precuneate gyrus* is bounded by the marginal and subparietal rami of the sulcus cinguli, the parietooccipital sulcus and the superior border. It is a medial extension of the superior parietal lobule. The triangular area between the parietooccipital sulcus and the posterior half of the calcarine sulcus is designated the *cuneate gyrus*. The cuneate gyrus and the *lingual gyrus* are continuous with the occipital lobe of the dorsolateral surface.

The *lingual gyrus* lies between the calcarine and collateral sulci. The *collateral sulcus* is on the medioinferior surface of the temporal lobe. The lingual gyrus is continuous anteriorly with the *parahippocampal gyrus* which lies between the collateral and hippocampal sulci. The parahippocampal gyrus terminates anteriorly by curving around the anterior end of the hippocampal sulcus. The resultant hook-shaped structure is known as the uncus (Figs. 129–131). It may be noted (Figs. 128, 129) that the cingulate gyrus is connected to the parahippocampal gyrus by a narrow convolution, the *isthmus of gyrus fornicatus*. The cingulate gyrus, isthmus, parahippocampal gyrus, and uncus comprise the *fornicate gyrus*.

Because of its obliquity the inferior surface of the temporal lobe is not sharply delimited from its medial surface; the inferior temporal sulcus therefore is visible from the medial side (Fig. 128). The area between it and the collateral sulcus is called the *occipitotemporal gyrus*, which may show a lateral and a medial division (Fig. 131). The rhinal fissure, when present, continues forward from the collateral sulcus and completes the separation of the parahippocampal and occipitotemporal gyri.

The inferior surface of the frontal lobe of the cerebral hemisphere (Figs. 130, 131) presents the *olfactory sulcus* about 1 centimeter lateral to its medial border; the olfactory tract lies in this sulcus. It may be noted that the olfactory tract divides into medial and lateral olfactory stria as it approaches the anterior perforated substance. The area medial to the sulcus is known as the *gyrus rectus* (Figs. 130, 131). Lateral to the sulcus the surface is irregularly convoluted and the convolutions are termed the *orbital gyri*.

Chapter 12

The Sensory and Associative Mechanisms
of the Cerebral Cortex

In the anterior part of the parietal lobe, the **posterior central gyrus** is the *general sensory* or *somatesthetic area* of the cortex (Figs. 124, 127). Sensory impulses from the contralateral half of the face, oral cavity, pharynx, and abdomen reach the lower part of the posterior central gyrus; impulses from the face and oral cavity are brought to this area from the posteromedial ventral thalamic nucleus by way of the posterior limb of the internal capsule. The area for reception of impulses from the upper extremity is immediately superior to that for the eye and above this area the head, neck, trunk, and lower extremity are represented in that order from below upward. The foot and the genitalia are represented in that part of the posterior central gyrus that extend into the paracentral lobule on the medial surface of the hemisphere (Fig. 132). General sensory impulses from the areas caudal to the head reach the somatesthetic area from the posterolateral ventral thalamic nucleus by way of the posterior limb of the internal capsule (Fig. 123). The posterior ventral nucleus of the thalamus (including posterolateral and posteromedial nuclei) may be assumed to be composed of a number of vertical laminae arranged serially in a lateromedial direction with each lamina receiving afferent impulses related to all modalities of general sensation from a specific region of the body. The impulses from the lower limbs and perineal region are received in the most laterally situated laminae and those from the head region in the most medially situated laminae with intervening laminae concerned with impulses from intermediate regions in a regular serial order.

In addition to being represented contralaterally there is considerable evidence to indicate that pain sense, to a limited degree, is conducted from receptors to the ipsilateral thalamus. At necropsy following hemispherectomy investigators have found complete degeneration of the posterolateral ventral nucleus of the human thalamus. Yet, while these patients lived, retention of sense of pain was observed. From these observations, ipsilateral thalamic representation has been postulated. In discussing the contralateral residual sensibility in hemispherectomized men and hemidecorticate monkeys other investigators suggested that the remaining crude sensation is due both to ipsilateral thalamic representation and to residual thalamic function on the operated side. Moreover, it has been reported that after destroying the ipsilateral thalamus in the totally hemispherectomized monkey, there was retention of pain sensibility. These preparations would seem to answer the

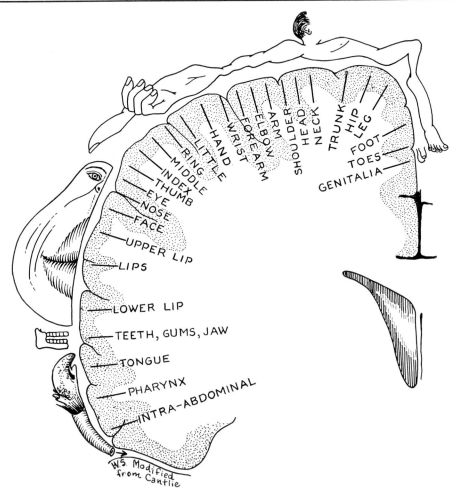

FIG. 132. Sensory homunculus showing representation in the sensory cortex (after Penfield and Rasmussen, *Cerebral Cortex of Man,* The Macmillan Co.).

problem in favor of ipsilateral sensory representation in the thalamus as the cause of retention of the sense of pain. Localization of pain remains poor in the totally hemispherectomized animals except in the face. The retention of painful reception and localization over the trigeminal area has been documented in man after hemispherectomy. Little difference was found in the degree of contralateral hypesthesia between hemidecorticate and totally hemispherectomized monkeys. Light touch, vibratory sensation, sense of position, and placing reactions were measurably absent in both.

Perception of a given sensory stimulus probably involves considerably more than a simple synaptic termination of thalamocortical fibers on a group of neurons in the sensory cortex. It has been reported from electroencephalographic studies that afferent impulses resulting from stimulation of peripheral receptors give rise, in the cortex, to periodically recurring cortical waves which were interpreted as the repetitive discharges of reverberating circuits between thalamic nuclei and the sensory cortex. A description of reverberating circuits as they probably exist within the brain appears on page 135; in addition to corticosubcortical there are intracortical and subcortical circuits. The

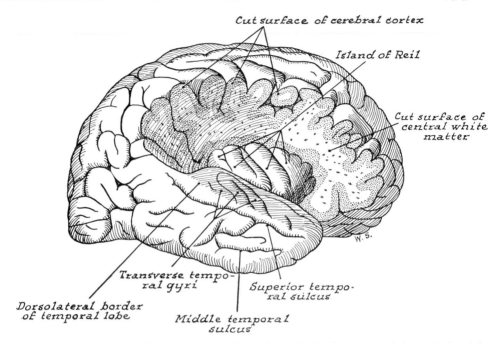

Cut surface of cerebral cortex

Island of Reil

Cut surface of central white matter

W.S.

Transverse temporal gyri

Superior temporal sulcus

Dorsolateral border of temporal lobe

Middle temporal sulcus

FIG. 133. Superior lateral view of the right cerebral hemisphere with the lower parts of the parietal and frontal areas removed to expose the superior surface of the temporal lobe and the insula in the depth of the lateral sulcus (in part after Sobotta-McMurrich).

repetitive discharges described were abolished by interruption of corticothalamic connections, indicating their dependence on a corticosubcortical reverberating circuit.

Parietal lesions which involve the somatesthetic area result in the patient's failure to perceive weak stimuli, inability to localize the point at which a perceptible stimulus is applied, and loss of ability to differentiate between one- and two-point stimulation. Stereognostic sense and the sense of position are also impaired. The probability that pain stimuli are perceived at the thalamic level has been noted (Chap. 6). That this is true is indicated by the fact that pain sensibility is altered to a lesser extent by lesions of the somatesthetic area than are tactile and proprioceptive senses. Moreover, it is reported that an increase in the pain threshold does not result from a cortical lesion. An increased threshold for pain or complete anesthesia in the presence of a cortical lesion has been attributed

to shock or to damage to subcortical structures.

It has been reported that lesions of the posterior ventral thalamic nuclei in cats account for supersensitivity of the sensory cortex. Such supersensitivity may play a role in the spontaneous pain and hyperpathia (*thalamic* or *Dejerine-Roussy syndrome*) seen in man following lesions of these nuclei. It may be noted, however, that ablation of the sensory cortex does not abolish thalamic pain.

Electrical stimulation of the posterior central gyrus evokes accurately localized sensory impressions in the conscious human subject. A number of workers have also reported that it is possible to elicit discrete and complex movements by stimulation of the area with strong currents. Such movements may be facilitated mainly by association neurons whose axons connect the somatesthetic area with the motor and premotor areas of the cortex.

The **auditory area** of the cortex is

buried in the posterior ramus of the lateral sulcus. The posterior half of the superior surface of the superior temporal gyrus, forming the lower boundary of the lateral fissure, presents two or three transverse gyri (Figs. 93, 133). The most anterior of these gyri is usually more prominent than the others; it is referred to as the *convolution of Heschl* and it constitutes the cortical center for hearing. Auditory impulses reach the area from the medial geniculate body by way of the sublentiform part of the internal capsule (Fig. 117). Both ears are represented in the auditory area of either side.

Tumors in either temporal lobe which impinge on the transverse gyri account for auditory symptoms; these include tinnitus and diminution of auditory acuity which are almost always manifested bilaterally, and auditory hallucinations. Such tumors are also likely to produce visual and olfactory symptoms. The visual symptoms are due to pressure on the geniculocalcarine fibers (Fig. 111). The olfactory disturbances result from involvement of the olfactory cortex on the medial side of the temporal lobe (uncus and parahippocampal gyrus).

Unilateral destruction of the auditory area does not cause deafness but when done on the left side in right-handed individuals may result in inability to associate the usual meaning with the sounds heard; this condition is referred to as *sensory aphasia* or, more specifically, as *auditory verbal agnosia*. In one reported study a sensory type of aphasia occurred in sixteen of a series of sixty-two individuals with temporal lobe tumors; fourteen of these were right-handed with left-sided tumors while two definitely left-handed patients had tumors on the right side. The tendency toward concentration of certain functions in the left hemisphere of right-handed individuals or *left cerebral dominance* is a distinguishing characteristic of the human brain. *Motor aphasia,* manifested by loss of the faculty of vocal expression, is due to destruction of the *motor speech area* which is in the inferior frontal gyrus of the left hemisphere in right-handed subjects; it is also an indication of left cerebral dominance.

Stimulation of the auditory area gives rise to roaring and buzzing sensations. Stimulation of the cortex adjacent to the auditory area gives rise to vertigo and thus indicates that vestibular impulses are also projected on temporal areas. The **vestibular area** has been described as lying just medial to the auditory gyrus. In the cat the area has been found to be adjacent to and actually overlapping the auditory area. Other investigators have reported the vestibular area to be anterior to the auditory area, to which predominantly crossed impulses were projected from the medial and spinal vestibular nuclei. Vertigo was a symptom in eleven of the sixty-two cases of temporal lobe tumor mentioned above; nystagmus appeared in only four.

The **visual area** of the cortex is located on both sides of the posterior half of the *calcarine sulcus* and on the ventral side of its anterior half (Figs. 128, 129). It may extend around the occipital pole on to the dorsolateral surface of the hemisphere. Visual impulses reach the calcarine area from the *lateral geniculate body* by way of the *geniculocalcarine tract* (Fig. 111). *Macular* or *central vision* is projected on the posterior limit of the calcarine area. Concentric zones, progressing anteriorly from this point, represent successively more peripheral areas of the retina. The peripheral limits of the retina therefore are represented at the anterior limit of the calcarine sulcus. Visual impulses originating in the upper quadrants of the retina are projected on the upper portion of the visual cortex and those originating in the lower quadrants are projected on the lower portion. Accordingly, the right upper quadrants of both retinae send impulses to the upper half of the right visual area; the right lower quadrants send them to its lower half. The former respond to visual stimuli from the left lower quadrants of the visual fields; the latter to those from the left upper quadrants.

Destruction of the calcarine cortex of one hemisphere results in contralateral homonymous hemianopia which differs from that due to a complete lesion of one optic tract (Fig. 111,7) in that macular or central vision is not lost. No satisfactory explanation has been advanced for the persistence of central vision in such cortical lesions. Bilateral representation of the macula has most frequently been presumed to be responsible for the phenomenon, but anatomical evidence of such representation is lacking. Some workers have asserted that the sparing of macular vision in cortical lesions is a misconception that has arisen because lesions interpreted as completely destroy-

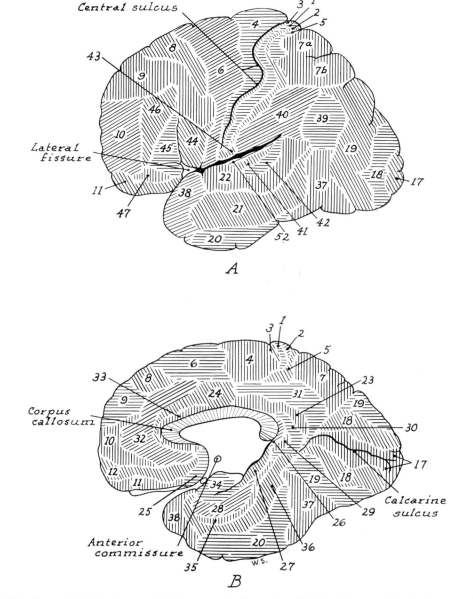

FIG. 134. Structurally distinctive areas of the human cerebral cortex (modified from Brodmann). A, Dorsolateral surface. B, Medial surface.

ing the calcarine cortex have not actually been that extensive. Cases of complete unilateral occipital lobectomy have been reported in which there was no macular sparing.

Brodmann and others have charted the various areas of the cerebral cortex on the basis of cytoarchitecture and have designated each area by number. The somatesthetic area, in Brodmann's chart (Fig. 134), comprises numbered areas 3, 1 and 2; the auditory area is 41 and the visual cortex is area 17. Perception of specific modalities has been demonstrated to be the function of these cortical areas; integration and association of similar and dissimilar sensory impulses are functions of association areas. General sensory impulses are integrated in the parietal cortex posterior to the posterior central gyrus with the result that the individual is enabled to differentiate between areas stimulated, between degrees of stimulation, and even between types of tactile, pain, or proprioceptive stimuli applied; areas 5 and 7 are particularly concerned with this discriminatory function (Fig. 134).

Auditory association areas include 41 and 22; on the dominant side these areas relate sounds (or words) heard at a given time with those heard at other times during the life of the individual and thus facilitate the interpretation of these sounds as they apply to the environment which obtains at any given moment in his existence. It has been reported that areas 42 and 22 on the right side of the brain were able to take over to some extent gnostic functions which were affected by a left-sided thrombosis which destroyed these areas on the dominant side.

Electrical *stimulation of the visual cortex* (area 17) in the conscious subject gives rise to impressions of pin-points of light in corresponding loci in the fields of vision; *stimulation of the peristriate area* (area 18, Fig. 134) produces integration of the more primitive impressions elicited from area 17 into geometric figures; *stimulation of area 19* (Fig. 134)

introduces color and definitive forms of familiar objects.

It has been suggested that retention of isolated sensory impressions within the brain that can be recalled at some later time and compared with current impressions, may be facilitated by *reverberating circuits* within the cortex and subjacent white matter. In such a circuit the first neuron would be fired by a sensory impulse and would in turn fire the second neuron which would then fire the third and so on until the original neuron was again fired by the last neuron in the circuit. Assuming that the time required for the nervous impulse to traverse the circuit is sufficient to permit each neuron to restore its energy through normal metabolic processes, the sensory impulse that originally fired the circuit may continue to exist within it unless and until the ability of one or all the neurons involved to restore energy between firings is interfered with by injury, vascular degeneration, or some toxic factor within the brain. The association of many sensory impressions of the same or different types (visual, tactile, pain, thermal) may probably be accounted for by the participation of a single neuron in more than one reverberating circuit.

Memory for past experiences, involving the simultaneous perception and integration of all types of environmental stimuli, appears to be concentrated in an area near the posterior limit of the temporal lobe. Electrical stimulation of this part of the dorsolateral surface of the cerebrum, which is essentially encircled by visual, general sensory, and auditory association areas, gives rise to integrated recall of previous experience or previous thinking. Recent studies suggest that for lesions of the temporal lobe to cause impairment of memory they must involve the hippocampal formation. Furthermore, reports indicate that temporal lobe lesions cause loss of memory only when they are bilateral and involve both the hippocampal formation and parahip-

10

pocampal gyrus. A further discussion of the hippocampus and related areas is given in Chapter 24.

Similarities between memory and the electronic computing machines have been emphasized which support the generally accepted concept that a neuron circuit can be set in action by an incoming single impulse and that the circuit may then go on reverberating as long as metabolism supports it or until it is modified by other incoming impulses.

A reasonable theory of *frontal lobe function* has been advanced which replaces the older theory that memory is dependent on the integrity of the frontal cortex and its connections with other cortical and subcortical centers. The concept is that the frontal lobes, which are without primary function such as mediation of sight or hearing, act secondarily through their connections to maintain or sustain emotional states, trends of association (judgment), and motor actions or the inhibition of such actions. The functions sustained by the frontal lobes are those which can be brought under voluntary control but may operate without the help of the frontal lobe. After frontal lobotomy, states of worry, fear, depression, tension, and negativism are relieved and may be replaced by states characterized by excessive intake of food, outspokenness, and lack of initiative.

The **cingulate gyrus,** on the medial aspect of the cerebral hemisphere (Fig. 134, areas 23, 24, 33), is an important link in the system of corticosubcortical reverberating circuits responsible for "emotional expression." Bilateral lesions of the cingulate gyri account for apathy, akinesia, mutism, urinary incontinence, indifference to pain, and, in the terminal stages, stupor and coma. Frontal lobotomies and leukotomies (section of white matter of frontal lobe) only minimally affect the afferent and efferent connections between the cingulate gyrus and the thalamohypothalamic nuclei; therefore, depressive states, apparently due to over-

activity of more anteriorly and laterally located circuits, may be relieved by such procedures with relative integrity of the circuits responsible for active emotional expression.

BIBLIOGRAPHY

Arnot, R., 1952: A theory of frontal lobe function. A.M.A. Arch Neurol. Psychiat., *67,* 487–495.

Austin, G. M., and Grant, F. C., 1955: Physiologic observations following total hemispherectomy in man. Surgery, *38,* 239–258.

Barris, R. W., and Schuman, H. R., 1953: Bilateral anterior cingulate gyrus lesions, syndrome of the anterior cingulate gyri. Neurology, *3,* 44–52.

Celesia, G. G., Broughton, R. J., Rasmussen, T., and Branch, C., 1968: Auditory evoked responses from exposed human cortex. Electroenceph. Clin. Neurophysiol., *24,* 458–466.

Chang, H. T., 1950: The repetitive discharges of corticothalamic reverberating circuit. J. Neurophysiol., *13,* 235–257.

Clark, W. E. L., and Powell, T. P. S., 1953: On the thalamo-cortical connexions of the general sensory cortex of *Macaca.* Proc. Roy. Soc. (London), B, *141,* 467–487.

Cobb, S., 1952: On the nature and locus of mind. A.M.A. Arch Neurol. Psychiat., *67,* 172–177.

Critchley, M., 1966: The enigma of Gerstmann's syndrome. Brain, *89,* 183–198.

Foerster, O., 1929: Beiträge zur Pathophysiologie der Sehbahn und der Sehsphäre. J. Psychol. Neurol., *39,* 463–485.

Fulton, J. F., 1949: *Physiology of Nervous System.* 3rd Ed. Oxford University Press, New York.

Geschwind, N., 1965: Disconnexion syndromes in animals and man. Brain, *88,* 237–294.

Halstead, W. C., Walker, A. E., and Bucy, P. C., 1940: Sparing and nonsparing of "macular" vision associated with occipital lobectomy in man. A.M.A. Arch. Ophthal., *24,* 948–966.

Head, H., 1918: Sensation and the cerebral cortex. Brain, Part II, *41,* 57–253.

Hubel, D. H., and Wiesel, T. N., 1968: Receptive fields and functional architecture of monkey striate cortex. J. Physiol. (London), *195,* 215–243.

Massopust, L. C., Jr., and Daigle, H. J., 1960: Cortical projection of the medial and spinal vestibular nuclei in the cat. Exp. Neurol., *2,* 179–185.

Mettler, F. A., 1943: Extensive unilateral

cerebral removals in primate: physiologic effects and resultant degeneration. J. Comp. Neurol., *79*, 185–245.

Mickle, W. A., and Ades, H. W., 1954: Rostral projection pathway of the vestibular system. Amer. J. Physiol., *176*, 243–246.

Millikan, C. H., and Darley, F. L. (Eds.), 1967: *Brain Mechanisms Underlying Speech and Language.* Grune & Stratton, New York.

Mountcastle, V. B., and Henneman, E., 1952: The representation of tactile sensibility in the thalamus of the monkey. J. Comp. Neurol., *97*, 409–439.

Mountcastle, V. B., and Powell, T. P. S., 1959: Neural mechanisms subserving cutaneous sensibility with special reference to the role of afferent inhibition in sensory perception and discrimination. Bull. Johns Hopkins Hosp., *105*, 201–232.

Nielsen, J. M., 1951: Anterior cingulate gyrus and corpus callosum. Bull. Los Angeles Neurol. Soc., *16*, 235–243.

Nielsen, J. M., 1953: Spontaneous recovery from aphasia: autopsy. Bull. Los Angeles Neurol. Soc., *18*, 147–148.

Northrop, F. S. C., 1948: The neurological and behavioristic psychological basis of the ordering of society by means of ideas. Science, *107*, 411–417.

Penfield, W., 1952: Memory mechanisms. A.M.A. Arch. Neurol. Psychiat., *67*, 178–198.

Penfield, W., and Rasmussen, T., 1950: *The Cerebral Cortex of Man. A Clinical Study of Localization of Function.* The Macmillan Co., New York.

Penfield, W., and Jasper, H. H., 1954: *Epilepsy and the Functional Anatomy of the Human Brain.* Little, Brown & Company, Boston.

Penfield, W., and Milner, B., 1958: Memory deficit produced by bilateral lesions in the hippocampal zone. A.M.A. Arch. Neurol. Psychiat., *79*, 475–497.

Piercy, M., 1967: Studies of the neurological basis of intellectual functions. Clinical studies. In *Modern Trends in Neurology,* D. Williams, Ed. Butterworths, London, Vol. 4, pp. 106–124.

Schuell, H., 1953: Aphasic difficulties understanding spoken language. Neurology, *3*, 176–184.

Scoville, W. B., and Milner, B., 1957: Loss of recent memory after bilateral hippocampal lesions. J. Neurol. Neurosurg. Psychiat., *20*, 11–21.

Sperry, R. W., 1966: Brain bisection and mechanisms of consciousness. In *Brain and Conscious Experience,* J. C. Eccles, Ed. Springer-Verlag, Berlin, Heidelberg, New York, pp. 298–308.

Spiegel, E. A., 1934: Labyrinth and cortex: the electroencephalogram of the cortex in stimulation of the labyrinth. A.M.A. Arch. Neurol. Psychiat., *31*, 469–482.

Spiegel, E. A., and Szekely, E. G., 1954: Cortical supersensitivity after lesions of the ventral thalamic nuclei. Fed. Proc., *13*, 143–144.

Spiegel, E. A., Kletzkin, M. S., Szekely, E. G., and Wycis, H. T., 1954: Role of hypothalamic mechanisms in thalamic pain. Neurology, *4*, 739–751.

Strobos, R. R. J., 1953: Tumors of the temporal lobe. Neurology, *3*, 752–760.

Walker, A. E., and Fulton, J. F., 1938: Hemidecortication in chimpanzee, baboon, macaque, potto, cat and coati. A study in encephalization. J. Nerv. Ment. Dis., *87*, 677–700.

Weinstein, E. A., Cole, M., Mitchell, M. S., and Lyerly, O. G., 1964: Anosognosia and aphasia. Arch. Neurol. (Chicago), *10*, 376–386.

White, R. J., Schreiner, L. H., Hughes, R. A., MacCarty, C. S., and Grindlay, J. H., 1959: Physiologic consequences of total hemispherectomy in the monkey. Neurology, *9*, 149–159.

Chapter 13

Histology of the Cerebral Cortex

The perceptive, integrative, and motor capabilities of the cerebral cortex are facilitated by surprisingly constant and logical laminar interrelationships among the several types of neurons located therein.

Although there is a great variety of neurons within the cerebral cortex, the cell types commonly recognized include pyramidal cells, stellate cells, horizontal cells (of Cajal), cells of Martinotti, and fusiform cells.

Pyramidal cells are the most numerous and range in size from about 10 to 100 μ in diameter. They are generally classified as small, medium, large, and giant pyramidal cells (cells of Betz). From the apex of the pyramidal cell the apical dendrite arises which extends toward the surface of the cortex and ends in numerous branches. Numerous smaller dendrites, which are termed basal dendrites, emerge from the base and sides of the pyramidal cells and extend into the adjacent layers.

The stellate cells are small in size; most are in the range of 5 to 10 μ in diameter. These cells have many branched dendrites which terminate near the cell of origin, and a short axon which also branches profusely. The stellate cells are often called granule cells on the basis of their appearance in Nissl preparations.

The horizontal cells are small with fusiform cell bodies. They are found in the most superficial layer of the cortex, and their processes course horizontally for considerable distances.

The cells of Martinotti are small triangular or rounded neurons and are multipolar in character. They are found throughout the various layers of the cortex. The axons of these cells extend toward the surface of the cortex and the dendrites spread in various directions. The connections of the processes are limited to intracortical neurons.

The fusiform cells are located primarily in the deepest layer of the cerebral cortex. The dendrites of these neurons extend into the upper cortical layers and the axons enter the white matter although the specific distribution is unknown.

Despite the lack of a uniform distribution of the respective cell types within the cerebral cortex, there is a characteristic lamination of neurons and fibers. The pattern of lamination may be observed in Nissl-stained sections (cytoarchitecture) or in preparations stained for myelin (myeloarchitecture).

The neopallial cortex, which comprises the major part of the cortex in man, has, according to the Brodmann scheme, six recognizable layers at some stage of development based on its cytoarchitecture. For this reason the neocortex may be referred to as the "homogenetic" type or as "isocortex." The phylogenetically older cortex, which developed in relation to the olfactory system, includes the archipallium (hippocampus) and paleopallium (pyriform cortex). Since these parts of the cortex do not show the six layers, they are designated "heterogenetic" in type, or "allocortex." These areas are considered further in Chapter 24, The Rhinencephalon.

Layers of the Neocortex

The six layers of neocortex according to the scheme of Brodmann (Figs. 135, 138) are from the surface inward:

I. Molecular layer (plexiform layer)
II. External granular layer
III. Pyramidal layer
IV. Internal granular layer
V. Ganglionic layer
VI. Polymorphic layer.

The **molecular layer** contains horizontal cells (Fig. 135), a few cells with short axons (Golgi type II), and the terminal ends of dendrites from cells of deeper layers.

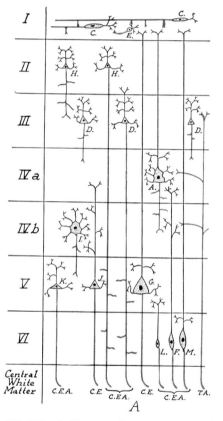 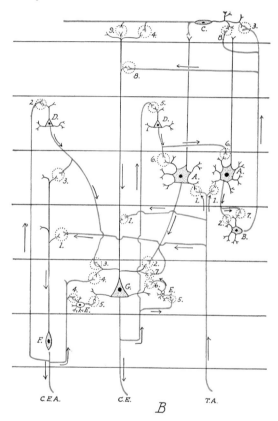

FIG. 135. *A,* Diagrammatic representation of the cell layers of the sensory areas of the cerebral cortex showing the distribution of the dendrites and axons of each type of neuron. Axons are colored red. *B,* Diagram illustrating some of the possibilities for neuron chains of varying lengths to bombard the large pyramidal cells with a given nervous impulse which enters the cortex over a thalamic afferent fiber (*T.A.*). Axons are colored red and, in order to avoid the confusion that would result from the use of several cells of a given type, the same cell has been utilized in two or more of the nine circuits depicted. A single impulse entering the cortex over the thalamic afferent fiber may be traced to one of the dendritic processes of the large pyramidal cell (*G*) through a single synapse (*1*) or through neuron chains containing two to nine synapses.

Letters in *A* and *B* indicate cell types as follows: *A,* star pyramidal cell; *B,* Golgi type I cell; *C,* horizontal cell; *D,* medium pyramidal cell of layer III; *E,* Golgi type II cell; *F,* medium spindle cell; *G,* large pyramidal cell; *H,* small pyramidal cell; *I,* stellate cell; *J,* medium pyramidal cell of layer V; *K,* short pyramidal cell; *L,* short spindle cell; *M,* long spindle cell.

Axons in the central white matter are indicated as follows: *C.E.,* cortical efferent (projection); *C.E.A.,* cortical efferent (association): *T.A.,* thalamic afferent.

Synapses in *B* are numbered *1, 2, 3,* and so on according to their position in a given neuron chain. The direction of nervous impulses is indicated by arrows placed alongside the axon or dendrite concerned. (After Lorente de Nó.)

The **external granular layer** contains many granule and small pyramidal cells and their dendrites. The dendrites of cells in the deeper strata pass through this layer and some of the dendrites of layer III terminate in it.

The **layer of pyramidal cells** has an outer zone containing chiefly medium-sized pyramids and an inner zone containing larger pyramidal cells. Some of the afferent fibers from the thalamic nuclei (Fig. 135, *T.A.*) terminate in relation to the dendrites of the medium-sized pyramids in the latter layer.

The **internal granular layer** contains a large number of small stellate cells and scattered small pyramids. This layer is characterized by dense fibrillar plexuses formed, in the parietal area, by afferent fibers from the thalamus and, in the temporal and occipital areas, by afferents from the medial and lateral geniculate

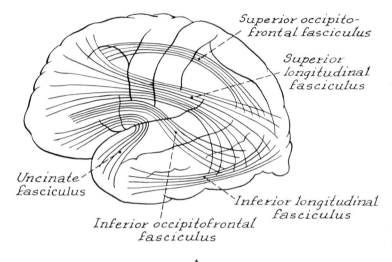

A

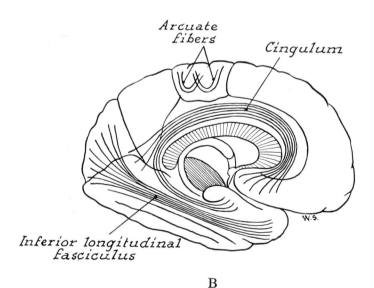

B

FIG. 136. Long and short association pathways within the cerebrum superimposed on a superior lateral view of the left hemisphere in A and on a medial view in B. (B after Sobotta-McMurrich.)

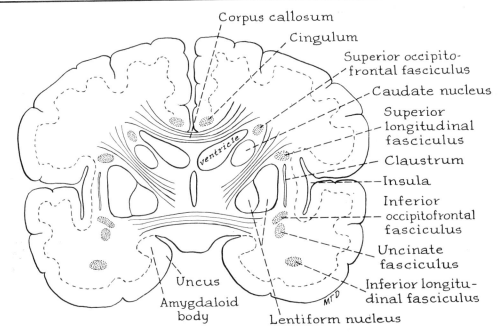

Corpus callosum

Cingulum

Superior occipito-
frontal fasciculus

Caudate nucleus

Superior
longitudinal
fasciculus

Claustrum

Insula

Inferior
occipitofrontal
fasciculus

Uncinate
fasciculus

Inferior longitu-
dinal fasciculus

ventricle

Uncus

Amygdaloid
body

Lentiform nucleus

FIG. 137. Coronal section of the brain illustrating the long association pathways in relation to other structures.

bodies (Fig. 135, *T.A.*). The outer line of Baillarger is in this layer.

Layer V contains large, medium, and short pyramidal cells (Fig. 135). The long dendrites of the large pyramids reach the plexiform layer whereas collaterals and basilar dendrites are distributed within layer V exclusively. The dendrites of the medium pyramids end in layer IV and therefore have numerous synapses with the thalamic and geniculate afferents. The dendrites of the short pyramids end within layer V. The internal line of Baillarger is in this layer.

Spindle cells of three types—long, medium, and short—are found in **layer VI** (Fig. 135). The long spindles have dendrites which give off collaterals in layer VI and then ascend undivided and without further collaterals to reach the plexiform layer. The dendrites of the medium spindles end in layer IV in relation to the thalamic afferents and those of the short spindles end in layer V.

Afferent fibers from the thalamus, as has been noted, chiefly terminate in relation to the star pyramids and stellate cells in layer IV. *Association fibers* from other cortical areas, including commissural fibers from the opposite hemisphere, give off collaterals in the deep layers, but their main areas of distribution are in layers I to IV; the majority end in layers II and III.

The axons of the pyramidal and stellate cells of layers I to IV ramify chiefly within the gray matter, but some of the axons of the former reach the underlying white matter and become association and commissural fibers. The pyramidal axons also give off numerous collaterals, particularly in layers V and VI. Axons of the large pyramids in layer V become projection or association fibers. Those of the short pyramids are largely commissural and pass through the corpus callosum. Axons of spindle cells in layer VI are distributed to other areas of the cortex as association fibers.

Association fibers may be short or long (Fig. 136). The short association fibers connect adjacent gyri and, because of their course around and deep to the intervening fissure or sulcus, are often referred to as *U-fibers* or *arcuate fibers.* The long association fibers are arranged in rather definite bundles and connect more widely separated areas of the cortex. The six such bundles which are more commonly recognized include the *cingulum,* the *uncinate fasciculus,* the *superior* and *inferior longitudinal fasciculi,* and the *superior* and *inferior occipitofrontal fasciculi* (Figs. 136, 137). The *cingulum* courses above the corpus callosum within the cingulate gyrus. It interconnects the orbitofrontal region with cortical areas throughout the extent of the fornicate gyrus. The *uncinate fasciculus* passes deep to the lateral fissure and interconnects the temporal pole region with the basal frontal cortex. The *superior longitudinal fasciculus* courses from the frontal area over the region of the insula and lentiform nucleus into the temporal, parietal, and occipital cortex. It contains many short fibers interconnecting these adjacent cortical regions. It is separated from the more medial and deeper coursing *superior occipitofrontal fasciculus* by fibers of the internal capsule as they continue into the corona radiata. The main bundle of fibers in the superior occipitofrontal fasciculus courses below the lateral border of the corpus callosum medial to the area at which callosal and internal capsule fibers interdigitate. This fasciculus interconnects frontal and occipital regions with temporal and insular cortex. The *inferior occipitofrontal fasciculus* lies above and adjacent to the uncinate fasciculus and courses below the lentiform nucleus and extreme capsule interconnecting occipital and frontal areas of the cortex.

The *inferior longitudinal fasciculus* extends from the temporal to occipital regions. Posteriorly, it is in relation to the more medially located system of visual radiations and considered to be a part thereof by some authors.

The **complex pattern of intracortical connections** is diagrammatically illustrated in Figure 135*B*. A thalamic affer-

ent fiber (*T.A.*) is shown entering the cortex from the subjacent white matter. Collaterals from this fiber synapse on the ascending dendrite of a large, deep pyramidal cell (*G*) and on that of a medium spindle cell (*F*) within layer IVb; its terminal divisions synapse on the dendrites of star pyramids in layer IVa. Numerous other possible connections with stellate cells and with Golgi types I and II cells have been omitted for the sake of simplicity. The axons of the large, deep pyramidal and medium spindle cells, respectively, enter the white matter as projection (*C.E.*) and association (*C.E.A.*) fibers; collaterals from them ascend through the cortex to synapse on the dendrites or Golgi type II (*E*), medium pyramidal (*D*), and large, deep pyramidal (*G*) cells. Through the medium of the various cells and synapses depicted in the diagram a nervous impulse entering the cortex over a single thalamic afferent fiber may reach the dendrites of a given large, deep pyramidal cell through neuron chains which include from one to nine synapses. Two or more circuits have been directed through some of the cells in order to avoid the confusion which would result from the inclusion in the diagram of several more of each type of cell. Actually, many more cells (spindle, medium pyramidal, horizontal, stellate, and Golgi types I and II) would probably function in the several neuron chains shown converging on the large, deep pyramidal cell.

On the average, each synapse accounts for a conduction delay of 0.6 millisecond; therefore, the same impulse may be delivered to the pyramidal cell several times and at fairly regular intervals, depending on the number of synapses crossed enroute. It has been proposed that many of the impulses arriving at the synapse of a cell (by way of specific thalamic and other afferents) fail to cross the synapse because they do not reach threshold, but may do so provided that the conditions necessary for summation are fulfilled.

Summation is accomplished through the neuron chains by a succession of impulses impinging on the cortical cells thus creating in them a constant state of facilitation, and eventually stimulating them to discharge into their axons.

It must be kept in mind that, in addition to the impulses from the thalamus to a given cortical area, there are also impulses arriving from all other areas of the cerebral cortex by way of associa-

tion and commissural fibers. As has been mentioned, these fibers largely terminate in the second and third layers of the cortex, but they may send collaterals to cells in any of the deeper layers that they traverse. Thus the afferent impulses from other cortical areas also reach the dendrites of the large pyramidal cells either directly or through neuron chains of varying lengths.

Feed-back, as applied to the nervous

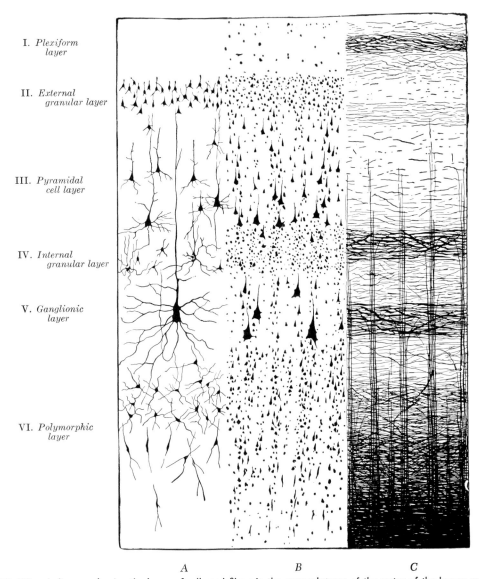

I. *Plexiform layer*

II. *External granular layer*

III. *Pyramidal cell layer*

IV. *Internal granular layer*

V. *Ganglionic layer*

VI. *Polymorphic layer*

A   B   C

FIG. 138. A diagram showing the layers of cells and fibers in the gray substance of the cortex of the human cerebral hemisphere, according to the histological methods of Golgi, Nissl, and Weigert. A, Stained by the method of Golgi; B, by that of Nissl; C, by that of Weigert. (After Brodmann: from Luciani's *Physiology*, Macmillan & Co., Ltd.) (From Gray's Anatomy, 28th ed., Charles Mayo Goss, Ed., Lea & Febiger, Philadelphia.)

system, means that the activity of the reverberating circuits is modified by the return of some of the output of the system as input. When the hand is extended toward an object a series of signals flow back through visual, tactile, and proprioceptive mechanisms to inform the central mechanism how far the hand is overshooting or undershooting. The amount of error determines the return input until the error becomes zero.

When stained with iron-hematoxylin the laminated character of the cortex is shown to be due to layers of myelinated fibers (Fig. 138). The concentrations of myelinated fibers have been given special designations. The *outer line of Baillarger* forms the outer part of layer IV; the *inner line of Baillarger* is in the inner half of layer V. The less prominent *band of Bechterew* is at the outer margin of layer III. Baillarger's inner line is absent in the calcarine cortex, but the outer line is especially well-marked. The prominent outer line in this area is called the *stria of Genarri* and, because of this prominent stria, the calcarine cortex is often referred to as the *striate area*.

BIBLIOGRAPHY

Bailey, P., Von Bonin, G., Garol, H. W., and McCulloch, W. S., 1943: Long association fibers in cerebral hemispheres of monkey and chimpanzee. J. Neurophysiol., *6,* 129–134.

Bailey, P., and Von Bonin, G., 1951: *The Isocortex of Man.* University of Illinois Press, Urbana.

Bonin, G. Von, and Bailey, P., 1947: *The Neocortex of Macaca mulatta.* University of Illinois Press, Urbana.

Brodmann, D., 1909: Vergleichende Lokalisationslehre der Grosshirnrinde in ihren Prinzipien dargestelt auf Grund des Zellenbaues. Barth, Leipzig.

Campbell, A. W., 1905: *Histological Studies on the Localization of Cerebral Function.* Cambridge University Press, Cambridge.

Cobb, S., 1952: On the nature and locus of mind. A.M.A. Arch. Neurol. Psychiat., *67,* 172–177.

Economo, C. Von, 1927: *Zellaufbau der Grosshirnrinde des Menschen.* Julius Springer, Berlin.

Kuypers, H. G. J. M., Szwarcbart, M.-K., Mishkin, M., and Rosvold, H. P., 1965: Occipitotemporal corticocortical connections in the rhesus monkey. Exp. Neurol., *11,* 245–262.

Lorente de Nó, R., 1949: The structure of the cerebral cortex. In Fulton's *Physiology of the Nervous System*, 3rd ed. Oxford University Press, New York, pp. 288–330.

Pakkenberg, H., 1966: The number of nerve cells in the cerebral cortex of man. J. Comp. Neurol., *128,* 17–20.

Pope, A., 1967: Microchemical architecture of human isocortex. Arch. Neurol., *16,* 351–356.

Rakic, P., and Yakovlev, P. I., 1968: Development of the corpus callosum and cavum septi in man. J. Comp. Neurol., *132,* 45–72.

Chapter 14

The Motor Cortex and Its Projections

The **motor area of the cortex,** also designated **area 4,** occupies the posterior half of the anterior central gyrus (Fig. 134). It is broader superiorly than inferiorly and, like the posterior central gyrus, extends into the paracentral lobule on the medial surface of the hemisphere. Representation is similar to that in the somatesthetic area; accordingly, the area having to do with the motor innervation of the lower limb is superiorly placed and extends on to the medial surface while the head region is represented in the lowermost part (Fig. 139).

The **motor cortex** differs structurally from the parietotemporooccipital sensory areas in that pyramidal cells are found in all layers except the outer or plexiform layer. In the posterior lip of the anterior central gyrus, layer V contains the *giant pyramidal cells of Betz* (Fig. 140). The axons of these cells along with those from other cortical pyramidal cells are distributed to motor neurons in the brain stem and spinal cord as *corticobulbar* and *corticospinal fibers* (Fig. 140). Corticobulbar fibers originate from the lateral and inferior portions of the motor cortex, whereas corticospinal fibers originate mainly from the more superior parts. The *motor neurons,* on which they synapse— either directly or through the medium of internuncial cells—are found in the motor nuclei of cranial nerves and in the anterior gray columns of the spinal cord.

When the motor centers in the brain evoke movement in muscle, descending nerve impulses may reach the muscles by either of two routes. In the first route, impulses course directly, or through intercalated neurons, to large (alpha) anterior gray column cells and so to the muscles. The second, or indirect, route is responsible for excitation of the "small nerve" or *gamma-efferents.* The latter route causes contraction of *intrafusal muscle fibers* (within the neuromuscular spindles) causing negligible tension as measured externally, but sufficing to stretch the primary sensory endings in the muscle spindles and, through the stretch reflex arc (Figs. 45, 46), to activate the main muscle fibers. This circuitous initiation of contraction introduces delay but has the advantage that, during shortening, the muscles are under the influence of the servoproperties of the stretch reflex. A constant rate of discharge over the *alpha route* sets up tension that is independent of length. The *gamma-efferent system,* however, is believed to operate a servomechanism that makes the main muscle follow length changes in the spindle. At a constant rate of gamma discharge the muscle will tend to maintain a fixed length independent of tension. The circumstances under which one or the other of these routes or various mixtures of the two are called into play are not known although it is probable that posture would

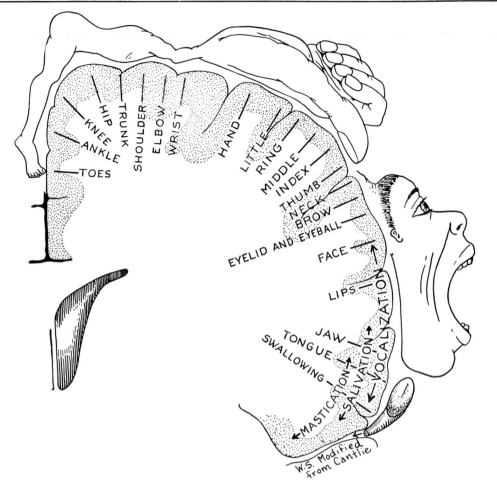

FIG. 139. Motor homunculus illustrating motor representation in area 4, anterior central gyrus. (After Penfield and Rasmussen, *Cerebral Cortex of Man*, The Macmillan Co.)

mainly employ the gamma route and that rapid movements with minimum reaction time traverse the alpha route.

Experiments indicate that the relation of descending fibers to motor neurons concerned with alpha-motor innervation of facial muscles and the distal muscles of the limbs is a monosynaptic one and that more than one synapse is involved in the alpha-motor pathway to proximal limb muscles.

The **corticobulbar fibers** traverse the genu of the internal capsule, and the **corticospinal fibers** pass through its posterior limb (Fig. 141). From the internal capsule both sets of fibers enter the basis pedunculi of the mesencephalon where,

except for a small medial bundle of corticobulbar fibers, they occupy its middle three-fifths (Fig. 142). Corticospinal, together with some corticobulbar, fibers are arranged in longitudinal bundles in the basilar part of the pons (Fig. 143). The bundles are intermingled with the pontile fibers and nuclei; collaterals from corticospinal fibers terminate in the pontile nuclei and thus provide for reverberating circuits through the cerebellum which return impulses to the motor cortex (Chap. 19).

Corticospinal fibers, after traversing the basis pontis, enter the pyramids of the medulla (Fig. 144). It should be noted that, throughout their course to

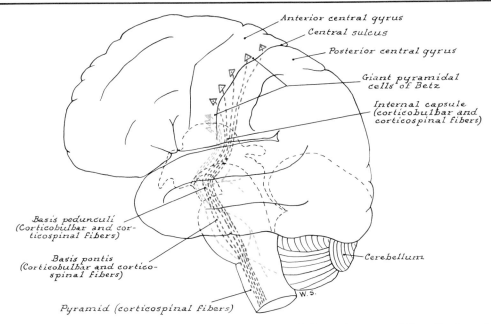

FIG. 140. Diagram showing the origin and course of some of the corticobulbar and corticospinal fibers. The descending fibers are superimposed on a lateral view of the brain in which the positions of the brain stem and cerebellum are indicated by dotted lines. Corticobulbar fibers are colored blue; corticospinal fibers, red.

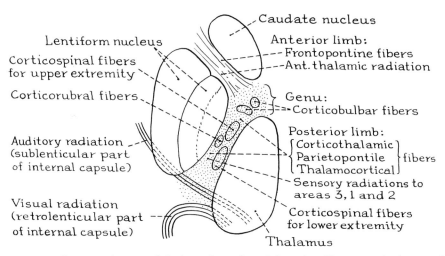

FIG. 141. Diagram illustrating the parts of the internal capsule and the various fiber systems in the respective parts as seen in horizontal section.

this point, they have remained on the side of their origin. At the caudal limits of the pyramids 80 to 90 per cent of them cross to the opposite side through the *motor* or *pyramidal decussation* and enter the *lateral corticospinal tracts* in the lateral funiculi of the spinal cord (Figs. 41, 145, 147). The lateral corticospinal tracts, like the sensory tracts, are specifically laminated; the most laterally placed fibers have the longest intramedullary course and end in the most caudal segments of the spinal cord.

Uncrossed corticospinal fibers (10 to 20 per cent) enter the anterior funiculi of the spinal cord where they form the

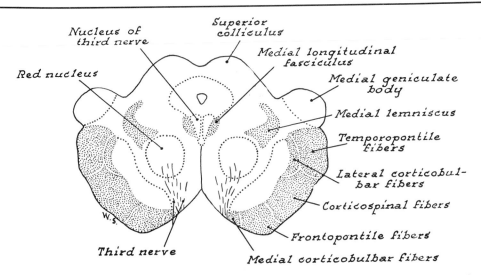

FIG. 142. Section through the mesencephalon showing the locations of the various types of fibers in the basis pedunculi.

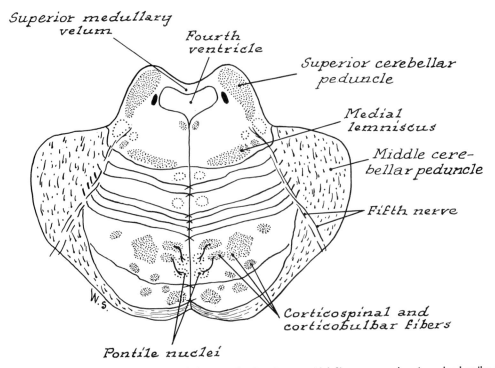

FIG. 143. Section through the rostral part of the pons showing the pyramidal fibers arranged as irregular bundles in its basilar part.

anterior corticospinal tracts (Figs. 146, 147). They also terminate in relation to anterior gray column cells, but may cross to the opposite side through the anterior white commissure just before doing so. The anterior corticospinal tracts do not extend below the thoracic levels of the cord.

The **corticospinal tracts** are often referred to as the *pyramidal tracts* because they pass through the medullary pyramids. The pyramidal tracts are by defi-

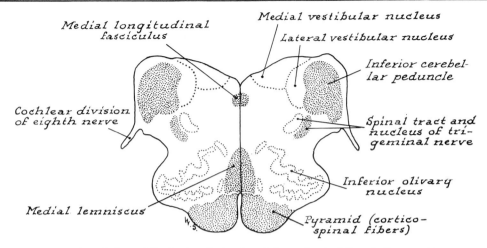

FIG. 144. Section through the medulla showing the location of the corticospinal fibers in the pyramids.

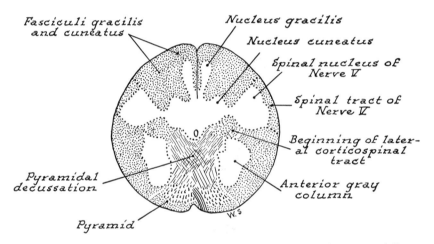

FIG. 145. Section through the lower end of the medulla showing the decussation of corticospinal fibers.

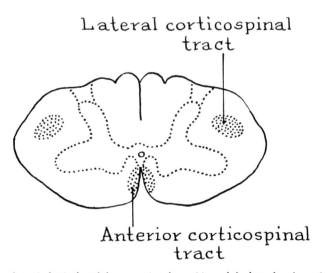

FIG. 146. Section through cervical spinal cord demonstrating the positions of the lateral and anterior corticospinal tracts.

nition the fibers that arise in the cortex and pass through the medullary pyramids to the spinal cord. It is to be emphasized that these fibers do not arise solely from the giant cells of Betz, nor do they arise exclusively from area 4. It has been shown that there are approximately 34,000 Betz cells in each cerebral hemisphere and that each pyramid contains about 1 million axons. About 30,000 of these fibers are of large diameter, 9 to 22 μ, which compares favorably to the number of Betz cells.

From the various estimates that have been made, it appears that about one-third of the pyramidal tract fibers originate in area 4 and that approximately 20 per cent arise from cells in the postcentral gyrus. Area 6 also has been reported to contribute pyramidal fibers, and studies in the monkey indicate an origin from areas 4, 6, 8, 3, 1, 2, 5, and 7. Threshold movements have been elicited from stimulating area 4 and areas 6 and 5 of the monkey under local anesthesia.

Evidence for fibers within the pyra-

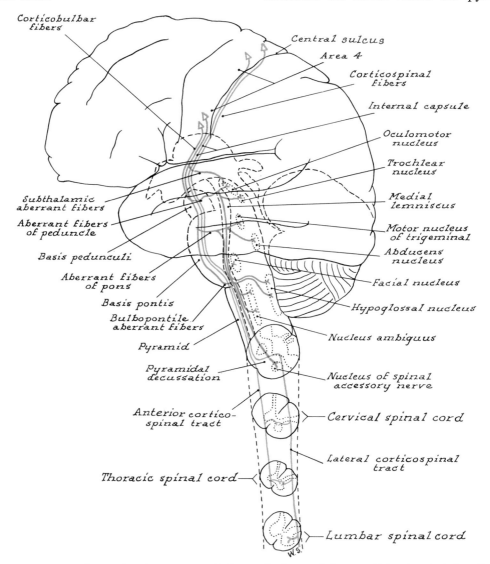

FIG. 147. Diagram showing the origin, course, and ultimate distribution of the pyramidal and corticobulbar fibers. Corticobulbar fibers are blue; corticospinal fibers, red.

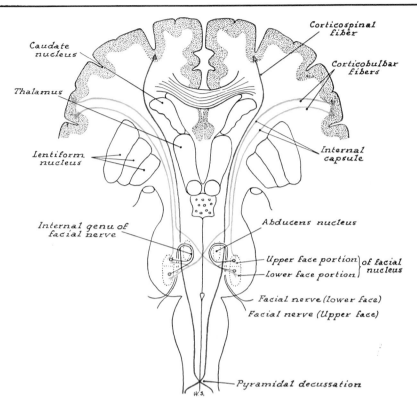

FIG. 148. Diagram illustrating the probable distribution of corticobulbar fibers to the facial nuclei. (In part after Villiger.)

midal tracts which subserve functions other than motor has been provided by a number of recent anatomical and physiological studies. The studies indicate that the pyramidal tracts contain many fibers of cortical origin which serve to modulate sensory input at subcortical levels. In cats and primates, direct cortical fibers coursing via the pyramidal tracts have been traced to the posterior column nuclei and to the spinal trigeminal nucleus. Significantly, these fibers have been shown to modify the excitability of the posterior column nuclei. Peripherally evoked activity of neurons in these sensory nuclei can be either facilitated or depressed by stimulating the sensorimotor cortex in cats having complete brain stem transections except for the pyramidal tracts.

The **corticobulbar fibers,** in gradually decreasing numbers, accompany the corticospinal fibers through the mesencephalon and pons (Fig. 147).

The fibers that accompany the corticospinals to the levels of the respective motor nuclei are considered as direct corticobulbars. Others that leave the corticospinal fibers at levels above the motor nuclei subserved and course caudally, generally in the medial lemniscus to their termination, are designated *aberrant corticobulbars*. The corticobulbar fibers are functionally like the corticospinals and most decussate (note exception below) at or near the level of the motor nucleus in which they terminate.

Three main bundles of aberrant corticobulbar fibers are recognized: *aberrant fibers of the peduncle, aberrant fibers of the pons,* and *bulbopontile aberrant fibers* (Fig. 147). A fourth and smaller bundle of corticobulbar fibers, given off in the subthalamic region, is designated *subthalamic aberrant*.

The **aberrant fibers of the peduncle** leave the posterior aspect of the basis pedunculi in the rostral part of the mesencephalon; they are distributed, by way of the medial lemniscus, to the nuclei of the contralateral third, fourth, and sixth nerves and to the cells of origin of the spinal portion of the spinal accessory nerve.

The **aberrant fibers of the pons** separate from the pyramidal system in the rostral part of the basis pontis and enter the medial lemniscus; they are distributed mainly to the motor nucleus of the contralateral fifth nerve, to the nucleus ambiguus, and to the hypoglossal nucleus. The *nucleus ambiguus* extends throughout the length of the medulla and gives origin to the branchial motor (special visceral efferent) fibers of the ninth, tenth, and eleventh nerves.

The **bulbopontile aberrant fibers** separate from the main mass of pyramidal fibers at the level of the junction of pons and medulla; they are distributed to the nuclei of the facial and hypoglossal nerves and to the nucleus ambiguus. The part of the facial nucleus that innervates the upper part of the face receives fibers from the motor areas of both hemispheres whereas that part from which the peripheral fibers to the lower muscles of the face originate, receives upper motor neuron fibers only from the contralateral motor cortex (Fig. 148). This is indicated by the observation that unilateral destruction of the lower part of the motor cortex or of the genu of the internal capsule results in paralysis of only the lower part of the face on the contralateral side. The orbicularis oculi and frontalis muscles still function bilaterally. Upper motor neuron paralysis of the facial muscles can thus be readily differentiated from lower motor neuron paralysis such as might result from destruction of the facial nerve in its canal; the latter type of paralysis involves all the facial muscles on the side of the lesion.

The **subthalamic aberrant fibers** are distributed to the rostral part of the oculomotor nucleus (Fig. 147).

BIBLIOGRAPHY

Bernhard, C. G., and Bohm, E., 1954: Cortical representation and functional significance of the corticomotoneuronal system. A.M.A. Arch. Neurol. Psychiat., *72*, 473–502.

Chambers, W. W., Everett, N. B., and Windle, W. F., 1948: Electrical stimulation of the cerebral cortex of the monkey under local anesthesia. Anat. Rec., *100*, 148.

Chambers, W. W., and Liu, C. N., 1957: Cortico-spinal tract of the cat. An attempt to correlate the pattern of degeneration with deficits in reflex activity following neocortical lesions. J. Comp. Neurol., *108*, 23–55.

Dejerine, J., 1914: *Semiologie des Affections du Systeme Nerveux*. Masson et Cie, Paris.

Evarts, E. V., 1968: Relation of pyramidal tract activity to force exerted during voluntary movement. J. Neurophysiol., *31*, 14–27.

Granit, R., Holmgren, B., and Merton, P. A., 1955: The two routes for excitation of muscle and their subservience to the cerebellum. J. Physiol., *130* 213–224.

Jabbur, S. J., and Towe, A. L., 1961a: The influence of the cerebral cortex on the dorsal column nuclei. Nervous Inhibitions—Proceedings of an Intern. Symposium. Pergamon Press, London, New York, pp. 419–423.

Jabbur, S. J., and Towe, A. L., 1961b: Cortical excitation of neurons in dorsal column nuclei of cat, including an analysis of pathways. J. Neurophysiol., *24*, 499–509.

Kuypers, H. G. J. M., 1958a: An anatomical analysis of cortico-bulbar connexions to the pons and lower brain stem in the cat. J. Anat., *92*, 198–218.

Kuypers, H. G. J. M., 1958b: Corticobulbar connexions to the pons and lower brainstem in man. An anatomical study. Brain, *81*, 364–388.

Kuypers, H. G. J. M., 1958c: Some projections from the peri-central cortex to the pons and lower brain stem in monkey and chimpanzee. J. Comp. Neurol., *110*, 221–251.

Lassek, A. M., 1940: The human pyramidal tract. II. A numerical investigation of the Betz cells of the motor area. A.M.A. Arch. Neurol. Psychiat., *44*, 718–724.

Lassek, A. M., 1942: The pyramidal tract. The effect of pre- and postcentral cortical lesions on the fiber components of the pyramids in monkey. J. Nerv. Ment. Dis., *95* 721–729.

Lawrence, D. G., and Kuypers, H. G. J. M., 1968: The functional organization of the motor system in the monkey. I. The effects of bilateral pyramidal lesions. Brain, *91,* 1–14.

Levin, P. M., 1949: Efferent fibers. In *The Precentral Motor Cortex,* P. C. Bucy, Ed., University of Illinois Press, Urbana, Chap. 5, pp. 135–148.

Levin, P. M., and Bradford, F. K., 1938: The exact origin of the cortico-spinal tract in the monkey. J. Comp. Neurol., *68,* 411–422.

Minckler, J., 1944: The course of efferent fibers from the human premotor cortex. J. Comp. Neurol., *81,* 259–277.

Penfield, W., and Jasper, H., 1954: *Epilepsy and the Functional Anatomy of the Human Brain.* Little, Brown and Company, Boston.

Phillips, C. G., 1967: Corticomotoneuronal organization. Projection from the arm area of the baboon's motor cortex. Arch. Neurol. (Chicago), *17,* 188–195.

Towe, A. L., and Jabbur, S. J., 1961: Cortical inhibition of neurons in dorsal column nuclei of cat. J. Neurophysiol., *24,* 488–498.

Towe, A. L., and Zimmerman, I. D., 1962: Peripherally evoked cortical reflex in the cuneate nucleus. Nature, *194,* 1250–1251.

Walberg, F., 1957: Corticofugal fibers to the nuclei of the dorsal columns. An experimental study in the cat. Brain, *80,* 273–287.

Woolsey, C. W., and Chang, H. T., 1947: Activation of the cerebral cortex by antidromic volleys in the pyramidal tract. Res. Publ. Ass. Res. Nerv. Ment. Dis., *27,* 146–161.

Chapter 15

Motor Neurons: Somatic and Branchial

Motor neurons, in relation to which corticobulbar and corticospinal fibers terminate, were briefly referred to in the preceding chapter. They are found in the motor nuclei of cranial nerves (Fig. 149) and in the anterior gray columns of the spinal cord.

The **oculomotor nuclei** are located in the central gray matter of the mesencephalon, anterior to the cerebral aqueduct, and at the level of the superior colliculi (Figs. 70, 150). Each nucleus gives origin to *somatic efferent fibers* which course anteriorly through the red nucleus and

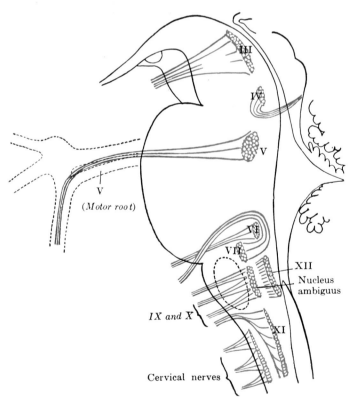

FIG. 149. Nuclei of origin of cranial motor nerves schematically represented, lateral view. (From Gray's Anatomy, 28th ed., Charles Mayo Goss, Ed., Lea & Febiger, Philadelphia.)

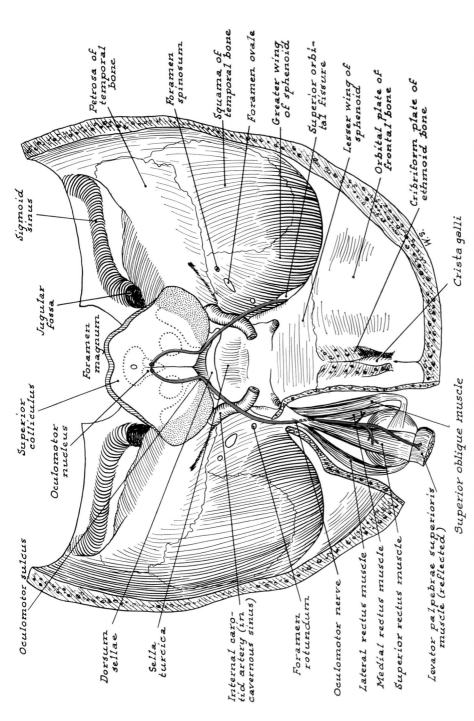

FIG. 150. Diagram of a part of the floor of the cranial cavity with a section of the mesencephalon in situ to show the origin and course of the oculomotor nerve. The orbital cavity and superior orbital fissure have been opened on the left by removal of portions of the orbital plate of the frontal bone and the lesser wing of the sphenoid. The distribution of the oculomotor nerve to the inferior rectus and inferior oblique muscles is not shown.

emerge from the mesencephalon through the oculomotor sulcus on the medial side of the basis pedunculi (Fig. 150). The fibers of the oculomotor nerve, like those of the trochlear and abducens nerves are classified as *somatic efferent* because they supply muscles that are derived from mesenchymal condensations homologous with head somites. *In its extramedullary course* the oculomotor nerve passes through the cavernous sinus and superior orbital fissure; within the orbit it is distributed to all the extrinsic muscles of the eye except the superior oblique and lateral rectus. Following removal of one or more eye muscles retrograde degeneration studies of the oculomotor nuclei have revealed a marked degree of segregation of the neurons innervating individual muscles. Of particular significance is the finding that the unpaired caudal central area is concerned with the innervation of the levators palpebraerum.

The **trochlear nuclei** are found directly caudal to the oculomotor nuclei, at the level of the inferior colliculi (Figs. 68, 151). The *somatic efferent fibers* from the trochlear nucleus course posteriorly and somewhat caudally around the central gray matter and decussate to the opposite side through the superior medullary velum. The *superior medullary velum* stretches between the superior borders of the superior cerebellar peduncles and forms the roof of the rostral part of the fourth ventricle (Fig. 143). The trochlear nerve, after its decussation, emerges from the lateral margin of the velum and encircles the mesencephalon to reach the cavernous sinus. It courses through the sinus and the superior orbital fissure and ends in the superior oblique muscle of the eye. It is probable that the corticobulbar fibers to the trochlear nucleus are uncrossed; if not, the superior oblique muscle receives its cortical innervation from the ipsilateral hemisphere.

The **motor nucleus of the trigeminal nerve** is in the pons just medial to the main sensory nucleus (Figs. 64, 152).

The fibers originating from it are classified as *special visceral efferent* (branchial motor) because they innervate striated muscles derived from the mesoderm of the visceral (branchial) arches. Together with the proprioceptive fibers from the mesencephalic nucleus, they form the *motor root* (portio minor) of the trigeminal nerve which, after emerging from the pons just rostral to the sensory root (portio major), crosses the superior border of the petrosa, passes posterior to the trigeminal ganglion, and emerges from the cranial cavity through the foramen ovale. The motor and proprioceptive fibers are distributed to the muscles of mastication, to the mylohyoid muscle and anterior belly of the digastric, and to the tensors palati and tympani; those to the last two muscles reach them by way of the otic ganglion.

The **nucleus of the abducens nerve** is situated in the caudal third of the pons beneath the floor of the fourth ventricle; it is more or less separated from the floor of the ventricle by the genu of the facial nerve (Figs. 153–155). The nucleus and the genu are responsible for an elevation in the floor of the ventricle known either as the *facial colliculus* or the *abducens eminence*. The *somatic efferent* fibers of the abducens nerve course anteriorly and caudally through the tegmentum and basis pontis and emerge from the brain stem through the sulcus formed at the junction of the medulla and pons (Fig. 56). At its point of emergence the nerve is just lateral to the rostral limit of the pyramid of the medulla. Its course from this point is forward through a notch formed at the junction of the temporal petrosa and the dorsum sellae and then through the cavernous sinus; it enters the orbit by way of the superior orbital fissure and innervates the lateral rectus muscle (Fig. 153).

The proximity of the motor ocular nuclei (oculomotor, trochlear, and abducens) to the medial longitudinal fasciculi (Fig. 101) has been noted. The vestibulo-

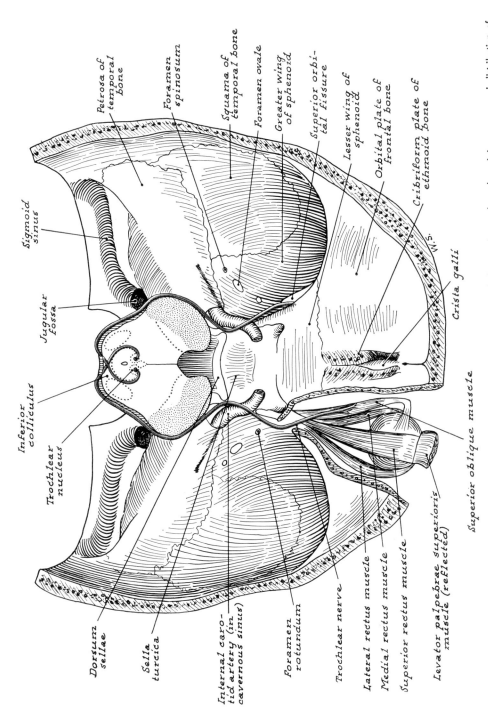

FIG. 151. Diagram of a part of the floor of the cranial cavity with a section of the mesencephalon in situ to show the origin, course, and distribution of the trochlear nerve.

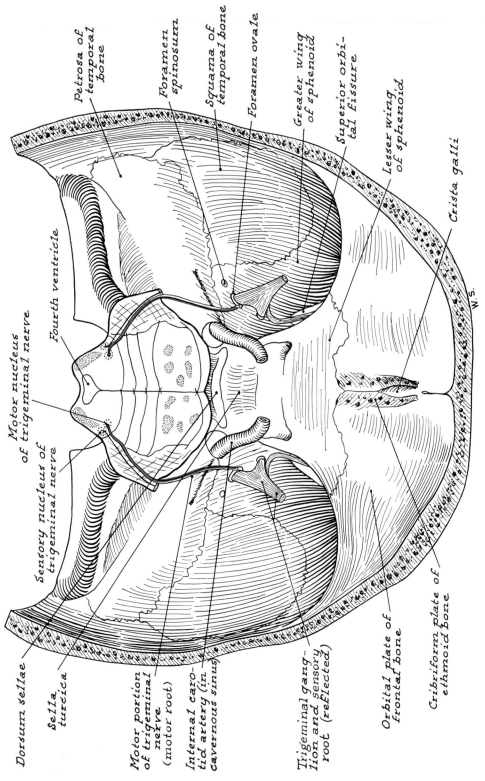

FIG. 152. Diagram of a part of the floor of the cranial cavity with a section of the pons in situ showing the origin and course of the motor fibers of the trigeminal nerve. The trigeminal ganglion has been reflected forward to show the exit of the motor root from the cranial cavity through the foramen ovale.

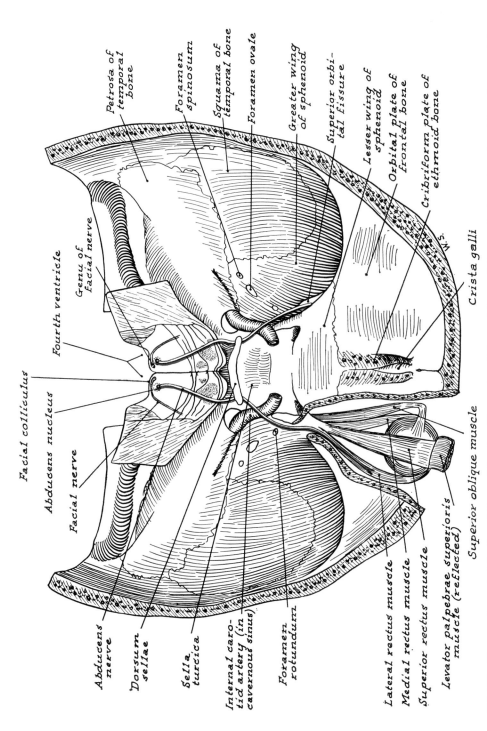

FIG. 153. Diagram of a part of the floor of the cranial cavity with a section of the caudal part of the pons in situ to show the origin and course of the abducens nerve.

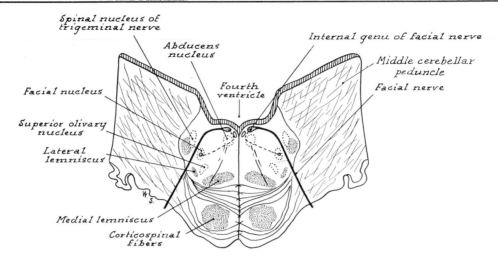

FIG. 154. Section through the caudal part of the pons diagrammatically showing the origin and course of the facial nerve fibers within the pons.

ocular connections by way of the fasciculi and their functions in eye reflexes and in the maintenance of tone in the eye muscles are discussed in Chapter 9.

The **nucleus of the facial nerve** is anterolateral and caudal to that of the abducens nerve (Figs. 154, 155). Its neurons are included in the *special visceral efferent* group. The fibers originating in the nucleus course posteromedially through the tegmentum of the pons and around the caudal limit of the abducens nucleus. They then turn sharply forward and continue in that direction beneath the floor of the fourth ventricle and posteromedial to the abducens nucleus for a distance of about ½ centimeter where they again change their course and pass laterally across the posterior aspect of the abducens nucleus. After crossing the nucleus they pass anterolaterally and caudally through the tegmentum and basis pontis; they finally emerge at the sulcus between pons and medulla, some distance lateral to the point of emergence of the abducens nerve. That portion of the facial nerve in relation to the abducens nucleus is designated as its *internal genu.*

The **facial nerve,** after its emergence from the brain stem, courses through the internal auditory and facial canals; it leaves the latter canal by way of the stylomastoid foramen and, after having divided into its terminal branches within the substance of the parotid gland, is distributed to the muscles of expression. The *external genu* of the nerve is in the facial canal at the point where the canal changes its direction from lateral to posterior.

The **nucleus ambiguus,** so-called because it is not clearly defined in sections of the medulla, occupies a position posterior to the inferior olivary nucleus (Figs. 156, 157). It extends throughout the length of the medulla and gives origin to *special visceral efferent fibers* of the glossopharyngeal and vagus nerves and to some of those of the spinal accessory. The fibers unite to form a series of filaments that emerge from the medulla along the line of the posterolateral sulcus. The ninth, tenth, and eleventh nerves emerge from the cranial cavity through the jugular foramen.

The **special visceral efferent fibers** of the *glossopharyngeal nerve* are distributed to the stylopharyngeus and superior constrictor muscles; those of the *vagus,* to muscles of the pharynx and larynx. Those of the *spinal accessory* (from the nucleus ambiguus) join the vagus and are also

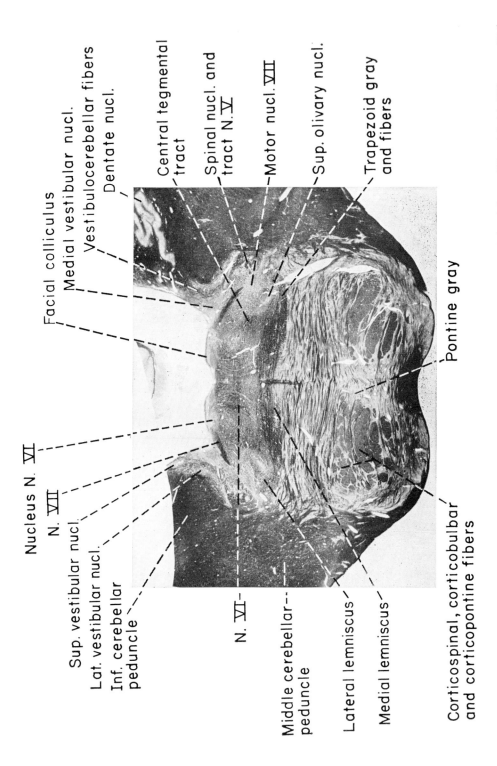

Nucleus N. VI

N. VII

Facial colliculus
Medial vestibular nucl.
Vestibulocerebellar fibers
Dentate nucl.

Central tegmental tract
Spinal nucl. and tract N. V
Motor nucl. VII
Sup. olivary nucl.
Trapezoid gray and fibers

Sup. vestibular nucl.
Lat. vestibular nucl.
Inf. cerebellar peduncle

N. VI

Middle cerebellar peduncle

Lateral lemniscus
Medial lemniscus

Pontine gray

Corticospinal, corticobulbar and corticopontine fibers

FIG. 155. Photomicrograph of a transverse section through the caudal pons at at the level of motor nuclei of the abducens (VI) and facial (VII) nerves. Weil stain.

distributed to the pharynx and larynx. Other special visceral efferent fibers of the spinal accessory nerve arise from cells in the lateral part of the anterior gray column of the upper five or six cervical segments of the spinal cord, enter the cranial cavity through the foramen magnum, join the cranial fibers, and after

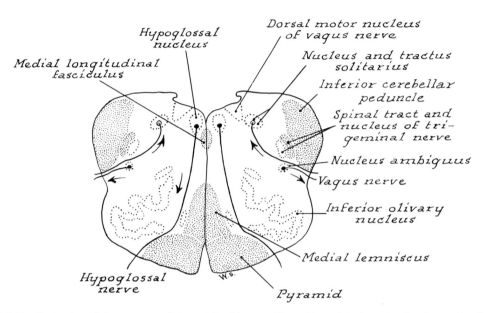

FIG. 156. Section through the open part of the medulla oblongata. The positions of the hypoglossal nucleus and nucleus ambiguus are indicated as are the routes of the efferent fibers arising from them. Sensory fibers of the vagus nerve are shown entering the medulla and terminating in the nucleus solitarius. Direction of conduction is indicatd by arrows.

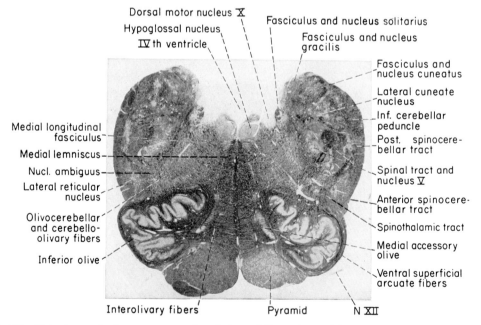

FIG. 157. Photomicrograph of a transverse section of the medulla at the caudal part of the fourth ventricle. Note the reduced pyramid on the right which is due to partial degeneration of pyramidal tract fibers resulting from hemorrhage into the internal capsule (see Chaps. 16 and 18). Weil stain.

passing through the jugular foramen, are distributed to the sternocleidomastoid and trapezius muscles.

The **nuclei of the hypoglossal nerves** are found in the medulla beneath the floor of the fourth ventricle, on both sides of the median raphé (Figs. 156, 157). They account for bilateral eminences in the floor of the ventricle known as the *hypoglossal trigones* (Fig. 40). The medial longitudinal fasciculi are immediately ventral to the nuclei. The fibers of the hypoglossal nerve (somatic efferent) course anteriorly and somewhat laterally from their origin in the nucleus and emerge from the medulla just lateral to the pyramid (Figs. 156, 157). The hypoglossal nerve leaves the cranial cavity through the hypoglossal canal and is distributed to the muscles of the tongue which are classified as somatic because of their derivation from occipital myotomes.

The **anterior gray column cells** in the spinal cord, with the probable exception of those that give origin to the spinal root of the spinal accessory nerve, are somatic efferent in function. Their axons emerge from the cord in the region of the anterolateral sulcus and enter the ventral roots of the spinal nerves (Fig. 5). After traversing the ventral root and trunk of a given spinal nerve they are distributed, by way of its ventral and dorsal divisions, to striated muscles of mesodermal somite origin.

Somatic and special visceral efferent nerve fibers terminate in motor end plates (Fig. 18B, C). Motor end plates are usually located near the midpoints of muscle fibers; they account for elevated areas on the fibers which are covered by sarcolemma. The neurilemmal sheaths of the nerve fibers appear to become continuous with the sarcolemma whereas the myelin sheaths terminate on reaching it. Underneath the sarcolemma the nerve fibers divide into fibrils which form a network in relation to the sarcoplasm.

BIBLIOGRAPHY

Courville, J., 1966: The nucleus of the facial nerve; the relation between cellular groups and peripheral branches of the nerve. Brain Res., *1,* 338–354.

Lawn, A. M., 1966: The localization, in the nucleus ambiguus of the rabbit, of the cells of origin of motor nerve fibers in the glossopharyngeal nerve and various branches of the vagus nerve by means of retrograde degeneration. J. Comp. Neurol., *127,* 293–305.

Liu, C.-N., and Chambers, W. W., 1964: An experimental study of the corticospinal system in the monkey *(Macaca mulatta)*. The spinal pathways and preterminal distribution of degenerating fibers following discrete lesions of the pre- and postcentral gyri and bulbar pyramid. J. Comp. Neurol., *123,* 257–284.

Nyberg-Hansen, R., and Brodal, A., 1963: Sites of termination of corticospinal fibers in the cat. An experimental study with silver impregnation methods. J. Comp. Neurol., *120,* 369–391.

Patten, B. M., 1968: *Human Embryology,* 3rd ed., Blakiston Div., McGraw Hill, New York.

Renshaw, B., 1946: Central effects of centripetal impulses in axons of spinal ventral roots. J. Neurophysiol., *9,* 191–204.

Szentágothai, J., 1949: Functional representation in the motor trigeminal nucleus. J. Comp. Neurol., *90,* 111–120.

Warwick, R., 1953: Representation of the extra-ocular muscles in the oculomotor nuclei of the monkey. J. Comp. Neurol., *98,* 449–503.

Chapter 16

Functions of the Motor Cortex and Motor Pathways

Cortical area 4 of Brodmann which extends mediolaterally along the precentral gyrus is known as the primary motor area (Figs. 158, 160). As discussed in Chapter 14, this area is no longer considered to be the exclusive site of origin for the pyramidal (corticospinal) tract, nor is it the only cortical area concerned with volitional or skilled movements. Nevertheless, numerous studies have shown that area 4 is most fundamentally involved in the execution of delicate movements. That electrical stimulation of the frontal lobe of man, particularly of the precentral gyrus, produced movements in the opposite limbs has been known for almost 100 years. However, the details of the representation of the body on the cortex as well as the functional implications of this somatotropic representation are still in

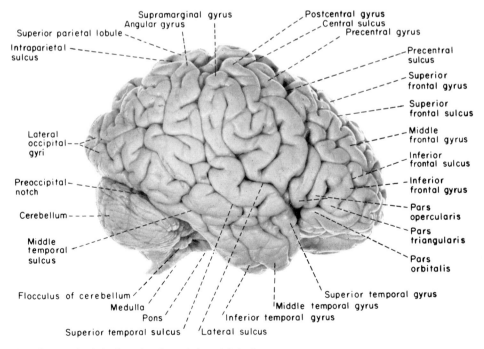

FIG. 158. Photograph of the lateral surface of the adult brain.

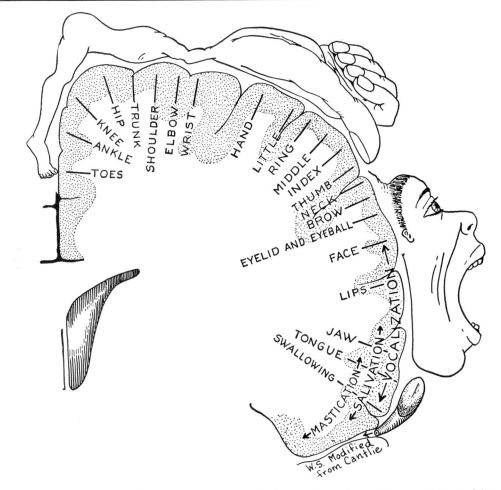

FIG. 159. Motor homunculus illustrating motor representation in area 4, anterior central gyrus. (After Penfield and Rasmussen, *Cerebral Cortex of Man*, The Macmillan Co.)

dispute. Figure 159 shows the pattern of motor representation together with an indication of the amount of cortex concerned with various bodily parts. It may be noted that, as in the case of the somatesthetic cortex, the body has an upside-down representation in the motor area. The leg area is represented in large part medially within the paracentral lobule and the face area is represented inferolaterally. The arm representation is between these areas. The larger areas of the cortex devoted to those parts of the body with the capacity for the finer and highly controlled movements reflects the increased number of underlying cortical cells which activate or govern these movements. With respect to the often disputed question of whether functional organization in the cortex is in terms of movements or muscles, recent studies have shown that it is the latter. It has, for example, been shown in the monkey motor cortex that there is a focus of neurons surrounded by a field for each muscle and that the foci for two muscles never overlap, even though the field of one muscle may overlap the field of another. These and other studies lead to the concept that the different movements are organized through the many connections of intracortical neurons with the Betz and other pyramidal cells in the deep layers rather than through the arrangement of these cells.

There is general agreement among the various investigators relative to the mediolateral extent and pattern of somatotropic localization within the primary motor cortex. There is less agreement, however, about the extent of the area anteriorly. According to some investigators, the axial musculature of the monkey is represented in cortical area 6; others include a part of the frontal eye fields, area 8, in the primary motor area.

A small second motor area of body representation has been described which is located in the part of the precentral gyrus which extends along the upper lip of the lateral fissure (Figs. 160, 161). A third somatotropic area of motor representation, the *supplementary motor area* (Figs. 160, 161), has been described for man and for the monkey. This area is located within the medial hemispheric portion of area 6 (Fig. 161). Little is known about the anatomical and physiological parameters of these lesser motor

areas. There is recent evidence, however, that the supplementary motor area of the monkey exerts its effects through the extrapyramidal system and contributes no fibers to the pyramidal tracts. No doubt much of the confusion which exists relative to primary motor areas is due to the overlapping of cortical areas related respectively to the pyramidal and extrapyramidal systems. (The extrapyramidal system is considered in Chapter 17.)

Capsular hemiplegia, owing to destruction of fibers in the internal capsule, is the most common lesion in man which damages or destroys the descending system of cortical fibers. The clinical signs of capsular hemiplegia are: *paralysis* or *paresis* on the contralateral side, *exaggerated deep reflexes* (knee jerk, ankle jerk, and others which constitute responses to lengthening of muscles); *absence* of *abdominal and cremasteric reflexes;* and the appearance of the *Babinski sign.* The paralysis is at first flaccid in character

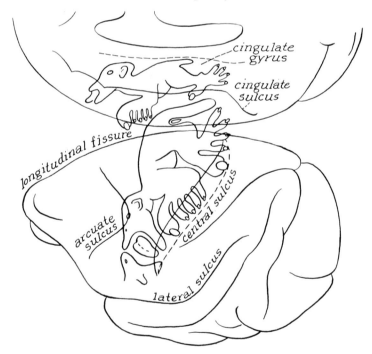

FIG. 160. Diagram illustrating the somatotropic organization of the primary, secondary, and supplementary motor areas in relation to the central sulcus and longitudinal fissure. The precentral and cingulate gyri have been rolled back to show the localization in the buried cortex. A dotted line represents the bottom and a solid line indicates the top of a sulcus. An ipsilateral face area is shown inferiorly. Note that much of the primary simunculus and the major part of the supplementary area extend into area 6 of the premotor area (after Woolsey et al., 1952).

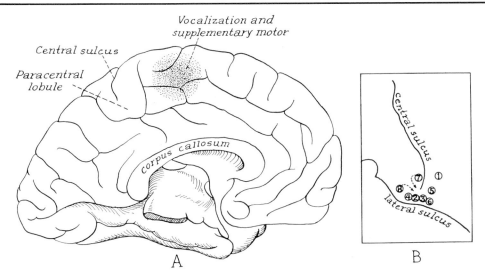

FIG. 161.   Diagram illustrating the secondary motor areas in the human cerebral cortex. A, Vocalization and supplementary motor area on the medial surface. B, The secondary motor in the opercular region. Stimulation at 1 produced movement in hand of opposite side; at 2, desire to move contralateral hand; at 3, movement of contralateral hand and foot; at 4, desire to move hand on side stimulated; at 5, desire to move and paralysis of contralateral hand; at 6, desire to move and paralysis of contralateral foot; at 7, subcortical stimulation produced movement of ipsilateral toe; at 8, subcortical stimulation produced movement of contralateral hand (after Penfield and Rasmussen, 1950).

and later becomes spastic. (Flaccid paralysis is characterized by lack of resistance to passive movement of an affected extremity and spastic paralysis by increased resistance. Absence of deep reflexes ordinarily is associated with flaccidity; an increased activity of these reflexes is associated with spasticity.)

The abdominal reflex consists of ipsilateral contraction of the anterior abdominal muscles in response to scratching the abdominal skin on one side. The contraction of the muscles produces deviation of the umbilicus toward that side. Unlike the deep reflexes, the abdominal reflex is thought to have a cortical arc. The afferent impulses arising in the receptors in the skin of the anterior abdominal wall reach the parietal cortex, and perhaps the frontal cortex as well. The efferent side of the arc is within or closely associated with the pyramidal tract and, for that reason, is interrupted by a lesion in the motor cortex or along the course of the pyramidal fibers. The reflex is either diminished or abolished, depend-

ing on the extent of the lesion and such alterations may be limited to the lower half of the abdominal wall in pyramidal tract lesions at midthoracic levels.

The cremaster reflex is also of the superficial variety and probably depends on a cortical arc. It consists of contraction of the cremaster muscle with consequent retraction of the testis in response to lightly scratching the skin of the inner side of the thigh.

The Babinski sign requires explanation; it is often referred to as a "positive Babinski sign," but this is a misnomer. When a blunt instrument is drawn across the lateral side of the plantar surface of the foot of a normal subject in a heel-to-toe direction, the toes are flexed (plantar flexion); the most striking degree of flexion is exhibited by the great toe. This is a normal reaction and it is correctly called the plantar reflex. When the same stimulus is applied in the case of upper motor neuron disease, there is an upward or dorsiflexion, particularly of the great toe, with or without fanning of the other toes. This is due to the contraction of physiologic flexors. This abnormal response is known as the *sign of Babinski.*

The Babinski sign occurs normally in infants in response to plantar stimulation. This may be due to the fact that the corticospinal fibers are not completely myelinated for a considerable period after birth (six to eighteen months or longer). Although absolute correlation between myelination and function of nerve tracts has not been proved, enough experimental evidence has been presented to warrant the assumption that incomplete myelination may be a factor in the dorsiflexion response in infants.

Exaggeration of the deep reflexes (hyperreflexia) has been explained in somewhat the same manner as the change in character of the plantar reflex. Deep reflexes include all stretch or myotatic ones of the phasic type. They are elicited by a sharp tap on the tendon or muscle. They function through spinal or brain stem arcs as has been previously explained. The knee jerk is described in detail in Chapter 5 and its arc is typical. Although an exaggeration of these reflexes may result from inflammation or irritation at the segmental level, a persistence of the hyperactivity is usually due to damage of descending fibers which are inhibitory to the reflex. Investigators have shown that in order for increased deep reflexes and spasticity to occur there must be an involvement of the cortically originating extrapyramidal fibers. A discussion follows in the immediate section and in Chapter 17.

Lesions of the motor cortex or of its projections in man seldom, if ever, occur in pure form. For example, a so-called upper motor neuron lesion, of which capsular hemiplegia is the most common, involves both pyramidal and extrapyramidal fibers as these are intermixed within the posterior limb of the internal capsule (Fig. 141). It follows that the only possibilities for interrupting pyramidal fibers

in pure culture are at the medullary pyramids (Fig. 156) or at the cortex, i.e., a lesion localized to the posterior part of the precentral gyrus, area 4. These localized interruptions of pyramidal tract fibers have been made in the monkey and chimpanzee and, in general, the results have been the same from removing area 4 as from sectioning the pyramidal tract. The results of area 4 ablation were a deficit of voluntary isolated or fine movements with flaccidity rather than spasticity. There was no evidence of exaggerated deep reflexes. The results were confirmed by pyramidal tract sectioning. Flaccidity was apparent in both the monkey and chimpanzee although less in the latter. There was an absence of abdominal reflexes and the Babinski sign appeared in the chimpanzee. The status of the cremasteric reflex has not been assessed in the pyramidectomized chimpanzee. Since it is a superficial reflex, like the abdominal, it can reasonably be assumed to be absent following pyramidectomy.

From these experiments, it would appear that the remaining signs of capsular hemiplegia are attributable to damage of cortically originating extrapyramidal fibers. These include *spasticity, exaggerated deep reflexes,* and some *paralysis* (gross movements).

Extrapyramidal pathways from the cortex to the brain stem and spinal cord include *corticopontine, corticonigral, corticorubral, corticostriate, corticopallidal, corticotegmental, corticosubthalamic, corticohypothalamic,* and *corticothalamic* fibers. Although some of these overlap in origin with the pyramidal tract fibers, they differ in that they are interrupted by one or more synapses in subcortical centers before neuronal contact is made at the segmental level. Another difference is that by definition these extrapyramidal fibers do not pass through the medullary pyramids. This system of fibers is considered in more detail in Chapter 17 with the subcortical components of the extrapyramidal system.

The basis for the recovery of voluntary activity that follows a lesion (e.g., in the internal capsule) that supposedly interrupts all corticospinal fibers to a limb or entire side of the body has been of considerable dispute. No doubt the return of voluntary movement is in part due to recovery of function in neurons impaired only temporarily by edema or related phenomena of the pathological process. As these tissue reactions subside, the neurons that were not permanently damaged could function normally. Additionally, since cortically originating extrapyramidal fibers support at least some complex voluntary movements, the nondamaged fibers of this system could be responsible for residual function.

Another consideration to be made relative to residual or so-called return of function is the extent of bilateral representation of muscles in the cortex.

All muscles may be represented to some extent in the ipsilateral motor cortex. Those of the eyelids, jaw, and trunk, which act bilaterally, have the greatest degree of bilateral representation. The proximal muscles of the limbs receive less innervation from the ipsilateral cortex and those of the fingers and toes least of all. So far as the eyelids and jaw are concerned, their ipsilateral innervation may be accounted for on the basis of uncrossed corticobulbar fibers. In attempting to account for ipsilateral innervation of the trunk and upper extremity the first possibility that suggests itself is the uncrossed or anterior corticospinal tract although it is usually conceded that its component fibers cross through the anterior commissure, just before their termination, and end in relation to anterior gray column cells on the side opposite that of their cortical origin (Fig. 147). Some anterior corticospinal fibers that failed to cross to the opposite side have been reported. Such uncrossed fibers, terminating in relation to ipsilateral anterior gray column cells, might account for ipsilateral (cortical) innervation of the muscles of the upper limbs and trunk. The presence of some uncrossed fibers in the lateral corticospinal tracts, which has been reported, could account for ipsilateral innervation of the lower extremities.

It has been shown in monkeys that monosynaptic relationships between upper and lower motor neurons are responsible for the individuality of movements in the distal hand muscles and that this monosynaptic system is only contralaterally represented in the motor cortex. Because stimulation studies on the human cerebral cortex indicated that only contralateral responses could be obtained by cortical stimulation, it has been assumed that a monosynaptic system with contralateral representation plays an even more important role in man than in the monkey for corticospinal activation of both distal and proximal muscles in the extremities. It seems probable that much of the ipsilateral innervation which has been attributed to area 4 is actually a function of extrapyramidal fibers with their origins in adjacent areas of the cortex. Support for such an assumption is provided by experiments which have shown that the cortical field from which monosynaptic responses in a given nerve can be elicited is more restricted than those from which polysynaptic (delayed) responses can be evoked, and that the cortical field from which polysynaptic facilitation of a certain group of motor neurons could be evoked had a greater expansion anteriorly (presumably into area 6) than the field from which monosynaptic responses in the same group of neurons were elicited.

The totally hemispherectomized monkey regains agility in standing, walking, and climbing, but no resumption of function for finer movements has been seen. The hemispherectomized animal may actively grasp a wire screen with the contralateral fingers or toes, but the contralateral extremities are never used for feeding, picking up objects, or other fine motions. Nevertheless, the restoration of motor function in the monkey after total hemispherectomy gives credence to the theory of bilaterality of motor innervation. Bilateral movements from cortical stimulation of the monkey have been observed by several investigators, and ipsilateral movements on stimulation of the medial surface of the human hemisphere have been reported. It is probable that the residuals of motor function observed after human hemispherectomy, as in the monkey, may be explained, at least in part, on the basis of ipsilateral cortical innervation traveling via the direct, uncrossed pyramidal tract although it is recognized that removal of a hemisphere in the human is not as complete as that accomplished in the monkey.

BIBLIOGRAPHY

Bates, J. A. V., 1953: Stimulation of medial surface of human cerebral hemisphere after hemispherectomy. Brain, 76, 405–447.

Bernhard, C. G., and Bohm, E., 1954: Cortical representation and functional significance of the corticomotoneuronal system. A.M.A. Arch. Neurol. Psychiat., 72, 473–502.

Bucy, P. C., and Fulton, J. F., 1933: Ipsilateral representation in motor and premotor cortex of monkeys. Brain, 56, 318–342.

Bucy, P. C., Ladpli, R., and Ehrlich, A., 1966: Destruction of the pyramidal tract in the monkey. The effects of bilateral section of cerebral peduncles. J. Neurosurg., 25, 1–20.

Chang, H. T., Ruch, T. C., and Ward, A. A., Jr., 1947: Topographical representation of muscles in motor cortex of monkeys. J. Neurophysiol., 10, 39–56.

DeVito, J. L., and Smith, O. A., Jr., 1959: Projections from the mesial frontal cortex (supplementary motor area) to the cerebral hemispheres and brain stem of the Macaca mulatta. J. Comp. Neurol., 111, 261–277.

Foerster, O., 1936: The motor cortex in man in the light of Hughlings Jackson's doctrines. Brain, 59, 135–159.

Fritsch, G., and Hitzig, E., 1870: Über die elektrische Erregbarkiet des Grosshirns, Arch. Anat. Physiol., 37, 300–332.

Fulton, J. F., and Kennard, M. A., 1934: A study of flaccid and spastic paralyses produced by lesions of the cerebral cortex in primates. Res. Publ. Ass. Res. Nerv. Ment. Dis., 13, 158–210.

Hines, M., 1937: The "motor" cortex. Bull. Johns Hopkins Hosp., 60, 313–336.

Hines, M., 1949: Significance of the precentral motor cortex. In The Precentral Motor Cortex. 2nd ed. P. C. Bucy, Ed. University of Illinois Press, Urbana.

Kuypers, H. G. J. M., 1960: Central cortical projections to motor and somatosensory cell groups. Brain, 83, 161–184.

Lawrence, D. G., and Kuypers, H. G. J. M., 1968: The functional organization of the motor system in the monkey. I. The effects of bilateral pyramidal lesions. Brain, 91, 1–14.

Lawrence, D. G., and Kuypers, H. G. J. M., 1968: The functional organization of the motor system in the monkey. II. The effects of lesions of the descending brain-stem pathways. Brain, 91, 15–36.

Lauer, E. W., 1952: Ipsilateral facial representation in motor cortex of macaque. J. Neurophysiol., 15, 1–4.

Lewandowsky, M., 1907. Die Functionen des zentralen Nervensystems. G. Fischer, Jena.

Marchiafava, P. L., 1968: Activities of the central nervous system: motor. Ann. Rev. Physiol., 30, 359–400.

Patton, H. D., and Amassian, V. E., 1954: Single—and multiple—unit analysis of cortical stage of pyramidal tract activation. J. Neurophysiol., 17, 345–363.

Patton, H. D., and Amassian, V. E., 1960: The pyramidal tract: its excitation and functions. In Handbook of Physiology, Vol. II, Sec. 1, Neurophysiology. John Field, Ed.-in-Chief. Williams & Wilkins Co., Baltimore, pp. 837–862.

Penfield, W., and Rasmussen, T., 1950: The Cerebral Cortex of Man; A Clinical Study of Localization of Function. The Macmillan Co., New York.

Penfield, W., and Welch, K., 1951: The supplementary motor area of the cerebral cortex. A clinical and experimental study. A.M.A. Arch. Neurol. Psychiat., 66, 289–317.

Ruch, T. C., Patton, H. D., Woodbury, S. W., and Towe, A. W., 1961: Neurophysiology. W. B. Saunders, Philadelphia.

Sugar, O., Chusid, J. G., and French, J. D., 1948: A second motor cortex in the monkey (Macaca mulatta). J. Neuropathol. Exp. Neurol., 7, 182–189.

Tower, S. S., 1940: Pyramidal lesion in the monkey. Brain, 63, 36–90.

Tower, S. S., 1949: The pyramidal tract. In The Precentral Motor Cortex. 2nd ed. P. C. Bucy, Ed. University of Illinois Press, Urbana.

Walker, A. E., and Richter, H., 1966: Section of the cerebral peduncle in the monkey. Arch. Neurol. (Chicago), 14, 231–240.

White, R. J., Schreiner, L. H., Hughes, R. A., MacCarty, C. S., and Grindlay, J. H., 1959: Physiologic consequences of total hemispherectomy in the monkey. Neurology, *9*, 149–159.

Woolsey, C. N., Settlage, P. H., Meyer, D. R., Sencer, W., Pinto-Hamuy, T., and Travis, A. M., 1952: Patterns of localization in precentral and "supplementary" motor areas and their relation to the concept of a premotor area. Res. Publ. Ass. Res. Nerv. Ment. Dis., *30,* 238–264.

Chapter 17

The Extrapyramidal System

Reference is made in the previous chapter to the fact that cortically originating extrapyramidal fibers support at least some complex voluntary movements and that damage to this system of fibers is responsible for some of the symptoms of capsular hemiplegia. It is further pointed out that these fibers, in contrast to the pyramidal, make synapses with subcortical centers before establishing contact with neurons at the segmental level. Another difference in these two systems concerns their medullary course, i.e., by definition the pyramidal fibers are those within the

Brodmann Areas

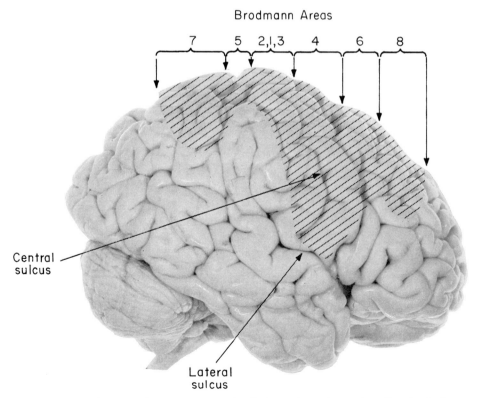

FIG. 162. Extrapyramidal regions of cerebral cortex. The shading indicates in rough outline the Brodmann areas usually considered as giving rise to extrapyramidal fibers. Note the extensive overlap with sites of origin of the pyramidal or corticospinal tract (see Chap. 14).

medullary pyramids. This chapter provides a more complete account of the extrapyramidal motor system which extends from the cortical and subcortical areas of origin to the segmental level. The system includes cortically originating fibers, several nuclei and fiber tracts in the basal telencephalic region, and many nuclei and fiber tracts in the diencephalon and more caudal levels of the neuraxis.

The cortical sites of origin of extrapyramidal fibers originally were considered to be outside the primary motor area (Brodmann area 4) or precentral gyrus. Widespread cortical areas were designated as extrapyramidal on the basis that

electrical stimulation of a site would cause movement, or that ablating a region would produce an impairment of motor function. More recently, it has been shown that the pyramidal and extrapyramidal cortical areas overlap extensively and even include sensory areas. (In fact, the appropriateness of dividing motor systems into pyramidal and extrapyramidal categories is now questioned.) Figure 162 illustrates the major regions of the cerebral hemisphere most frequently referred to as extrapyramidal.

The basal telencephalic nuclei, the basal ganglia, will be considered together with an account of related structures, such

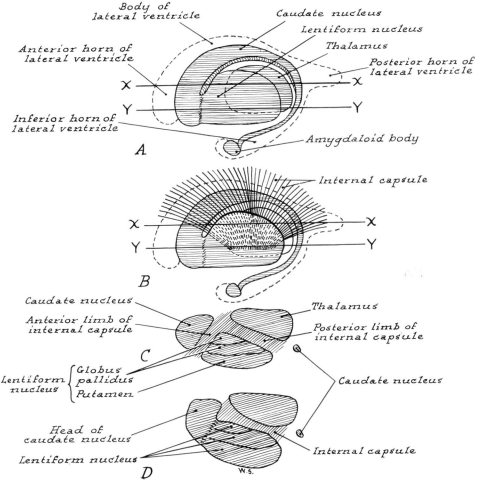

FIG. 163. A, Diagram of basal ganglia (not including the claustrum) as seen from the lateral side. The relationship of the lateral ventricle to the nucleus is indicated. B, Diagram of the basal ganglia showing the relationship of the internal capsule to its component nuclei. C, Horizontal section through the basal ganglia and thalamus at the level designated "X" in A and B. D, Horizontal section at level "Y" in A and B (modified from Jackson-Morris).

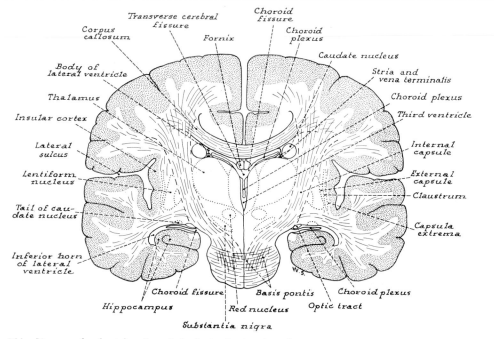

FIG. 164. Diagram of a frontal section of the brain showing the relations of the insula, basal ganglia, and dien-cephalon.

as the substantia nigra, red nucleus, and reticular formation of the brain stem. The basal ganglia of both sides, as classically described, include the *lenti-form* and *caudate nuclei, amygdaloid body,* and the *claustrum* (Fig. 163).

The claustrum and lentiform nucleus are directly medial to the insula with the claustrum the more superficially placed (Figs. 164, 166, 168). The layer of white matter between the insular cortex and the claustrum is called the capsula ex-trema. The insular part of the cerebral cortex or *island of Reil* can be readily exposed by removal of the opercular portions of the frontal, parietal, and temporal lobes of the cerebrum (Figs. 93, 133). The insular cortex, overgrown by the adjacent neopallial areas of the cortex, is buried in the depth of the lateral sulcus. The lentiform nucleus and claustrum are separated from one another by the *external capsule,* and the internal capsule is closely applied to the inner surface of the lentiform nucleus. The *internal capsule* fills the interval developed be-

tween the lentiform nucleus and the body of the caudate nucleus (Figs. 163, 166, 167).

The **lentiform nucleus** rests on the anterior perforated substance which is lateral to the optic chiasm (Fig. 130). When sectioned, the lentiform nucleus is seen to be divided into lateral and medial portions (Figs. 163, 166–168) by the *external medullary lamina;* the lateral portion is designated the *putamen* and the medial portion, the *globus pallidus.* The globus pallidus is subdivided into external and internal parts by an *internal medullary lamina.*

The **putamen** contains small triangular or polygonal cells with short axons and larger cells with long axons and multi-directional dendrites. The small neurons participate in internuclear connections between putamen, caudate nucleus, and globus pallidus. The long axons of the larger neurons contribute to the efferent pathways from the lentiform nucleus.

The **globus pallidus** is the main effer-ent center of the basal ganglia. It con-

Body of corpus callosum   Cave of septum pellucidum

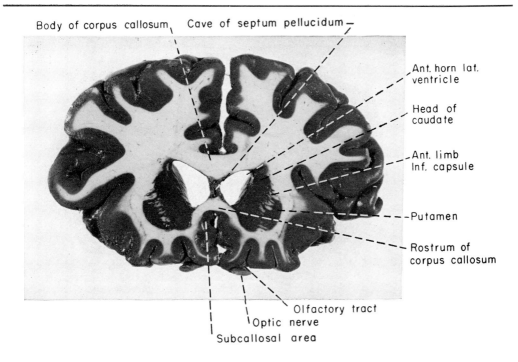

Ant. horn lat.
ventricle

Head of
caudate

Ant. limb
Inf. capsule

Putamen

Rostrum of
corpus callosum

Olfactory tract
Optic nerve
Subcallosal area

FIG. 165. Coronal section at the level of the rostrum of the corpus callosum (anterior view).

Anterior commissure   Superior frontal gyrus   Middle frontal
gyrus

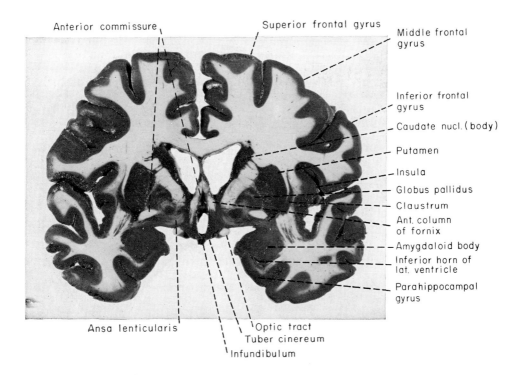

Inferior frontal
gyrus

Caudate nucl.(body)

Putamen

Insula

Globus pallidus

Claustrum

Ant. column
of fornix

Amygdaloid body

Inferior horn of
lat. ventricle

Parahippocampal
gyrus

Ansa lenticularis   Optic tract
Tuber cinereum
Infundibulum

FIG. 166. Coronal section at the level of the anterior columns of the fornices (posterior view).

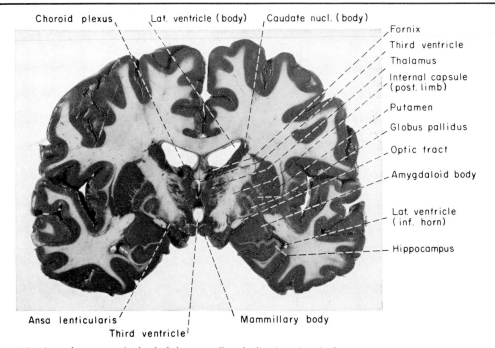

Choroid plexus   Lat. ventricle (body)   Caudate nucl. (body)

Fornix
Third ventricle
Thalamus
Internal capsule (post. limb)
Putamen
Globus pallidus
Optic tract
Amygdaloid body
Lat. ventricle (inf. horn)
Hippocampus

Ansa lenticularis   Mammillary body
Third ventricle

FIG. 167. Coronal section at the level of the mammillary bodies (anterior view).

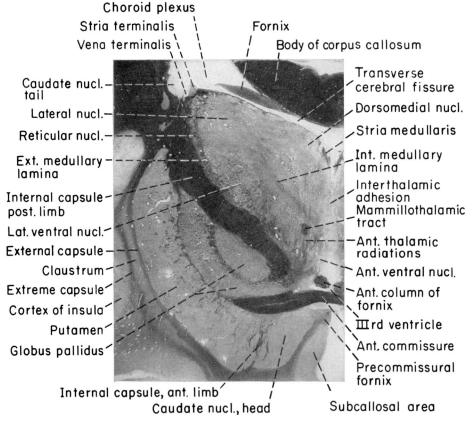

Choroid plexus
Stria terminalis
Vena terminalis   Fornix
                         Body of corpus callosum

Caudate nucl. tail
Lateral nucl.
Reticular nucl.
Ext. medullary lamina
Internal capsule post. limb
Lat. ventral nucl.
External capsule
Claustrum
Extreme capsule
Cortex of insula
Putamen
Globus pallidus

Transverse cerebral fissure
Dorsomedial nucl.
Stria medullaris
Int. medullary lamina
Interthalamic adhesion
Mammillothalamic tract
Ant. thalamic radiations
Ant. ventral nucl.
Ant. column of fornix
IIIrd ventricle
Ant. commissure
Precommissural fornix

Internal capsule, ant. limb
Caudate nucl., head   Subcallosal area

FIG. 168. Photomicrograph of an oblique section through the diencephalon and basal telencephalon illustrating the thalamus and basal ganglia. Weil stain.

tains neurons of the motor type—large, multipolar and pyramidal- or spindle-shaped.

The **caudate nucleus** consists of head, body, and tail. The head is continuous with the anterior end of the lentiform nucleus (Figs. 163, 165, 168) and also rests on the anterior perforated substance. The body begins at the level of the rostral end of the thalamus and, gradually becoming reduced in circumference, arches upward and caudally over the thalamus and internal capsule. The still more attenuated tail continues around the poste-

rior limit of the thalamus and enters the temporal lobe of the cerebrum where it courses downward and forward in the roof of the inferior horn of the lateral ventricle finally ending at the amygdaloid body. Small stellate cells in the caudate nucleus send their axons to the putamen and globus pallidus of the lentiform nucleus. Axons of larger multipolar cells scattered among the stellate cells are distributed exclusively to the globus pallidus.

The **amygdaloid body** is buried within the tip of the temporal lobe, above the rostral limit of the lateral ventricle (Figs.

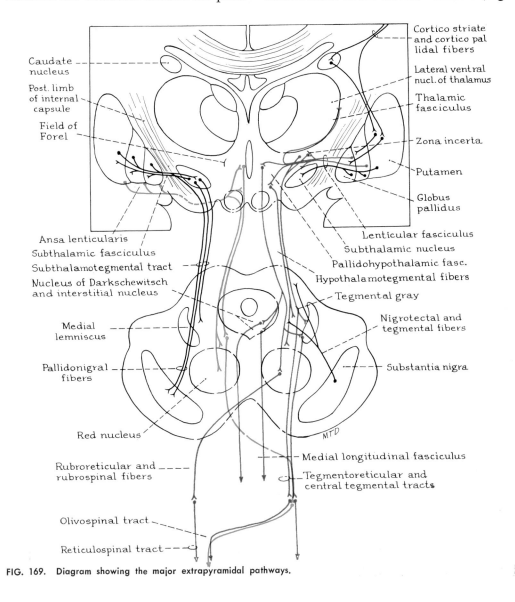

FIG. 169. Diagram showing the major extrapyramidal pathways.

163, 166, 167). Although it is included as one of the classical basal ganglia, it has no known motor functions and is related instead to the olfactory system and limbic lobe. Thus, discussion of the amygdaloid body is deferred to Chapter 24 which treats the rhinencephalon.

The **claustrum,** although included as a part of the basal ganglia, usually is considered to be a detached portion of the insular cortex. Little is known about the connections and functions of the claustrum, although it has been reported to have direct connections with Brodmann areas 9, 11, and 22, and with the insular cortex.

The **corpus striatum** is the combination of caudate nucleus and lentiform nucleus with the intervening fibers of the internal capsule. Strands of gray matter connecting the two nuclei through the anterior limb of the internal capsule are responsible for its striated appearance (Figs. 119, 120, 165, 168). The *striatum* includes only the caudate nucleus and the putamen of the lentiform nucleus. The phylogenetic terms—archistriatum, paleostriatum, and neostriatum—often are used and should be defined. The *archistriatum* includes only the amygdaloid body; the *paleostriatum* is the globus pallidus; the term *neostriatum* is synonymous with *striatum* and refers to the combination of putamen and caudate nucleus which are phylogenetically newer than the other parts and are histologically similar. The globus pallidus is often referred to as *pallidum.*

It is apparent that the terminology with respect to the basal ganglia is very confusing, complicated by the inclusion of the claustrum and amygdaloid body, which seem not to be related functionally to caudate and lentiform nuclei. Thus it is more meaningful to use a functional terminology and to apply the term "basal ganglia" to the caudate and lentiform nuclei and to the related gray (e.g., substantia nigra and subthalamic nucleus). Nuclei of the subthalamus that are re-

lated to the striatum and pallidum and are also a part of the extrapyramidal system include the *subthalamic nucleus, zona incerta, nucleus of the field of Forel,* * and the rostral extensions of the *red nucleus* and *substantia nigra* (Figs. 165, 168, 169). The **subthalamic nucleus** lies above the cerebral peduncle and medial to the internal capsule. It is surrounded by fascicles of fibers and is in relation to the rostral extent of the substantia nigra. The *zona incerta* is a small grouping of cells dorsal to the subthalamic nucleus and is separated from it by fibers of the lenticular fasciculus. The nucleus of the field of Forel (H field) consists of scattered cells which lie medial to the zona incerta and is in relation to the lenticular fasciculus and ansa lenticularis (Fig. 169). The red nucleus, prominent in the tegmentum at the superior collicular level of the midbrain, extends into the caudal and medial subthalamic area (Figs. 165, 169). The **substantia nigra,** conspicuous throughout the midbrain tegmentum, has a rostral extension into the subthalamus which lies embedded in the dorsal part of the cerebral peduncle (Figs. 70, 169).

In addition to and surrounding the red nucleus of the midbrain tegmentum at the superior collicular level is an extensive accumulation of reticular neurons, the tegmental gray (deep tegmental nucleus) of the midbrain (Figs. 70, 169). This nucleus extends caudally through the level of the inferior colliculus and has many connections with the above-mentioned subtelencephalic and subthalamic nuclei as well as with extrapyramidal areas of the cortex. The conspicuous *central tegmental tract* (Figs. 68, 169, 170) is believed to arise in large part from the

* Forel, whose name is applied to certain areas of the subthalamus, used the German word *Haube* to designate the "cap" of fibers rostral to the red nucleus. As a result, the letter H is used with reference to groups of fibers in this area. The prerubral field is the H field of Forel, the thalamic fasciculus is equivalent to the H_1 field, and the H_2 field designates the lenticular fasciculus.

deep tegmental nucleus, the periaqueductal gray, and the red nucleus. It serves as a descending motor pathway to reticular neurons in more caudal brain stem levels. Many of the fibers in the central tegmental tract are short; others extend to the medulla (e.g., to the inferior olivary nucleus); and some have been traced to upper cord levels.

Many cortically originating extrapyramidal fibers impinge on these nuclei. Although there is no general agreement relative to the cortical areas that contribute extrapyramidal fibers to the respective basal telencephalic and brain stem nuclei, the majority of fibers arise from areas 4, 6, and 8. The cortically originating extrapyramidal pathways are listed in Chapter 16. Although some of these are treated in greater detail elsewhere, all are briefly considered here.

The **corticopontine fibers** that synapse in the basal pontine gray comprise a large system which relates the cerebral cortex to the cerebellum. This system includes frontopontocerebellar fibers that are known to arise primarily from areas 4 and 6, temporopontocerebellar, and occipitopontocerebellar fibers. This system of fibers is discussed in connection with the cerebellum in Chapter 19.

Corticonigral fibers originate in areas 4, 5, and 6 (Fig. 171) and prefrontal areas 9, 10, 11, and 12. The fibers originating more rostrally synapse on the more rostral part of the substantia nigra and the others in the more caudal parts.

It seems best to consider the cortical fibers to caudate and lentiform nucleus together, i.e., the **corticostriate** and **corticopallidal.** It is generally agreed that these have a widespread origin, although anatomical support for the extent and details of origin in man is limited. There is, however, good evidence that in the monkey fibers reach the caudate-lentiform complex from areas 4, 6, and 8 and from orbital cortex of the frontal lobe. Others

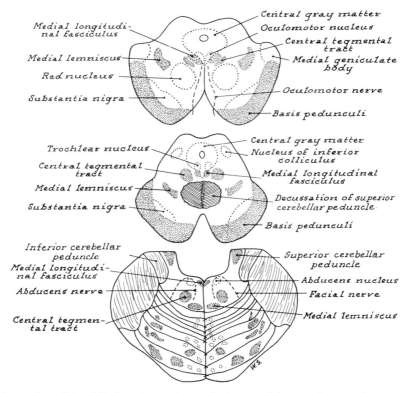

FIG. 170.   Cross-sections of the midbrain and pons showing the location of the central tegmental tract.

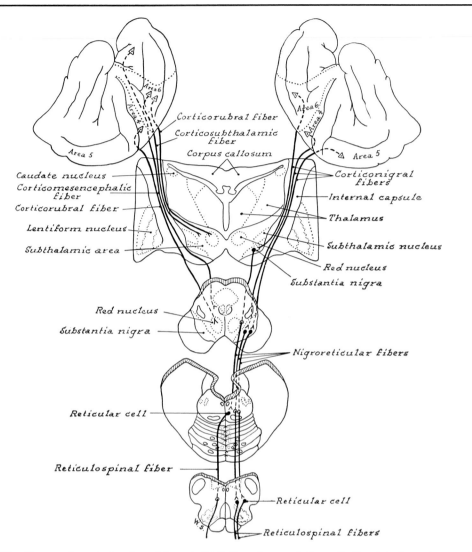

FIG. 171. Diagram demonstrating the origin and distribution of some of the cortically originating extrapyramidal projection fibers.

arise from areas 2, 5, and 7 of the parietal lobe, from the insula, from temporal pole cortex, and from the cingulate gyrus (areas 23 and 24). Although the globus pallidus is believed to receive some direct cortical fibers, the major input into this large nuclear mass (caudate-lentiform) is via the caudate and putamen (Fig. 169). The efferent fibers arise primarily in the globus pallidus.

Corticorubral and **corticosubthalamic fibers** are believed to arise from areas 4 and 6 (Fig. 171). From these same areas,

corticotegmental (corticomesencephalic) fibers reach the tegmental gray of the midbrain. It was noted above that the subthalamic area is continuous with the midbrain tegmentum and actually constitutes a rostral extension of the tegmentum into the diencephalon. Furthermore, the medial reticular area of the more caudal brain stem is related to the tegmental area of the midbrain and, significantly, these related areas receive fibers, at least in part, from comparable cortical areas. With respect to medial reticular

area of the medulla, physiological neuron-
ographic studies (strychnine stimulation
and recording) indicate cortical input
from the anterior part of the precentral
gyrus.

Corticohypothalamic fibers that arise
from components of the rhinencephalon
are quite numerous (see Chaps. 21 and
24). In addition, many cortical fibers
pass directly to the hypothalamus from
different parts of the frontal lobe, more
particularly from the orbital cortex.

Corticothalamic fibers originate from
many areas of the cortex and are considered in connection with the thalamus
(see Chap. 21). It is pertinent to men-
tion, however, that corticothalamic fibers
have been described originating in area
6 which project to the lateral ventral
nucleus.

In relation to the considerations here,
the cortically originating extrapyramidal
fibers to the thalamus seem important in
that the lateral ventral nucleus has been
shown to send projections to the globus
pallidus. In fact, there are many fibers
from the nuclei of the dorsal thalamus to
the caudate and lentiform nucleus.
Notably the putamen and caudate have
afferent connections with the centro-
medial nucleus, and globus pallidus receives fibers from the intralaminar nuclei.
Other afferent fibers of the pallidum include *nigropallidal* from the substantia
nigra which have been described by several investigators. They form a bundle
that extends forward from the rostral
limit of the substantia nigra, beneath
the subthalamic nucleus; fascicles pass
through the internal capsule, enter the
medial tip of the internal part of the
globus pallidus, and are distributed to
both parts of this structure and possibly
to the putamen.

In summary, the considerations of the
extrapyramidal system to this point have
called attention to a number of subtelencephalic and upper brain stem nuclei
which have a copious input of cortically
originating fibers and, in addition, other

afferent fibers to these nuclei have been
mentioned. Of the great number of extrapyramidal cortical areas mentioned, areas
of the frontal lobe are considered the
primary centers of origin for the extrapyramidal motor pathways which synapse
in the basal ganglia and related nuclei
before reaching the motor nuclei of the
cranial and spinal nerves. The motor
pathways from these basal nuclei to the
motor cells of the cranial and spinal
nerves remain to be considered. In addition, other efferent pathways of the subtelencephalic and related nuclear groups
are to be considered. The majority of
efferent fibers of the basal ganglia have
their origin in the lentiform nucleus. Only
a few fibers originate in the putamen; a
relatively larger number come from the
external division of the globus pallidus;
and the greatest number originate from
cells in its internal division (Fig. 169).
The main efferent pathways from the
lentiform nucleus are contained in or intimately related to three major fiber paths,
the *lenticular fasciculus,* the *ansa lenticularis,* and the *subthalamic fasciculus* (Fig.
169). The *pallidohypothalamic* and *thalamic fasciculi* branch off from the lenticular fasciculus. The *pallidonigral* fibers
are closely associated with the subthalamic fasciculus.

The **lenticular fasciculus** courses medially from its origin in the globus pallidus, pierces the internal capsule, and
enters the region of the zona incerta.
Some of the fibers synapse with cells
in this zone. From the zona incerta, fibers
course to the tegmentum of the midbrain
and enter the central tegmental tract
directly or after synapse in the tegmental
gray. The majority of fibers in the lenticular fasciculus continue medially in the
H_2 field of Forel and many synapse in the
nucleus of the field of Forel. With or without synapse in this nucleus, fibers pass
caudally to the midbrain and end in the
red nucleus, tegmental gray around the
red nucleus, *nucleus of Darkschewitsch,*
and the *interstitial nucleus of the medial*

longitudinal fasciculus. From the latter two nuclei, fibers arise that comprise the medial longitudinal fasciculi. These continue caudally to the motor nuclei of the cranial nerves. From cells in the red nucleus and tegmental gray which receive the lenticular fasciculus, fiber tracts arise that continue to the more caudal reticular areas of the brain stem and to the motor nuclei of origin for the cranial nerves. Motor neurons in the cervical spinal cord also receive an input from these fibers. The major descending fiber systems from the red nucleus and surrounding tegmental gray or nuclei include the *rubroreticular* and *rubrospinal, tegmentoreticular* and *central tegmental tracts* (Fig. 169). The reticulospinal tracts serve as the most important relays to the spinal neurons. *Olivospinal tracts* also provide a link in the caudal projection.

The **Pallidohypothalamic fasciculus** (Fig. 169), which arises from the globus pallidus, separates from the lenticular fasciculus in the H₂ field and courses ventromedialward and rostrally to enter the hypothalamus where it terminates in the ventromedial nucleus. This termination in the ventromedial nucleus is significant in that a relation is established for conduction from the pallidum to hypothalamus to the tegmentum of the midbrain through hypothalamotegmental fibers.

The **thalamic fasciculus** (pallidothalamic fibers, Fig. 169) courses medially in the dorsal part of the lenticular fasciculus to the H field where it curves sharply dorsalward and laterally in the H₁ field to the lateral ventral nucleus of the thalamus.

The **ansa lenticularis** (Fig. 169) arises from all divisions of the lentiform nucleus. It may also contain fibers from the temporal and insular cortices. These fibers accumulate below the lentiform nucleus to form the ansa. It courses medially, looping around the ventral border of the posterior limb of the internal capsule, into the region of the H field of Forel where some fibers synapse. Fascicles of the ansa,

together with fibers originating in the nucleus of the field of Forel, continue to the red nucleus and to the more caudal portions of the tegmental nuclei of the midbrain. Descending fibers from these midbrain centers and their relations with neurons at more caudal levels of the brain stem and upper cord were mentioned in relation to the lenticular fasciculus. Fascicles from the ansa have been traced to the hypothalamus and to the ventral thalamus.

The **subthalamic fasciculus** (Fig. 169) interconnects the lentiform nucleus with the subthalamic nucleus, and it is generally agreed that the fasciculus contains both afferent and efferent components. The efferent component (*pallidosubthalamic*) arises from both divisions of globus pallidus and a few fibers originate from the putamen. The fibers traverse the internal capsule ventral to the lenticular fasciculus and pass medially to the subthalamic nucleus. The afferent component (*subthalamostriate*) passes through the internal capsule and globus pallidus to the putamen.

From the subthalamic nucleus the **subthalamotegmental tract** descends into the midbrain, synapsing in the lateral tegmental gray. From the tegmental gray, tegmentobulbar and tegmentospinal tracts descend to the caudal reticular areas and to the cranial and spinal nerve motor nuclei.

Pallidonigral fibers (Fig. 169) are closely associated with the subthalamic fasciculus; they separate from the pallidosubthalamic fibers and swing caudalward along the ventrolateral border of the subthalamic nucleus to enter the substantia nigra. The pallidonigral fibers are joined by fine fascicles that appear to originate from the subthalamic nucleus and that also appear to enter the substantia nigra. Many fibers from substantia nigra project to the tegmental gray of the midbrain. Efferent fibers from the nigra to the pallidum also have been described.

To **summarize** the pattern of extrapyramidal projections from cortical levels to motor neurons of the brain stem and cord, it is important to note that generally the system is comprised of a multineuron chain. The cortically originating fibers feed into the basal ganglia which, through one or more neuronal links, project to the tegmental and/or reticular nuclei of the brain stem. An important pathway from the tegmental nuclei of the midbrain to reticular nuclei of more caudal brain stem levels is the central tegmental tract. The rubrospinal, rubroreticular, and reticulospinal fibers are important final links in the spinalward projection. The *rubrospinal* and *rubroreticular tracts* originate from the red nuclei; immediately after their emergence from the nuclei, the tracts decussate to the opposite side through the *ventral tegmental decussation (of Forel).*

After its decussation, the **rubrospinal tract** courses caudally through the tegmentum of the pons and reticular formation of the medulla. The tract is anteriorly and medially placed in the pontile tegmentum, and it lies immediately posterior

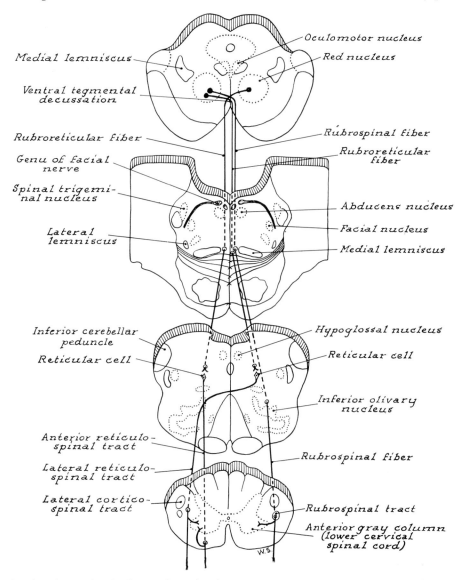

FIG. 172. The rubrospinal and rubroreticulospinal pathways.

13

to the olivary nucleus in the medulla (Fig. 172). Within the spinal cord the rubrospinal fibers are found in the lateral funiculus immediately anterior to the lateral corticospinal tract. Rubrospinal fibers terminate in relation to anterior gray column cells.

Rubroreticular fibers are more numerous in the human brain than are rubrospinal fibers. They synapse on cells in the reticular formation whose axons, as reticulospinal fibers, are also distributed to anterior gray column cells (Fig. 172). The ratio of rubroreticular to rubrospinal fibers is reversed in the cat and in some other animals.

Reticulospinal fibers (Fig. 172) form *anterior* and *lateral reticulospinal tracts* in the spinal cord; the former is found in the anterior funiculus, and the latter in the lateral funiculus. Each contains crossed and uncrossed fibers with crossings at both brain stem and spinal cord levels.

Despite a great amount of experimental work on animals and a vast number of clinical studies, we have no clear-cut appreciation of the functional interrelations of the extrapyramidal system with the other motor systems. This is particularly true with respect to the basal ganglia. It should be kept in mind that the pyramidal system is present only in mammals. Furthermore, birds and lower vertebrates have very little cerebral cortex and the basal ganglia are the highest centers of motor coordination. In general, the movements supported in these lower forms are stereotyped or automatic, repetitive, and gross in character with an absence of precise or specific movements. This is the pattern of movements in the infant, before mature structural and functional relations are established in the pyramidal tracts and in related descending cortical fibers. It is indicated in Chapter 16 that in the case of damage or destruction of the pyramidal system there is a great amount of residual or restored motor activity. This is probably largely due to intact components of the ontogenetically and phylogenetically primitive system (extrapyramidal).

In general, stimulation of the basal ganglia has not been very effective in producing movement nor has stimulation or the placement of lesions in the basal ganglia been very effective in clarifying their function. Nevertheless, a few clues to their function have emerged from these procedures. Stimulating the caudate nucleus of unanesthetized cats with implanted electrodes has given results indicating efferent projections from the nucleus to lower centers. The reactions to stimulation were manifested contralaterally, were stereotyped, and lacked the range of those elicited by stimulation of the motor cortex. They consisted of turning the head to the contralateral side and flexion of one or both contralateral extremities. These movements have also been obtained after removal of the motor cortex. A more active response to stimulation in cats with intact frontal cortices has led to the suggestion that facilitation of lower motor mechanisms by the cortex, and particularly the motor cortex, plays an important part in movements elicited from stimulation of the caudate nucleus. Moreover, it has been reported that caudate and pallidal stimulation was inhibitory to cortically induced movement.

Generally, experimental lesions in the basal ganglia have caused little motor dysfunction unless these were in conjunction with injury to the frontal cortex. For example, bilateral lesions have been placed in the basal ganglia of monkeys and chimpanzees with no apparent effect on motor activity. However, bilateral lesions of the pallidum in animals with bilateral lesions of the motor cortex resulted in increased resistance to passive movement (rigidity), tremor, and some motor weakness. Rigidity and tremor are common characteristic symptoms of basal ganglia disease in man. A third symptom is poverty of movement or a loss of associative movements which has been reported in monkeys following bilateral destruction of the ansa lenticularis and unilateral interruption of other efferent fibers of the globus pallidus.

Clinical Considerations

It is appropriate to consider the common clinical disorders attributable to damage of the basal ganglia and to discuss the resultant disturbances of posture and movement. It should be kept in mind, however, that these disorders are usually due to rather widespread or diffuse pathological processes, and it is difficult to associate the lesions with damaged structures which underlie the motor disturbances.

Parkinson's disease, also known as **paralysis agitans** or **Parkinson's syndrome,** is characterized by a variety of symptoms, the chief ones being rigidity, alternating tremor, slowness and poverty of movement, mask-like facies, and diminution of associated movements. Despite the name paralysis agitans there is no paralysis, but a disturbance of movement. The rigidity is apparent in the resistance offered in the passive movement of a limb. The rigidity is present in both flexor and extensor muscles and has the cogwheel or "lead pipe" quality. Thus rigidity is different from the spasticity which accompanies damage to the cortically originating extrapyramidal fibers.

The tremor of paralysis agitans is regular and rapid (often 4 to 8 per second) due to alternating contractions of agonist and antagonist muscles. It may be limited to the fingers, called "pill-rolling tremor," or it may involve the entire hand or limb. It occurs at rest and disappears during sleep and when the limb is moved voluntarily.

The substantia nigra in particular and the pallidum are generally considered to be the most common or consistent sites of pathology in the Parkinson syndrome. Evidence has been presented, however, which suggests that the tremor results from the loss of corticopallidal and corticostriatal fibers and that lesions of sub-

stantia nigra appear to be associated with more restricted bulbar spasms such as yawning and respiratory and lingual compulsions.

Tremor like that of Parkinson's disease has been produced in monkeys by experimental lesions placed in the ventrolateral part of the midbrain tegmental area.

Huntington's chorea, also known as **hereditary chorea,** is a degenerative disorder of middle age affecting the basal ganglia; it is characterized by jerky involuntary movements and progressive loss of mental function. In successive generations the age of onset usually decreases. The motor signs appear to be due to reduction in the number of cells in the corpus striatum, especially in the caudate nucleus, and to progressive degeneration of those which remain. The mental symptoms are explained by diminution in the number of cells in the cerebral cortex, especially in the inner three layers of the frontal, parietal, and temporal lobes.

Hemiballismus (hemichorea) results from unilateral lesions of the subthalamic nucleus. The jerky choreiform movements are likely to become violent; their appearance when there is a lesion of the nucleus suggests that the pallidosubthalamotegmental system normally exercises a check or steadying influence on one or another of the corticospinal, corticopontocerebellar, or dentatorubrothalamopallidal systems. It has been shown that hemiballismus may result from lesions in the globus pallidus or in the subthalamotegmental fibers as well as in the subthalamic nucleus itself. Hemiballismus may be ipsilateral or contralateral to the side of the lesion, depending on whether the location of the lesion involves pathways which subsequently cross, or interrupt subthalamotegmental fibers which have already crossed. Interruption of recurrent fibers from the subthalamic nucleus to globus pallidus appears to release the latter to abnormal activity with resultant contralateral hemiballismus of moderate degree.

Wilson's disease (hepatolenticular degeneration) is another degenerative disease associated with an error in body copper metabolism which appears in younger persons (ten to twenty-five years of age). The condition is characterized by tremor, rigidity, impairment of voluntary motion (including speech), and loss of facial expression. There may be causeless and uncontrollable laughing and crying. Softening and cavitation of the lentiform nucleus often can be seen macroscopically on postmortem examination of the brain from an individual having had this disease. Degeneration of nerve cells is more pronounced in the putamen than in the globus pallidus. The red nucleus, thalamus, cerebellum, and cerebral cortex may show associated involvement. Cirrhosis of the liver, for some unknown reason, usually is associated with the lenticular degeneration of Wilson's disease.

Athetosis is a symptom complex found either bilaterally or unilaterally, usually of congenital origin. It may be due to either congenital maldevelopment or birth injury. The extrapyramidal system may be affected in various ways, but the lesions appear to be primarily in the basal ganglia. The facial muscles move in a grimacing manner and the tongue writhes and protrudes spasmodically. There is difficulty in speaking and swallowing. The arm is adducted and internally rotated; the elbow is in semiflexion and the wrist and lesser digits are markedly flexed. The thumb is adducted and extended. The foot is turned inward and the great toe is extended. The upright position is accompanied by writhing movements. At rest, the limbs are hypotonic and movements cease during sleep.

Involvement of the basal ganglia in brain tumors has not generally been considered responsible for extrapyramidal symptoms. Cases of intracranial tumor, however, have been reported with signs of extrapyramidal involvement; these signs included tremor, athetosis, rigidity, decrease in associated movements, slowness, mask-like facies, and rhythmic alternating tremor.

In summary, it has been established that the major signs of damage to the cortically originating extrapyramidal fibers are spasticity and exaggerated reflexes, whereas the signs of basal ganglia disease are tremor, rigidity, and poverty of movement. Although there are no completely satisfactory explanations of the physiological mechanisms underlying these signs, it is readily apparent that a damaged or destroyed fiber tract or nucleus could not be responsible for such phenomena as tremor, spasticity, and rigidity. This suggests that the components of the extrapyramidal system may be more concerned with the regulation of movement than with its initiation. This concept, in fact, has become progressively more firmly established.

Facilitatory or inhibitory influences can be superimposed on a wide range of motor performances, depending on the site of stimulation within the reticular formation. The motor activities affected include flexor or extensor reflexes, decerebrate rigidity, and muscular responses evoked by stimulation of the motor cortex. Although there appears to be some overlap between the inhibitory area of the reticular formation and the facilitatory area, the general relationship is such that the facilitatory areas are more rostrally placed, extending forward from the medulla through pons and mesencephalon into the diencephalon. Specifically, there are several descending fiber tracts which can reciprocally influence spinal reflexes (mainly via interneurons) by facilitating or inhibiting alpha and gamma motoneurons. There is evidence that *rubrospinal* and *medullary reticulospinal fibers* facilitate motoneurons innervating flexor muscles and inhibit those innervating extensor muscles. *Vestibulospinal* and *pontine reticulospinal fibers* appear to do the converse, that is, inhibit flexor and facilitate extensor motoneurons. Also, contrasting effects may be exerted on similar muscle groups in the two halves of the body.

If cerebral cortical and cerebellar regions which project on the bulbar reticular regions are ablated, a pronounced exaggeration of stretch reflexes ensues. This exaggeration of reflexes, whereas initially marked and generalized, becomes attenuated with the passage of time and is limited to the antigravity (extensor) musculature. This is accounted for by the hypothesis that the inhibitory components of descending systems depend on excitation from cortical areas. In the absence of inhibitory influences a tonic check on postural spinal reflexes is lacking. Further, the excitatory action of the vestibulospinal fibers on extensor motoneurons is normally inhibited by the cerebellum. Thus with the cerebellum removed, the facilitatory drive on extensors is enhanced. Elucidation of this positive factor has been accomplished by transection of the thoracic spinal cord in animals exhibiting chronic spasticity; this is followed by loss or marked reduction of exaggerated stretch reflexes (extensor) in the lower extremity whose spinal innervation had been severed from the brain, but such reflexes in the upper extremity, whose spinal segments were still connected with the brain, maintained or increased their exaggeration. In accordance with reciprocal effects of descending fibers on motoneurons supplying antagonistic muscles, there is the converse increase of *flexor* reflexes in the lower extremity. Such flexor hyperreflexia which may come to characterize the lower extremity of chronic paraplegic man, in spite of the fact that the lower part of the spinal cord is separated from all descending influences, indicates the presence of intrinsic spinal cord mechanisms which are still in operation.

In summary, it appears that the stretch hyperreflexia associated with spasticity cannot be attributed simply to loss of an inhibitory influence, but is probably due to continued and unopposed presence of facilitation which proceeds downward by reticulospinal and vestibulospinal connections from the brain stem to motor neurons.

The gamma-efferent supply to the muscle spindle (Chap. 5), comprising as much as one-third of the ventral root outflow at some spinal levels, contributes to a recurrent loop by which the central nervous system can regulate its own proprioceptive input and, in this way, reflexly modify alpha-motor discharge responsible for both postural and phasic contractions of muscle. Descending influences can markedly increase or reduce the firing of the gamma-efferent supply to muscle spindles and so alter input from them. Thus, rubrospinal, reticulospinal, and vestibulospinal tracts possess an additional means of modifying motor activity over and above those effects exerted directly on alpha-motor outflows or on internuncial neurons influencing them. These in turn are influenced by extrapyramidal projections from the cerebral cortex and from the cerebellum.

This account of the inhibitory and facilitatory mechanisms provides a general framework for explaining some of the symptoms of extrapyramidal disease. Normally, it would appear that a balance exists in these two mechanisms, providing for the appropriate efferent output to the cranial and spinal motor neurons for smooth and orderly motor activity. The mechanisms allow appropriate adjustments at various levels of the neuraxis, although there is uncertainty relative to the level at which some of the adjustments are made. Through disease or experimental lesions, the balance is distributed which would allow for overactivity of either the facilitatory or inhibitory mechanism, resulting in inappropriate discharge of alpha and gamma motoneurons with subsequent impairment of spinal reflexes and movement.

BIBLIOGRAPHY

Bebin, J., 1956: The central tegmental bundle. An anatomical and experimental study in the monkey. J. Comp. Neurol., *105*, 287–332.

Bucy, P. C., 1949: Relation to abnormal involuntary movements. In *The Precentral Motor Cortex,* 2nd ed., P. C. Bucy, Ed. University of Illinois Press, Urbana, Chap. 15, pp. 395–408.

Bucy, P. C., Ladpli, R., and Ehrlich, E., 1966: Destruction of the pyramidal tract in the monkey. The effects of bilateral section of the cerebral peduncles. J. Neurosurg., *25,* 1–20.

Cajal (Ramon y), S., 1909–1911: *Histologie du Systeme Nerveux de l'Homme et des Vetébrés.* A. Maloine, Paris.

Carey, J. H., 1957: Certain anatomical and functional interrelations between the tegmentum of the midbrain and the basal ganglia. J. Comp. Neurol., *108,* 57–89.

Carpenter, M. B., and Strominger, N. L., 1967: Efferent fibers of the subthalamic nucleus in the monkey. A comparison of the efferent projections of the subthalamic nucleus, substantia nigra and globus pallidus. Amer. J. Anat., *121,* 41–72.

Carpenter, M. B., Fraser, R. A. R., and Shriver, J. E., 1968: The organization of pallido-subthalamic fibers in the monkey. Brain Res., *11,* 522–559.

Denny-Brown, D., 1962: *The Basal Ganglia and Their Relation to Disorders of Movement.* Oxford University Press, New York.

Forman, D., and Ward, J. W., 1957: Responses to electrical stimulation of caudate nucleus in cats in chronic experiments. J. Neurophysiol., *20,* 230–244.

Jansen, J. K. S., 1962: Spasticity—functional aspects. Acta Neurol. Scand., *38,* Suppl. 3, 41–51.

Jung, R., and Hassler, R., 1960: The extrapyramidal motor system. In *Handbook of Physiology,* Vol. II, Section 1, Neurophysiology, John Field, Ed.-in-Chief. Williams & Wilkins Co., Baltimore, Chap. 35, pp. 863–927.

Kennard, M. A., 1944: *Autonomic Function, The Precentral Motor Cortex.* The University of Illinois Press, Urbana, pp. 293–306.

Kennard, M. A., and Fulton, J. F., 1942: Corticostriatal interrelations in monkey and chimpanzee. Res. Publ. Ass. Res. Nerv. Ment. Dis., *21,* 228–245.

Lawrence, D. G., and Kuypers, H. G. J. M., 1968: The functional organization of the motor system in the monkey. II. The effects of lesions of the descending brain-stem pathways. Brain, *91,* 15–36.

Laursen, A. M., 1955: An experimental study of pathways from the basal ganglia. J. Comp. Neurol., *102,* 1–25.

Lindsley, D. B., Schreiner, L. H., and Magoun, H. W., 1949: An electromyographic study of spasticity. J. Neurophysiol., *12,* 197–205.

Magoun, H. W., 1958: *The Waking Brain.* Charles C Thomas, Springfield, Ill.

Magoun, H. W., and Rhines, R., 1946: An inhibitory mechanism in the bulbar reticular formation. J. Neurophysiol., *9,* 165–171.

Magoun, H. W., and Rhines, R., 1947: *Spasticity: The Stretch-Reflex and Extrapyramidal Systems.* Charles C Thomas, Springfield, Ill.

Marchiafava, P. L., 1968: Activities of the central nervous system: motor. Ann. Rev. Physiol., *30,* 359–400.

Marshall, W. H., and Essig, C. F., 1951: Relation of air exposure of cortex to spreading depression of Leão. J. Neurophysiol., *14,* 265–273.

Mettler, F. A., 1947: Extracortical connections of the primate frontal cerebral cortex. II. Corticifugal connections. J. Comp. Neurol., *86,* 119–166.

Mettler, F. A., Ades, H. W., Lipman, E., and Culler, E. A., 1939: The extrapyramidal system. A.M.A. Arch. Neurol. Psychiat., *41,* 984–995.

Meyer, M., 1949: A study of efferent connexions of the frontal lobe in the human brain after leucotomy. Brain, *72,* 265–296.

Niemer, W. T., and Magoun, H. W., 1947: Reticulo-spinal tracts influencing motor activity. J. Comp. Neurol., *87,* 367–379.

Papez, J. W., 1926: Reticulo-spinal tracts in the cat. Marchi method. J. Comp. Neurol., *41,* 365–399.

Papez, J. W., Bennett, A. E., and Cash, P. T., 1942: Hemichorea (hemiballismus). A.M.A. Arch. Neurol. Psychiat., *47,* 667–676.

Pollack, M., and Hornabrook, R. W., 1966: The prevalence, natural history and dementia of Parkinson's disease. Brain, *89,* 429–448.

Rae, A. S. L., 1954: The connections of the claustrum. Confinia Neurol., *14,* 211–219.

Ranson, S. W., Ranson, S. W., Jr., and Ranson, M., 1941: Fiber connections of corpus striatum as seen in Marchi preparations. A.M.A. Arch. Neurol. Psychiat., *46,* 230–249.

Rhines, R., and Magoun, H. W., 1946: Brain stem facilitation of cortical motor response. J. Neurophysiol., *9,* 219–229.

Rundles, R. W., and Papez, J. W., 1937: Connections between the striatum and the substantia nigra in a human brain. A.M.A. Arch. Neurol. Psychiat., *38,* 550–563.

Schreiner, L., MacCarty, C. S., and Grindlay, J. H., 1958: Production and relief of tremor in the monkey. In *Pathogenesis and Treatment of Parkinsonism,* William S. Fields, Ed. Charles C Thomas, Springfield, Ill., Chap. V, pp. 118–137.

Ward, A. W., Jr., and McCulloch, W. S., 1947: The projection of the frontal lobe on the hypothalamus. J. Neurophysiol., *10,* 309–314.

Ward, A. W., Jr., McCulloch, W. S., and Magoun, H. W., 1948: Production of an alternating tremor at rest in monkeys. J. Neurophysiol., *11,* 317–330.

Woodburne, R. T., Crosby, E. C., and McCotter, R. E., 1946: The mammalian midbrain and isthmus regions. Part II. The fiber connections. A. The relations of the tegmentum of the midbrain with the basal ganglia in *Macaca mulatta.* J. Comp. Neurol., *85,* 67–92.

Chapter 18

Lesions of the Motor Pathway

The middle cerebral artery gives off internal and external striate branches near its origin from the internal carotid. These branches enter the brain through the anterior perforated substance, just lateral to the optic chiasm (Fig. 173). They supply the basal ganglia and the internal capsule. One of these, supposedly larger than the others, has been referred to as the lenticulostriate artery. This vessel has been designated the "artery of cerebral hemorrhage" because it was believed to be most prone to rupture and to release of blood into the brain substance. Anatomically, there is no single vessel that meets these criteria. It is true, however, that these striate branches from the middle cerebral artery are frequently the sites of cerebral hemorrhage and thrombosis.

Such a hemorrhage is likely to destroy the genu and anterior part of the posterior limb of the internal capsule with resultant paralysis of the opposite side of the body. The degree of paralysis in the head region depends on how extensively the genu is involved by the hemorrhagic process. The upper part of the face will be spared because the motor neurons that supply it receive fibers from the motor cortices of both sides (Fig. 148). It was pointed out that the contralateral trunk muscles are unlikely to be much affected by a unilateral lesion of the internal capsule since they are ipsilaterally innervated in some manner. Transient paresis of the contralateral trunk muscles, however, has been reported following section of the basis pedunculi in monkeys.

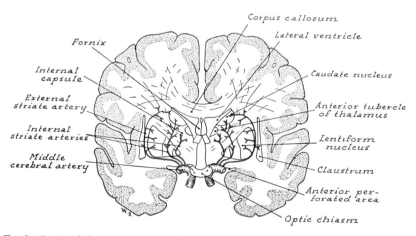

FIG. 173. The distribution of the striate branches of the middle cerebral artery (in part after Villiger).

Hemiplegia, as the term is ordinarily used, actually refers only to paralysis of the upper and lower extremities of one side; in lesions of the internal capsule, it may include the facial and other muscles of the head region, but paralysis of the trunk muscles is not ordinarily implied. When hemiplegia develops as the result of unilateral hemorrhage into the internal capsule the paralyzed limbs soon become spastic and the deep reflexes are increased. The abdominal reflex is lost on the side of the paralysis, and the Babinski sign usually appears on that side (Chap. 16).

Tumors developing in the interpeduncular space of the mesencephalon may destroy one or both oculomotor nerves (Fig. 174*A*). Destruction of either nerve results in ipsilateral ptosis of the upper eyelid and outward and downward deviation of the eye. Tumors of the inter-

peduncular space, if they expand laterally, may destroy one or both bases pedunculi (Fig. 174*B, C*). Unilateral involvement of the basis pedunculi interrupts corticospinal fibers and some extrapyramidal fibers and eventually results in hemiplegia of the opposite side with the usual signs. Bilateral destruction of the bases pedunculi results in quadriplegia or paralysis of all four extremities.

Observations indicate that unilateral interruption of the basis pedunculi in the monkey results in a syndrome that is "intermediate between spastic and hypotonic paresis." It is characterized by hypotonicity of all muscle groups, except the extensors of the digits, and by hyperactive deep reflexes. These observations are explained by the assumption that inhibitory pathways from the cerebral cortex do not course entirely within the basis pedunculi. (See Chap. 17 in relation to

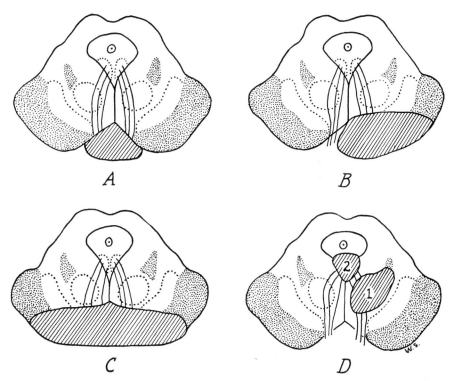

A

B

C

D

FIG. 174. Sections through the mesencephalon at the level of the superior colliculi showing the locations of lesions that interfere with voluntary motor functions. *A*, Tumor of the interpeduncular space destroying both oculomotor nerves. *B*, Unilateral expansion of a tumor of the interpeduncular space with encroachment on the basis pedunculi. *C*, Bilateral expansion of interpeduncular tumor with partial destruction of both bases pedunculi. *D*, Lesions in the mesencephalic tegmentum (1) and in the gray matter (2).

inhibitory and facilitatory mechanisms.) For the most part, the fibers whose interruption is responsible for the phenomenon of hypertonicity have separated from the corticospinal projection system prior to reaching the basis pedunculi; whereas those whose interruption is responsible for hyperreflexia accompany that system through the mesencephalon.

A surprising lack of spasticity has been noted in the totally hemispherectomized monkey. What spasticity is observed is limited to the affected upper extremity and is manifested by flexion. The lower extremity exhibits no evidence of resistance to passive movement and assumes a position of loose extension. Since slight hyperreflexia persists contralaterally and the affected leg is flaccid, the findings are comparable to the results of unilateral section of the basis pedunculi but would require an explanation different from that hypothesized as indicated above. Apparently, inhibitory fibers originate both ipsi- and contralaterally with at least part of those responsible for inhibition of muscle tone coming from the ipsilateral cerebral cortex.

A lesion of the central gray matter of the mesencephalon at the superior collicular level (Fig. 174D2) causes bilateral oculomotor paralysis. Such a lesion may extend caudally and also destroy the trochlear nuclei; then there will be bilateral paralysis of all the muscles of the eyes except the external recti, which are supplied by the abducens nerves. Pupillary reflexes (light and accommodation) are absent in subjects with lesions of the central gray matter because of destruction of the Edinger-Westphal nuclei, and in individuals with peripheral oculomotor lesions because of interruption of the efferent fibers from these nuclei.

Tegmental lesions of the mesencephalon (Fig. 174D1) are likely to involve the oculomotor fibers, the red nucleus, and the medial lemniscus. They may extend ventrally to involve the basis pedunculi. The symptoms arising from tegmental lesions may therefore include—in addition to oculomotor paralysis—contralateral loss of tactile and proprioceptive sensibility and, due to interruption of the cerebellorubrospinal pathway (centered in the red nucleus), asynergia of the contralateral limbs (see Chap. 19); if the basis pedunculi is encroached on, weakness or paralysis of the contralateral limbs will develop.

Tumors arising in either half of the basis pontis (Fig. 175A) produce contralateral hemiplegia with increased deep reflexes and spasticity. The abducens fibers, as they course through the caudal part of the basis pontis, are often destroyed by such tumors; the interruption of these fibers results in internal deviation of the ipsilateral eye. Paralysis of the lower face on the side opposite the lesion is likely to be one of the symptoms arising from this type of involvement since the corticobulbar fibers to the facial nuclei are still within the main "pyramidal" system at this level; they separate from the corticospinal fibers at the level of junction of pons and medulla and course to the facial nuclei by way of the bulbopontile aberrant pyramidal bundle (Fig. 147). Some lesions of the basis pontis extend laterally far enough to involve the emerging fibers of the facial nerve (Fig. 175B). In this event the entire face on the side of the lesion is paralyzed in association with contralateral hemiplegia and ipsilateral internal strabismus. The contralateral hemiplegia may include the lower half of the face as indicated above.

Spastic paralysis of the eye muscles, the muscles of mastication, the tongue muscles, and the muscles of the pharynx and larynx may result from *tegmental lesions* in the pons and caudal part of the midbrain, which interrupt corticobulbar fibers. Involvement of the medial lemniscus in the pontile tegmentum (Fig. 175C) destroys corticobulbar fibers destined for contralateral motor nuclei at levels caudal to the lesion (Fig. 147).

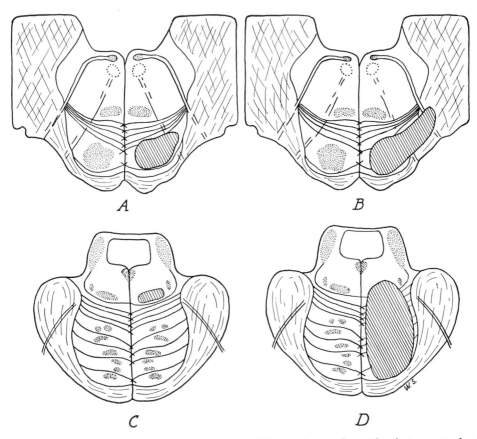

FIG. 175. Sections through the pons showing the locations of lesions that interfere with voluntary motor functions. A and B, Unilateral lesions of the basis pontis. C, Tegmental lesion that interrupts corticobulbar fibers in the medial lemniscus. D, Combined basilar and tegmental lesions.

A **pontile syndrome** of particular interest results from tumor or extensive hemorrhage in the rostral part of the pons with unilateral involvement of both basilar and tegmental areas (Fig. 175D). Such a lesion may damage the corticospinal and corticobulbar tracts and the medial lemniscus. The findings in this syndrome include contralateral hemiplegia, loss of tactile and proprioceptive sensibility on the contralateral side of the body, and paralysis of conjugate deviation of the eyes away from the side of the lesion. The contralateral hemiplegia includes the lower half of the face, the muscles of mastication, and the tongue. The paralysis of conjugate deviation of the eyes toward the side opposite that of the lesion is accounted for by destruction of the corticobulbar fibers in the medial lemniscus, which terminate in the contralateral abducens nucleus (Fig. 147). The abducens nucleus of either side, through connections with the other motor ocular nuclei by way of the medial longitudinal fasciculi, is believed to serve as the pacemaker for ipsilateral conjugate deviation of the eyes. In a lesion such as has been described, the abducens nucleus on the side opposite the lesion fails to receive cortical impulses and the subject is therefore unable to turn the eyes toward that side voluntarily.

Tegmental lesions of the pons, which destroy the abducens nucleus unilaterally, produce conjugate deviation of the eyes toward the opposite side and paralysis of deviation toward the side of the lesion.

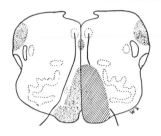

FIG. 176. Section through the medulla showing a common type of vascular lesion due to thrombosis of one or more branches of the anterior spinal artery.

These symptoms are due to interruption of the pacemaker mechanism. A small-celled portion of the abducens nucleus, termed "para-abducens" has sometimes been credited with the pacemaker function, but this has not been substantiated clinicopathologically.

Thrombosis of branches of the anterior spinal artery may result in unilateral destruction of the pyramid, adjacent extrapyramidal fibers, the medial lemniscus, and the hypoglossal nerve (Fig. 176). The paralysis in the contralateral extremities in such cases is of the spastic type; that in the ipsilateral half of the tongue, due to destruction of the axons of cells in the hypoglossal nucleus, is flaccid in character and there is atrophy of the paralyzed musculature. Atrophy of the tongue on the ipsilateral side in the presence of unilateral lesions of the hypoglossal nerve is usually observable. The diagnosis of lingual paralysis is easily made by having the patient protrude his tongue. The protruded tongue deviates toward the side of the paralysis.

The effects of traumatic spinal cord transections are flaccid paralysis, absence of sensation and suppression of reflexes, both skeletal and visceral, below the level of the lesion. The suppression or abolition of all reflexes is known as spinal shock, which is due to the functional interruption of the spinal tracts and not to the trauma of the lesion. The period of shock varies—some reflex activity may appear in three to five days, or it may not return for six weeks. The first reflexes to return are flexor movements, which are followed by the appearance of the Babinski sign, indicating damage to the cor-

ticospinal tracts (see Chap. 16). Several weeks or months following transection, the flexor reflexes usually become greatly exaggerated and spasms (mass reflexes) may appear. The next phase, beginning six months or more after injury, is characterized by a return of extensor reflexes.

It is generally agreed that spinal shock develops owing to the sudden interruption of the facilitatory pathways from supraspinal levels. The recovery or return of reflexes is less readily explainable, although it has been suggested that the recovery of function is a return of spinal motoneurons from a decreased excitability state to the normal "shock state."

Complete transection of the cord in man seldom occurs except on the battlefield. More common are partial transections produced by knife or bullet wounds, which may be hemisections giving rise to the classical Brown-Séquard syndrome. On the side of the hemisection, after the acute phase of the injury has passed, the pyramidal and extrapyramidal signs appear below the level of the lesion. They include the loss of voluntary movements and the sign of Babinski (damage to corticospinal tracts) and spasticity and exaggerated deep reflexes (damage to inhibitory extrapyramidal tracts). The facilitatory pathways also are interrupted, but the loss of this effect is surpassed by the loss of inhibitory mechanisms that normally dampen the segmental facilitatory mechanisms. Autonomic effects also may be apparent after hemisection, e.g., reduced sweating on the involved side below the level of the lesion. The sensory deficits include the loss of positional, vibratory, proprioceptive, and discriminatory tactile sensibility on the side of the lesion below the level of involvement owing to severance of the posterior columns. Pain and temperature sensibility are lost on the opposite side, beginning about two segments below the level of the lesion.

Not infrequently, intramedullary or extramedullary spinal cord tumors develop that produce various combinations of the motor signs and sensory deficits described for spinal cord transections. Although a tumor may produce a complete functional transection, the signs and symptoms usually appear gradually and progress with time. Additionally, in the early stages of growth, the signs may be associated with the segmental level of development, e.g., involvement of spinal roots.

Complete transverse lesions of the

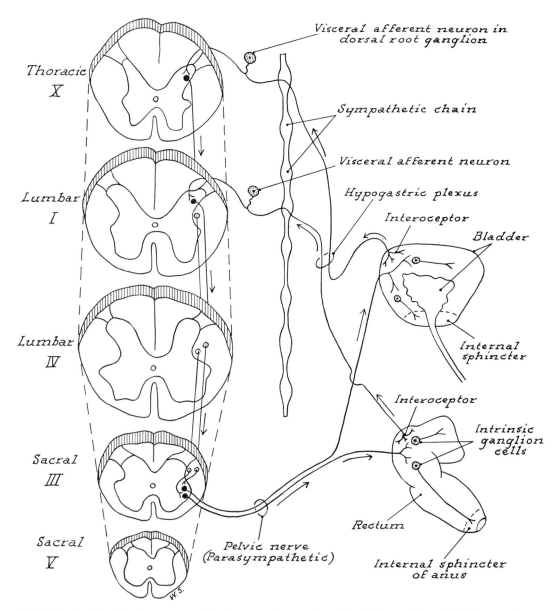

FIG. 177. The visceral reflex arc responsible for automatic emptying of the bladder and bowel following complete transection of the spinal cord in the thoracic region.

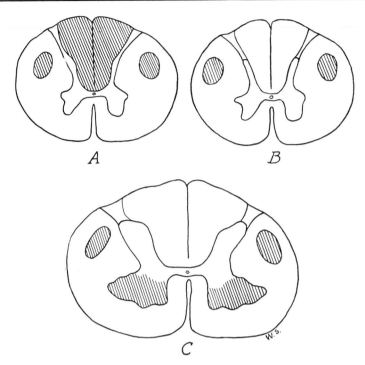

FIG. 178. *A,* Section through thoracic spinal cord showing the areas affected by subacute combined degeneration in pernicious anemia. *B,* Section through thoracic spinal cord showing the areas of degeneration in lateral sclerosis. *C,* Section through lower cervical spinal cord showing the sites of the degenerative process in amyotrophic lateral sclerosis.

spinal cord account for paralysis of the external sphincters of the bladder and bowel. At first there is likely to be acute retention of bowel and bladder contents due to spasm of the internal sphincters, but, after some time, so-called "cord bladder and bowel" usually develop. The cord bladder or bowel empties automatically when it is sufficiently distended. Automatic function depends on stimulation of visceral receptors in the wall of the viscus or in the peritoneum overlying it; afferent impulses thus set up enter the spinal cord (below the level of transection) over visceral afferent fibers that make direct or indirect connections with visceral efferent neurons in the intermediolateral gray column of the sacral region (Fig. 177). The axons of the efferent neurons reach the bladder or bowel by way of the pelvic nerves and plexuses and produce relaxation of the internal sphincter together with contraction of the smooth musculature of the wall of the viscus.

Subacute combined degeneration as it occurs in pernicious anemia has been described and the resulting sensory disturbances have been enumerated. The sensory disturbances were attributed to degeneration in the posterior funiculi. The associated degeneration in the lateral funiculi involves the lateral corticospinal tracts (Fig. 178*A*). In addition to loss of vibratory and position senses, the sense of movement, and two-point discrimination, the patient may exhibit gradually increasing stiffness and weakness of his limbs and hyperactive deep reflexes. The motor symptoms are particularly evident in the lower extremities or may be confined to them. The abdominal reflex usually is absent or diminished, and the Babinski sign is likely to be present bilaterally. The external sphincters are eventually involved unless the disease is controlled, which results in varying degrees of incontinence. A flaccid type of motor loss with decreased deep reflexes is also described as occurring in pernicious anemia and is attributed to peripheral neuritis.

Lateral sclerosis is a condition of unknown etiology in which the lateral corticospinal tracts are selectively and progressively involved in a degenerative process (Fig. 178*B*). There are no sensory disturbances but the limbs, and particularly the lower limbs, are eventually paralyzed with increased deep reflexes and spasticity.

Anterior poliomyelitis, resulting in partial or complete destruction of anterior gray column cells, is a common cause of flaccid paralysis. In this condition muscles whose motor neurons have been completely destroyed are markedly atrophied. Loss of deep reflexes is associated with the atrophy. In the bulbar type of poliomyelitis the gray matter of the medulla is affected with the result that vital functions are interfered with. Although referred to as "bulbar poliomyelitis," this type of involvement might better be termed "polioencephalitis." The use of the former term arises from the fact that the bulbar syndrome is caused by the same virus that is responsible for the more common involvement of the spinal cord. Spasticity of the muscles (increased resistance to passive movement) and exaggerated deep reflexes are observed during the earlier stages of poliomyelitis. These manifestations have been attributed to irritation of the anterior horn cells by the poliomyelitis virus or to destruction of internuncial cells within the spinal gray matter; the latter explanation is based on the hypothesis that the normal inhibitory effects, transmitted from reticulospinal and proprioceptive pathways to anterior horn cells by the internuncial cells, are interrupted. It has been demonstrated, in monkeys inoculated with poliomyelitis virus, that neither virus activity nor lesions in the spinal cord are necessary for

the production of the spasticity of acute poliomyelitis; it was concluded, on the basis of serial sections of the brains of these monkeys, that brain lesions were responsible for the spasticity observed. It was suggested, since lesions were present in the reticular formation of the hindbrain, that destruction of these areas may be responsible, at least in part, for generalized spasticity because of elimination of many "inhibitor" neurons.

Transection of the cauda equina accounts for flaccid paralysis of the lower extremities. It is important to remember that the roots of the cauda equina form peripheral nerves and that they will regenerate if they are sutured. Tumors arising in the lower part of the spinal canal also cause paralysis through pressure on the cauda equina; removal of such a tumor relieves the pressure and permits regeneration and return of function of the nerves.

The cauda has been sectioned in dogs and the effects of the procedure on the bladder have been studied. It was found that the bladder was "atypically" autonomous, i.e., due to loss of normal motor innervation, it functions through its intrinsic nerve plexuses independent of the central nervous system. In spite of dilatation and flaccidity of its musculature, the bladder is at least partially evacuated when the intravesical pressure is sufficiently increased.

Amyotrophic lateral sclerosis, of unknown etiology, affects the lateral funiculi and the anterior column cells (Fig. 178*C*). In typical cases, signs of involvement of descending motor fibers—spasticity, hyperactive deep reflexes, and the Babinski sign—are observed in the lower extremities. In the upper extremities muscle atrophy is seen in paradoxical conjunction with hyperactive reflexes. The muscle atrophy usually appears first in the intrinsic muscles of the hands. As muscle atrophy progresses the hyperactive reflexes give way to flaccidity and loss of deep reflexes; when this occurs, it indicates that the motor neurons have been irreparably damaged and the effects of degeneration in the lateral descending tracts can therefore no longer be seen in the muscles. Bulbar paralysis (soft palate, pharynx, larynx, and tongue), owing to involvement of motor neurons in the nuclei of the medulla, is a serious and constant complication of the disease and contributes significantly to its fatal termination.

BIBLIOGRAPHY

Bodian, D., 1946: Experimental evidence on the cerebral origin of muscle spasticity in acute poliomyelitis. Proc. Soc. Exp. Biol. Med., 61, 170–175.

Cannon, B. W., Magoun, H. W., and Windle, W. F., 1944: Paralysis with hypotonicity and hyperreflexia subsequent to section of the basis pedunculi in monkeys. J. Neurophysiol., 7, 425–437.

Carpenter, M. B., McMasters, R. E., and Hanna, G. R., 1963: Disturbances of conjugate horizontal eye movements in the monkey. I. Physiological effects and anatomical degeneration resulting from lesions of the abducens nucleus and nerve. Arch. Neurol. (Chicago), 8, 231–247.

Fisher, C. M., and Curry, H. B., 1965: Pure motor hemiplegia of vascular origin. Arch. Neurol. (Chicago), 13, 30–44.

Guttmann, L., 1952: Studies on reflex activity of the isolated cord in the spinal man. J. Nerv. Ment. Dis., 116, 957–972.

Hagbarth, K. E., and Kerr, D. I. B., 1954: Central influences on spinal afferent conduction. J. Neurophysiol., 17, 295–307.

Jacobson, C. E., Jr., 1942: Neurogenic vesical dysfunction: an experimental study. Proc. Staff Meet. Mayo Clin., 17, 286–288.

Kuhn, R. A., 1950: Functional capacity of the isolated human spinal cord. Brain, 75, 1–51.

Lawrence, D. G., and Kuypers, H. G. J. M., 1968: The functional organization of the motor system in the monkey. I. The effects of bilateral pyramidal lesions. II. The effects of lesions of descending brain-stem pathways. Brain, 91, 1–36.

Ruch, T. C., 1936: Evidence of the non-segmental character of spinal reflexes from an analysis of the cephalad effects of spinal transection (Scheff-Sherrington phenomenon). Amer. J. Physiol., 114, 457–467.

Ruch, T. C., Patton, H. D., Woodbury, S. W., and Towe, A. W., 1961: Neurophysiology. W. B. Saunders Co., Philadelphia.

Sherrington, C. S., 1906: The Integrative Action of the Nervous System. Yale University Press, New Haven, Conn.

Walshe, F. M. R., 1947: Diseases of the Nervous System. 5th ed. Williams & Wilkins Co., Baltimore.

White, R. J., Schreiner, L. H., Hughes, R. A., MacCarty, C. S., and Grindlay, J. H., 1959: Physiologic consequences of total hemispherectomy in the monkey. Neurology, 9, 149–159.

Chapter 19

The Cerebellum

The **cerebellum** ("little cerebrum") is a massive, organized accumulation of neurons located above the medulla oblongata and pons (Fig. 179) and is covered superiorly by the cerebral hemispheres (Fig. 1). It is a suprasegmental apparatus that is connected with the brain stem by three distinct bundles of nerve fibers, the *inferior, middle,* and *superior cerebellar peduncles* (Fig. 55). It will be recalled that these three peduncles also are known as the restiform body, brachium pontis, and brachium conjunctivum respectively. The cerebellum plays important roles in the regulation of reflex tonus of skeletal musculature, in the control of voluntary activity, and in the maintenance of equilibrium. In fact, it has been considered as the head ganglion of the proprioceptive

system. Situated posterior to the brain stem and between the spinal cord and cerebral hemispheres and having many afferent and efferent connections with these parts, it is in a favored position to serve in the control of muscle tonus and in the regulation of movement. The major subdivisions of the cerebellum are the median unpaired vermis and the paired lateral hemispheres (Fig. 180). This division into median and lateral parts is more apparent on the underside. The surface of the cerebellum is comprised of numerous folia with intervening sulci and fissures that extend transversely across the hemispheres and vermis (Figs. 179, 180). The deeper transverse depressions (fissures) have been employed for making secondary subdivisions of the vermis and

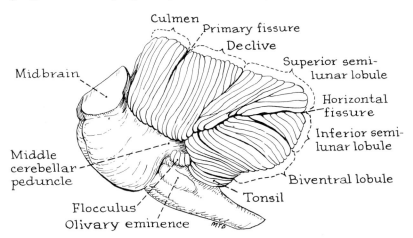

FIG. 179. Drawing of the cerebellum and the pons and medulla from the left side, inferolateral view.

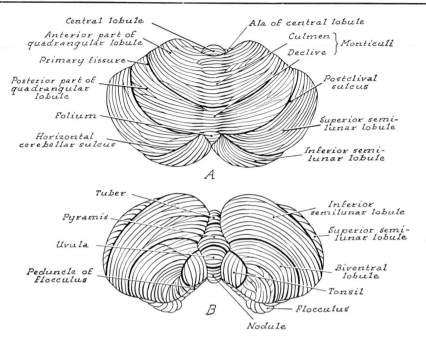

FIG. 180. A, Superior surface of the cerebellum; B, inferior surface of the cerebellum so oriented with relation to A as to indicate the continuity of folium and tuber (modified from Sobotta-McMurrich).

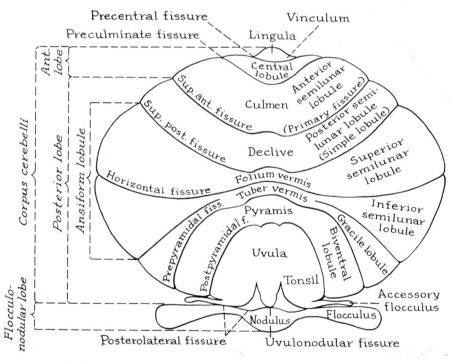

FIG. 181. Diagram of the human cerebellum (modified from Larsell, 1951).

hemispheres. The names given these parts by earlier investigators were based on their shape and have no functional significance. Furthermore, there was little agreement among these investigators in naming the parts, with the resultant confusion that exists in cerebellar terminology. One of the more common systems of terminology applied to the lobules of the cerebellum is given on the right side of Figure 181. This diagram, used in conjunction with the sagittal section (Fig. 182) and with the superior and inferior views of the cerebellum (Fig. 180*A, B*), serves to establish appropriate landmarks and boundaries of the larger gross divisions (lobes) that are shown on the left side of Figure 181. To identify the various lobules and fissures, perhaps it is most satisfactory to begin with the sagittal section and trace the fissures laterally. The postnodular fissure and its lateral extension (the posterolateral fissure) are the first to appear in embryonic development, and they separate the *flocculonodular* lobe from the remainder of the cerebellum or *corpus cerebelli*. The flocculonodular lobe, which has predominantly vestibular connections, is often called *archicerebellum,* denoting its early phylo-

genetic appearance. The superior anterior fissure (primary fissure) divides the corpus cerebelli into anterior lobe and posterior lobe. The *anterior lobe* and the *pyramis* and *uvula* comprise the *paleocerebellum,* which primarily receives proprioceptive and exteroceptive information from the head and body. The *posterior lobe,* except for the pyramis and uvula, is considered as *neocerebellum.* The neocerebellum developed phylogenetically in conjunction with the cerebral cortex, which is reflected in its extensive cortical connections through the corticopontile system. (See page 216 for a further consideration of this subdivision based on the phylogenetic concept.)

Sections of the cerebellum show that, like the cerebrum, it consists of a cortex, a core of white matter, and deeply buried nuclei (Figs. 183, 184). The cerebellar cortex, however, has a uniform structure throughout, and there are no described cytoarchitectonic subdivisions. The cerebellar nuclei are buried in the core of white matter. The largest and most laterally placed nucleus, on both sides, is the *dentate* (Fig. 184); it is similar in appearance to the inferior olivary nucleus. The *emboliform nucleus* is located in the

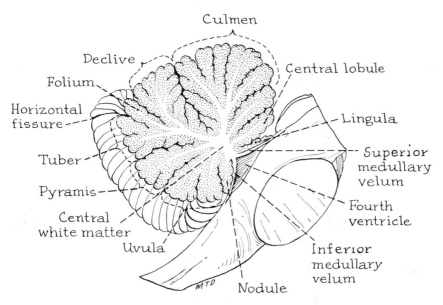

FIG. 182. Sagittal section of the cerebellum illustrating the lobules of the vermis.

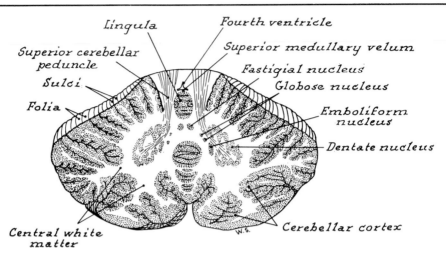

FIG. 183. Horizontal section of the cerebellum showing the arrangement of the cortical gray matter, and the locations of the central nuclei within the white matter (after Sobotta-McMurrich).

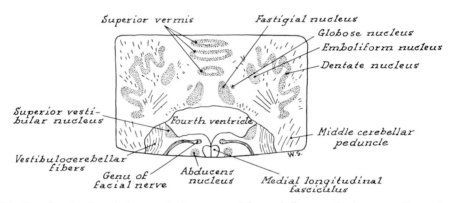

FIG. 184. Frontal section through the central white matter of the cerebellum at a level corresponding to that of the abducens nucleus in the pons showing the position and relations of the cerebellar nuclei (modified from Braus).

medially directed hilus of the dentate nucleus, and the *globose nucleus* is medial to it. The *fastigial* or *tectal nuclei* lie on both sides of the midline, in the roof of the fourth ventricle. Together the globose and emboliform nuclei are often called *nucleus interpositus,* particularly in lower mammals.

Histologically, the cerebellar cortex consists of two layers: the outermost, the *molecular;* and the innermost, the *granular* (Fig. 185). The molecular cell layer has many processes from neurons located in the deeper cerebellar layers and therefore is primarily a region of synapses. There are a few scattered stellate cells in the upper levels of the molecular layer

and more numerous, deeply placed ones that are called *"basket cells."* The axons of the basket cells course above the Purkinje cells in a plane at right angles to the long axis of the *folia* and give off many collaterals. The most conspicuous are the descending collaterals that form the synaptic networks or "baskets" about the **Purkinje cells.**

The Purkinje cells are large neurons arranged in a single cell layer within the deepest part of the molecular layers. These cells are the efferent neurons of the cerebellar cortex and their axons project to the cerebellar nuclei. Recurrent collaterals arise from the axons and some are believed to terminate on other Pur-

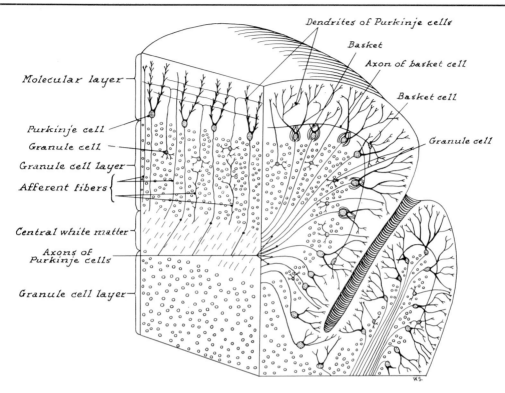

FIG. 185. Diagrammatic representation of a longitudinal section of a cerebellar folium (*left*) and of cross-sections of two adjacent folia (*right*) showing histologic and synaptic details (modified from Braus).

kinje cells. The dendrites of the Purkinje cells extend into the molecular layer where they branch profusely, always in the transverse plane of the folium. Thus, their extent of branching is observed only in sections cut at right angles to the long axis of the folium.

The inner layer of the cerebellar cortex is called the *granular layer* because of the numerous small, closely packed cells—the granule cells (Fig. 185). A typical granule cell has three to six short, slender dendrites that end in claw-like terminals. The axon is longer and extends into the molecular layer where it exhibits a T-shaped bifurcation giving rise to *parallel fibers*. These terminals course parallel to the long axis of the folium and synapse with spines on the dendritic branches of the Purkinje cells. The relations of the numerous parallel fibers with dendrites of many Purkinje cells provide the anatomical substrate for

the diffusion or spread of incoming impulses as well as for convergence. It has been estimated that a parallel fiber, 3 mm. in length, may contact the spines of 460 Purkinje cells.

Afferent fibers to the cerebellum usually are considered to be of two types, *mossy* and *climbing fibers*. Mossy fibers synapse with the claw-like terminals of three or more granule cells. There has been considerable uncertainty relative to the origin of the climbing fibers, but recent studies confirm that they arise from the inferior olivary complex of nuclei. Except for the system of olivocerebellar fibers, it appears that all incoming cerebellar fibers are of the mossy type.

The climbing fibers follow the dendritic arborization of the Purkinje cells and make synaptic contact with the smooth branches of the dendrites that are excitatory connections. Collateral branches of climbing fibers are reported to make connections with other cell types in the cerebellar cortex.

In addition to the granule cells, less numerous large stellate cells are present in the granule cell layer. Their dendritic terminals are in the molecular layer, and their axonic terminals synapse with the claw-shaped endings of the granule cells.

The **primary intrinsic circuits** of the cerebellum may be summarized as follows: Afferent mossy fibers synapse with terminals of granule cells which, through their parallel fibers, make contact with dendritic terminals of the Purkinje cells as well as with the dendrites of basket and stellate cells. The basket cells synapse with many Purkinje cells in the transverse plane, and the stellate cells are believed to activate other granule cells. The Purkinje cells provide the output from the cerebellar cortex through their axons to the cerebellar nuclei. This output may be modified by the recurrent collaterals of the Purkinje cells. Additionally, association fibers have been described that interconnect different regions of the cerebellar cortex.

The **major afferent pathways** of the cerebellum from the spinal cord and brain stem include *vestibulocerebellar fibers,* the *posterior* and *anterior spino-* *cerebellar tracts, superficial arcuate fibers,* the *spinoolivocerebellar system, reticulocerebellar* and *trigeminocerebellar fibers* (Figs. 186–188). Except for the vestibulocerebellar system, these tracts largely transmit proprioceptive impulses, although some carry, in addition, tactile and probably other sensory information as will be indicated. Other cerebellar afferents include *tectocerebellar fibers* from the tectum of the midbrain. The largest group of cerebellar afferents is the *corticopontocerebellar system* (Fig. 189).

Vestibulocerebellar fibers (Fig. 62), including both direct vestibular root fibers and secondary ones from the vestibular nuclei, end in the flocculonodular lobe and to a lesser extent in the lingula and uvula (Fig. 181). Some vestibular fibers terminate directly in the fastigial nuclei; others end in relation to granule cells. The course of the vestibulocerebellar fibers to the cerebellum through the medial part of the inferior cerebellar peduncle has been described (Chap. 9).

The *posterior spinocerebellar tract (of Flechsig)* is largely an uncrossed tract, which is made up of the axons of neurons whose cell bodies are in the *thoracic nucleus* (dorsal nucleus) (Figs. 35, 186). This column of nerve cells is found at the

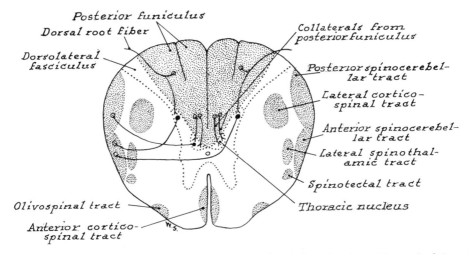

FIG. 186.   Diagram of a cross-section through upper thoracic spinal cord illustrating the positions and relations of the spinocerebellar tracts. Collaterals from the dorsal root fibers to posterior horn cells and from the posterior funiculi to the thoracic nucleus are shown. The components of the spinocerebellar tracts are traced from their cells of origin.

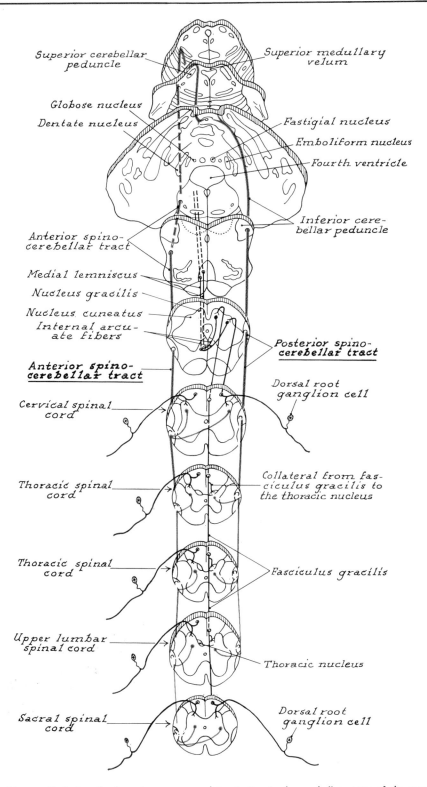

FIG. 187. Diagram illustrating the formation, course, and termination in the cerebellar cortex of the posterior and anterior spinocerebellar tracts.

point of junction of the posterior gray column with the posterior gray commissure in the upper two lumbar and in all of the thoracic segments of the spinal cord. Its cells receive collaterals from the posterior funiculi and, as stated above, send their axons into the posterior spinocerebellar tracts. The uncrossed component of the posterior spinocerebellar tract is greater than its crossed component. The tract occupies a position in the lateral funiculus of the cord between the lateral corticospinal tract and the periphery. In the medulla it migrates posteriorly and enters the inferior cerebellar peduncle through which it terminates in the cerebellum (Fig. 187). Proprioceptive impulses from the lower extremities and trunk reach the cerebellum by way of this tract.

The *anterior spinocerebellar tract* is composed of axons from the contra- and ipsilateral dorsal funicular gray (Fig. 187). In the lower lumbar and sacral regions a column of cells, similar in appearance and location to the thoracic nucleus at more rostral levels, has been designated Stilling's nucleus; it appears to contribute fibers to the anterior spinocerebellar tract. The number of crossed fibers in the anterior spinocerebellar tract is greater than the number of uncrossed fibers. The tract is situated peripherally in the lateral funiculus immediately ventral to the posterior spinocerebellar tract (Fig. 186). The anterior spinocerebellar tract and the spinotectal and lateral spinothalamic tracts constitute what is sometimes called *Gowers' tract*. The posterior horn cells, whose axons contribute to the formation of the anterior spinocerebellar tract, receive collaterals from the medial divisions of the dorsal roots at all levels of the spinal cord. The electrical activity in the tract, produced by stimulation of peripheral nerves, indicates representation of the four limbs (monkey and cat) as follows: contralateral hind limb maximally, ipsi- and contralateral

forelimbs less and approximately equally, and ipsilateral hind limb minimally.

The topographical pattern of localization in the anterior spinocerebellar tract is similar to that in the lateral spinothalamic tract with those fibers arising at sacral and lumbar levels most posterolaterally placed, those from thoracic levels in an intermediate position, and those from cervical spinal cord segments most anteromedially located. In the caudal medulla the anterior spinocerebellar tract maintains its anterior position with relation to the posterior spinocerebellar tract, but when the latter tract curves posteriorly in the inferior cerebellar peduncle, the anterior spinocerebellar fibers continue rostrally through the medulla and the tegmentum of the pons to the level of the junction of pons and midbrain. At this point they turn posteriorly around the lateral side of the superior cerebellar peduncle and enter the superior medullary velum through which they course to the cerebellum (Fig. 187). The anterior spinocerebellar tract is often referred to as the *indirect spinocerebellar tract,* because it doubles back on itself and enters the cerebellum from its rostral side. Proprioceptive impulses reach the cerebellum from the trunk as well as from all four extremities by way of the anterior spinocerebellar tracts.

Spinocerebellar fibers terminate chiefly in the vermis and paravermal portions of the anterior lobe. Most *anterior spinocerebellar fibers* end in the central lobule and culmen. The anterior spinocerebellar fibers from the lumbar regions terminate anteriorly to those from the cervical levels of the spinal cord. The *posterior spinocerebellar tracts* distribute fibers to the *central lobule, culmen, pyramis, uvula,* and *declive*. Spinocerebellar fibers end in relation to granule cells (Fig. 185). It is probable that the spinocerebellar tracts transmit exteroceptive impulses as well as proprioceptive information.

The **dorsal external arcuate fibers** (Fig. 188) are axons of cells in the *lateral*

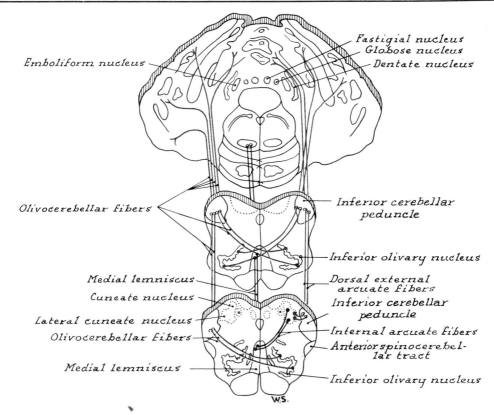

Emboliform nucleus

Fastigial nucleus
Globose nucleus
Dentate nucleus

Olivocerebellar fibers

Inferior cerebellar peduncle

Inferior olivary nucleus

Medial lemniscus
Cuneate nucleus
Lateral cuneate nucleus
Olivocerebellar fibers

Dorsal external arcuate fibers
Inferior cerebellar peduncle
Internal arcuate fibers
Anterior spinocerebellar tract

Medial lemniscus

Inferior olivary nucleus

W.S.

FIG. 188.   Diagram of the connections from the lateral cuneate and olivary nuclei to the cerebellum.

cuneate nucleus. The lateral cuneate nucleus, characterized by large cells like those in the thoracic nucleus, lies immediately lateral to the rostral part of the main cuneate nucleus (Fig. 43). The dorsal external arcuate fibers enter the cerebellum by way of the inferior cerebellar peduncle and probably are concerned particularly with proprioceptive and exteroceptive impulses from the neck. It will be remembered that proprioceptive and tactile impulses reach the main and lateral cuneate nuclei by way of the fasciculus cuneatus, and that those reaching the main nucleus are relayed upward to the thalamus through the internal arcuate fibers and the contralateral medial lemniscus. It now becomes evident that the impulses from the neck region at least, and possibly those from the upper extremities and upper part of the trunk, are also relayed to the cerebellum from

these nuclei. The ventral superficial arcuate fibers (Fig. 52) arise from the *arcuate nucleus* (Fig. 43) (probably a caudal extension of the pontine gray) and from reticular cells in the lateral part of the medulla. These fibers also enter the cerebellum through the inferior cerebellar peduncle.

As classically described, the **spinoolivary tract** originates in the spinal cord, probably from posterior horn cells of the opposite side. It lies in the anterior funiculus where its fibers are intermingled with olivospinal fibers (Fig. 186); the latter arise in the olivary nucleus and end in relation to anterior horn cells. The spinoolivary tract terminates in the inferior olivary nucleus.

Olivocerebellar fibers originate in the *main* and *accessory olivary nuclei;* practically all of them cross to the opposite side through the median raphé of the medulla and enter the cerebellum by way of the inferior cerebellar peduncle of that side (Fig. 188). The decussating olivocerebellar fibers are intermingled with those from the nuclei gracilis and cuneatus and therefore are included in the category of internal arcuate fibers. Olivocerebellar fibers are distributed to all parts of the cerebellar cortex. Afferent impulses from the spinal cord thus may reach the paleo- and neocerebellum through the combined system of *spinoolivary* and *olivocerebellar fibers* (Fig. 188).

Reticulocerebellar fibers from both the medial and lateral reticular areas of the brain stem have been described. In the cat these fibers have been shown to be quite extensive. In addition to the lateral reticular nucleus (Fig. 52) and the lateral tegmental area of the pons in such a system, a "paramedian reticular nucleus" (medial to the middle-third of the olivary nucleus) has been described that projects to the cerebellum through both uncrossed and crossed fibers with the uncrossed contingent being the more extensive. There is evidence that the paramedian reticular nucleus receives afferent fibers from the spinal cord as well as descending afferents from higher brain stem centers.

Trigeminocerebellar fibers are believed to arise from the chief sensory and mesencephalic nuclei of the trigeminal nerve and enter the cerebellum with the anterior spinocerebellar fibers. *Tectocerebellar fibers* from the midbrain tectum have

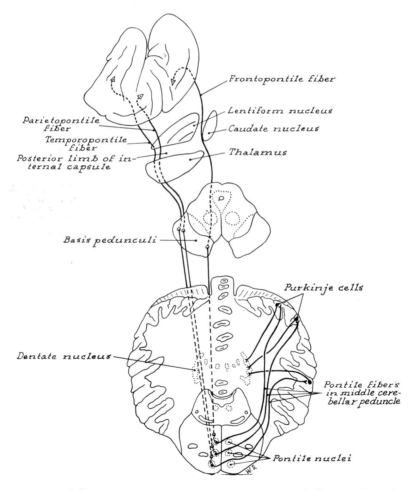

FIG. 189. Corticopontocerebellar connections. The origin and course of corticopontile fibers are shown diagrammatically.

been described that course to the cerebellum along the medial aspect of the superior cerebellar peduncle.

The **corticopontocerebellar system** of fibers is primarily related, both phylogenetically and ontogenetically, to the development of the neocortex and cerebellar hemispheres (neocerebellum). Thus, it is most highly developed in man. Corticopontine fibers arise particularly from the motor and premotor areas of the frontal lobe, and lesser numbers arise from the temporal, parietal, and occipital lobes (Fig. 189). *Frontopontile fibers* course caudally through the anterior limb of the internal capsule and the medial one-fifth of the basis pedunculi, whereas the *temporo-, parieto-, and occipitopontile fibers* traverse the posterior limb of the internal capsule and the lateral one-fifth of the basis pedunculi (Fig. 189). On reaching the basilar part of the pons, all corticopontile fibers synapse on the neurons whose cell bodies form the pontile nuclei. Pontocerebellar fibers originate in the pontile nuclei, decussate to the opposite side, and enter the cerebellum by way of the middle cerebellar peduncle (Figs. 62, 189). The great majority of these pontile fibers terminate in the neocerebellar cortex and some project to the paleocerebellum. It has been reported that all parts of the vermis except the nodule receive pontocerebellar fibers.

It is now well established that, in addition to proprioceptive stimuli, the cerebellum receives projections from tactile, auditory, and visual systems. These sensory-receiving areas are shown in Figures 190 and 191. It is believed that the reticulocerebellar system of fibers is involved in the relay of exteroceptive information as well as proprioceptive stimuli from the brain stem reticular substance to the cerebellar cortex. This seems likely since, for example, it is known that the ascending sensory systems of the cord give collaterals to the reticular nuclei of the brain stem. That the brain stem centers serve as relay stations for exteroceptive sensory information to the cerebellum is in accord with studies that show that the fifth nerve with its brain stem nuclei is responsible for a tactile projection from the face

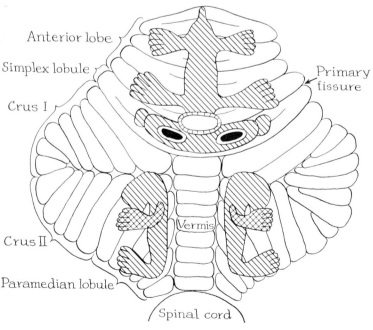

FIG. 190.   Schematic drawing illustrating the areas of projection of tactile impulses on the cerebellum of the cat (from Snider, 1952).

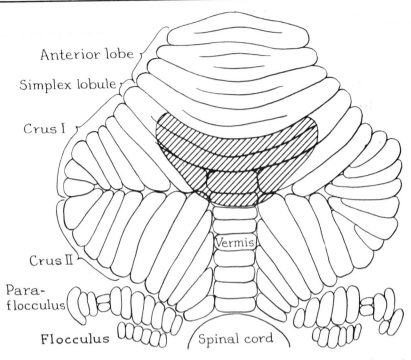

FIG. 191. Schematic drawing showing the area of projection of auditory and visual impulses on the cerebellum of the cat (from Snider, 1952).

to cerebellum. Additionally, the visual and auditory systems have been shown to use brain stem nuclei for relay of stimuli to cerebellum, the superior colliculus for visual, and the inferior colliculus and/or dorsal cochlear nucleus for auditory.

Reference was made to the fact that the *Purkinje cells* are the efferent neurons of the cerebellar cortex and that these project to the cerebellar nuclei. Recent studies have shown that the pattern of projection as well as the arrangement of nuclei in relation to the cortex is such that the cerebellum can be divided into a series of *longitudinal zones: medial, intermediate,* and *lateral* (Fig. 192). It may be noted that the medial, or *vermal cortex,* projects to the *fastigial* (medial) *nuclei* and to the *vestibular nuclei.* The intermediate, or *paravermal cortex,* projects to the *interpositus nuclei (globose and emboliform),* and the lateral cortical zone projects to the *dentate* (lateral) *nuclei.* The functional significance of these anatomical zones has been estab-

lished in the cat. These studies have shown that median zone (vermal cortex and fastigial nuclei) are concerned with postural tone, equilibrium, and movement of the entire body, and that the whole body is represented in each half of the vermis. The intermediate zone (paravermal cortex and nucleus interpositus) is concerned with discrete movements and postural reflexes of the ipsilateral limbs. These two cerebellar mechanisms were considered to fall into the functional classifications of motor activity known respectively as extrapyramidal and pyramidal.

It is apparent that the fastigial nuclei (Fig. 192) receive projections from all divisions of the vermian cortex, areas of the paleocerebellum in which the spinocerebellar tracts end. They also receive some fibers from the vestibular nerve and nuclei. The fastigial nuclei give origin to the fastigiobulbar tracts, which contain both crossed and uncrossed fibers—chiefly the latter. The *fastigiobulbar tract* (of both sides) descends in the medial part of the inferior cerebellar peduncle, where its component fibers are intermingled with vestibulocerebellar fibers; it is distributed to the lateral and spinal vestibular nuclei and to cells in the reticular formation (Fig. 193). This system of fibers includes cerebelloolivary fibers to the inferior olivary nuclei. One bundle of fastigiobulbar fibers winds around the superior cerebellar peduncle before joining the main tract and is designated the *uncinate fasciculus* (*of Russell*). Efferent impulses, on reaching the vestibular nuclei and reticular formation by way of the fastigiobulbar tract, may be relayed to anterior horn cells of the spinal cord through the *vestibulospinal* and *reticulo-* *spinal tracts* or may be returned to the cerebellum by way of vestibulocerebellar or reticulocerebellar fibers and thus participate in closed (reverberating) circuits. The close functional interrelationship between the reticular formation and the anterior lobe of the cerebellum, in the cat, is indicated by the observation that stimulation of the lateral reticular formation of the nucleus interpositus, or of the lateral cortical area of the anterior lobe results in ipsilateral extension and contralateral flexion. Stimulation of the medial reticular formation, fastigial nucleus, or medial cortical area produces a reciprocal type of reaction—ipsilateral flexion and contralateral extension.

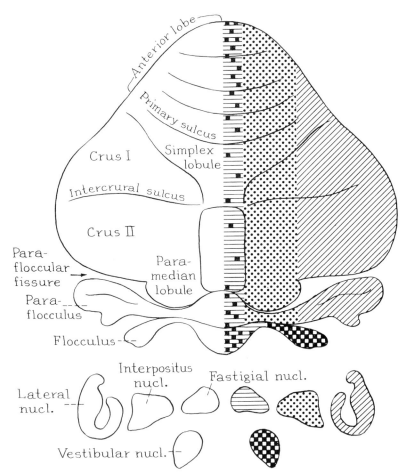

FIG. 192. Diagram of the corticonuclear zones in the primate cerebellum. The medial or vermal zone (horizontal lines) projects to the fastigial nucleus and to the vestibular nuclei; the intermediate or paravermal zone (stippled) projects to the interpositus nucleus; and the lateral zone (diagonal lines) projects to the dentate nucleus (from Jansen and Brodal, 1954).

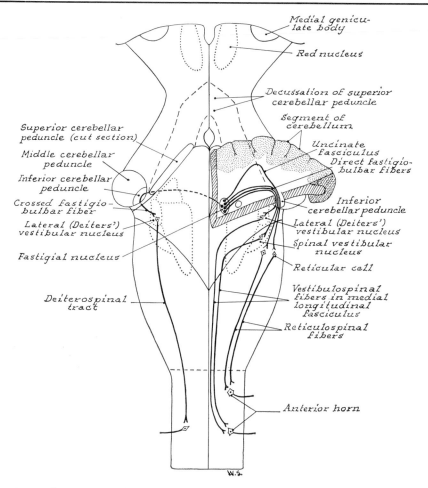

FIG. 193. Diagram of portions of the brain stem and spinal cord with a segment of cerebellum superimposed showing the fastigiovestibulospinal and fastigioreticulospinal connections.

The literature is controversial relative to the contribution of the fastigial nucleus to fibers in the superior cerebellar peduncle. It has been reported that in the cat there is a fastigial component to the superior peduncle. From studies on the monkey, hcwever, it was concluded that few, if any, fibers from the fastigial nuclei enter the superior cerebellar peduncle.

The cerebellar reflex arc, beginning with proprioceptors in muscles and contributed to by the posterior and anterior spinocerebellar tracts, the cerebellar cortex, the fastigial nucleus, and the vestibulospinal and reticulospinal tracts, aids in the maintenance of bilaterally balanced tonicity between extensor and flexor muscles of the neck, trunk, and lower extremities, which is essential to the upright posture. The arc may also participate in the regulation of muscular activity by controlling the tone of the muscles antagonistic to those furnishing the positive force in a given voluntary or reflex act; overaction of the agonists and protagonists is thereby prevented and smooth movements are facilitated.

Efferent fibers from the flocculus are distributed exclusively to the superior and lateral vestibular nuclei, and those from the *nodule* and *uvula* go to the fastigial nucleus, the dorsal reticular formation of the medulla, all the vestibular nuclei, and a few to the medial longitudinal fasciculi.

A cerebellar arc, involving these areas of cerebellar cortex, is thus seen to be superimposed on the simple vestibulospinal and vestibuloocular reflex arcs previously described (Chap. 9). It has been noted that unilateral destruction of the lateral vestibular nucleus, in the decerebrate animal, results in ipsilateral flexion and contralateral extension of the limbs similar to that following a fastigial lesion.

Nucleus interpositus (the combined globose and emboliform nuclei) receives Purkinje axons predominantly from the paravermian cortical zone (Fig. 192). It is apparent that this nucleus serves as the primary efferent nucleus for the paleocerebellum, although it receives fibers from the medial part of the neocerebellum. Fibers from the interpositus and dentate nuclei enter the superior cerebellar peduncle (Fig. 194). In the monkey, the dorsal two-thirds of the superior peduncle is reported to contain fibers from nucleus interpositus and the dorsal part of the dentate nucleus, and the ventrolateral third contains fibers from the ventral and lateral portion of the dentate nucleus. The superior cerebellar peduncle exits from the cerebellum through the isthmus region of the pons, lateral to the

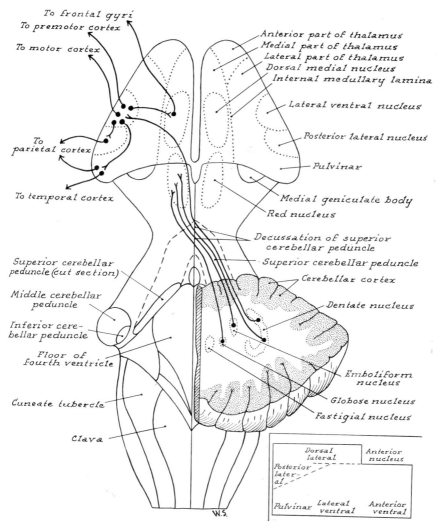

FIG. 194. Diagram showing the connections between the cerebellar nuclei and the red nucleus, and those between the cerebellar nuclei and the thalamus. Inset (after Ranson) is a lateral projection of thalamic nuclei.

superior medullary velum (Figs. 66, 194). It courses anteriorly and medially into the tegmentum of the midbrain and decussates at the level of the inferior colliculi (Figs. 68, 94, 170). After decussating, a smaller descending and a larger ascending limb are recognized. In the monkey, fibers from the descending limb are reported to arise mainly, if not exclusively, from the interposed and dorsal part of the dentate nucleus. These fibers have been followed into the medial longitudinal fasciculus, to tegmental and reticular nuclei of the brain stem, to the inferior olivary nuclei, and a few fibers to the cervical segments of the cord. The ascending limb, composed of fibers from the ventral and lateral parts of the dentate nucleus and from nucleus interpositus, has been traced to the contralateral red nucleus, lateral ventral nucleus of the thalamus, and to globus pallidus.

From the **red nucleus, inferior olivary nucleus, tegmental and reticular nuclei** of the brain stem, the descending pathways for the relay of cerebellar impulses to other brain stem centers and the spinal cord include the rubrospinal, olivospinal, and reticulospinal tracts. They were considered in Chapter 17 in relation to the extrapyramidal system.

The lateral zone of the cerebellum in particular, and the intermediate zone to a lesser extent, can influence motor activity at the level of the cerebral cortex. As indicated, these zones project to the interpositus and dentate nuclei (Fig. 192) that, in turn, provide a major input into the *lateral ventral nucleus* of the thalamus via the superior cerebellar peduncle (the major component coming from the dentate nucleus). Fibers from the red nucleus also reach the lateral ventral nucleus. The lateral ventral nucleus sends fibers through the internal capsule to the motor and premotor areas of the cerebral cortex (Fig. 194). Through this nucleus the neocerebellum, and the paleocerebellum to a lesser extent, can influence motor activity at the level of the cortical neurons.

Through internuclear connections within the thalamus, cerebellar impulses may be conducted from the lateral ventral nucleus to the lateral part of the *dorsal medial nucleus* in the medial part of the thalamus, to the *dorsal lateral* and *posterior lateral nuclei* in the lateral part of the thalamus, and to the *pulvinar* (Fig. 194). The lateral ventral nucleus sends fibers to the frontal gyri of the cerebrum. The dorsal and posterior lateral nuclei send fibers to the parietal lobules, and the pulvinar projects on the parietal and temporal lobes. It will be recalled that all these cortical areas give origin to extrapyramidal fibers (Chap. 17).

In the foregoing discussion of cerebellar structure and function, brief references have been made relative to the projection of impulses other than proprioceptive to the cerebellum. During recent years, a number of studies have shown that tactile areas exist in the cerebellar cortex. In accord with these studies, the conduction of tactile impulses has been demonstrated from the hairs around the foot pads of cats to the *paramedian lobules* of the cerebellum by way of both posterior and anterior spinocerebellar tracts. The projection of tactile impulses is ipsilateral with a somatotropic pattern of localization (Fig. 190). The body surface is represented in the anterior lobe and bilaterally in the posterior lobe. Auditory and visual areas in the cerebellum have also been demonstrated (Fig. 191). Significantly, there is evidence that motor, tactile, auditory, and visual areas in the cerebrum project to these same cerebellar areas, which in turn project back on the cerebral areas.

In **summary,** it may be said that the cerebellum receives a great variety of sensory impulses that are there monitored and/or coordinated. In turn, the cerebellum projects the synthesized or appropriate impulses to the motor centers of the brain stem, spinal cord, and cerebral cortex to control the motoneurons (Fig. 195). The expression of control is in the

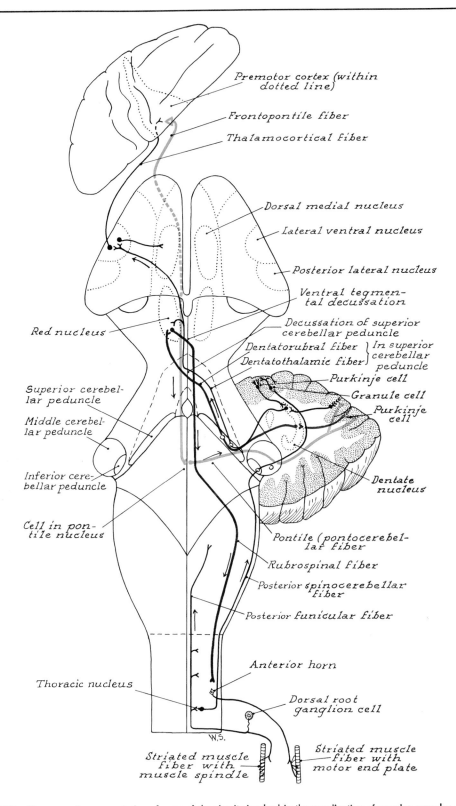

FIG. 195. Diagrammatic representation of some of the circuits involved in the coordination of complex muscular activity.

15

maintenance of equilibrium; in the maintenance of muscle tone (e.g., necessary for standing); and in the control of voluntary movements. The flocculonodular lobe primarily is concerned with vestibular mechanisms. The medial (vermal-fastigial) zone is concerned with postural mechanisms—equilibrium and movement of the entire body. The intermediate zone (paravermal-interpositus) is concerned with discrete movements and postural reflexes of the ipsilateral limbs. The lateral-dentate zone, which is most highly developed in primates, is particularly concerned with the control of discrete voluntary movements of the limbs. The signs of cerebellar disease are given in the next chapter and should serve to clarify these control mechanisms.

It is appropriate to add a few remarks relative to the more conventional division of the cerebellum into transverse zones versus the longitudinal division that has been given and that is based on recent anatomical and physiological studies.

The transverse division separating the flocculonodular lobe (archicerebellum) from the corpus cerebelli is justified, since the flocculonodular lobe is apparently concerned with vestibular phenomena only. However, for the *corpus cerebelli* division into the three longitudinal zones is more meaningful, as is indicated above. This is further supported by the signs and symptoms of cerebellar lesions in man. It should be emphasized, however, that there are no sharp boundaries between these longitudinal zones. Additionally, it may be said that, with respect to the phylogenetic considerations of the cerebellum, the medial zone of corpus cerebelli is roughly comparable to the parts long considered as paleocerebellum, and the intermediate and lateral zones are comparable to the neocerebellum. On the basis of fiber connections however, these subdivisions are not distinguishable, since pontocerebellar connections are distributed to paleocerebellum as well as neocerebellum. The advisability of upholding the terms paleo- and neocerebellum due to the difficulty of defining them precisely has been questioned.

The potential circuits involving the cerebellum and other brain and cord centers (Fig. 195) provide prime examples of neural loops that are involved in control mechanisms that may be compared with *servomechanisms*. This is particularly well illustrated in the case of reciprocal cerebellocerebral connections.

BIBLIOGRAPHY

Adrian, E. D., 1943: Afferent areas in the cerebellum connected with the limbs. Brain, *66,* 289–315.

Angevine, J. B., Jr., Mancall, E. L., and Yakovlev, P. I., 1961: *The Human Cerebellum, An Atlas of Gross Topography in Serial Sections.* J. & A. Churchill, Ltd., London.

Brodal, A., 1967: Anatomical studies of cerebellar fibre connections with special reference to problems of functional localization. In *Progress in Brain Research,* Vol. 25, *The Cerebellum.* C. Fox and R. S. Snider, Eds. Elsevier, Amsterdam, pp. 135–173.

Carpenter, M. B., and Stevens, G. H., 1957: Structural and functional relationships between the deep cerebellar nuclei and the brachium conjunctivum in the rhesus monkey. J. Comp. Neurol., *107,* 109–163.

Carrea, R. M. E., and Grundfest, H., 1954: Electrophysiological studies of cerebellar inflow. I. Origin, conduction and termination of ventral spino-cerebellar tract in monkey and cat. J. Neurophysiol., *17,* 208–238.

Chambers, W. W., and Sprague, J. M., 1955a: Functional localization in the cerebellum. I. Organization in longitudinal corticonuclear zones and their contribution to the control of posture, both extrapyramidal and pyramidal. J. Comp. Neurol., *103,* 105–129.

Chambers, W. W., and Sprague, J. M., 1955b: Functional localization in the cerebellum. II. Somatotopic organization in cortex and nuclei. A.M.A. Arch. Neurol. Psychiat., *74,* 653–680.

Cohen, D., Chambers, W. W., and Sprague, J. M., 1958: Experimental study of the efferent projections from the cerebellar nuclei to the brain stem of the cat. J. Comp. Neurol., *109,* 233–259.

Combs, C. M., 1956: Bulbar regions related to localized cerebellar afferent impulses. J. Neurophysiol., *19,* 285–300.

Dow, R. S., 1938: Efferent connections of the flocculonodular lobe in *Macaca mulatta*. J. Comp. Neurol., *68*, 297–305.

Dow, R. S., 1939: Cerebellar action potentials in response to stimulation of various afferent connections. J. Neurophysiol., *2*, 543–555.

Dow, R. S., 1942: The evolution and anatomy of the cerebellum. Biol. Rev., *17*, 179–220.

Eccles, J. C., Ito, M., and Szentágothai, J., 1967: *The Cerebellum as a Neuronal Machine*. Springer-Verlag, Berlin.

Fox, C. A., and Barnard, J. W., 1957: A quantitative study of the Purkinje cell dendritic branchlets and their relationship to afferent fibers. J. Anat. (London), *91*, 299–313.

Fox, C. A., Hillman, D. E., Siegesmund, K. A., and Dutta, C. R., 1967: The primate cerebellar cortex: A Golgi and electron microscope study. In *Progress in Brain Research*, Vol. 25, *The Cerebellum*. C. Fox and R. S. Snider, Eds., Elsevier, Amsterdam, pp. 174–225.

Hamori, J., and Szentágothai, J., 1966: Participation of Golgi neuron processes in the cerebellar glomeruli. An electron microscope study. Exp. Brain Res., *2*, 35–48.

Jansen, J., and Brodal, A. ,1940: Experimental studies on the intrinsic fibers of the cerebellum. II. The cortico-nuclear projection. J. Comp. Neurol., *73*, 267–321.

Jansen, J., and Brodal, A., 1954: *Aspects of Cerebellar Anatomy*. J. Jansen and A. Brodal, Eds. Gunderson, Oslo.

Jansen, J., and Jansen, J., Jr., 1955: On the efferent fibers of the cerebellar nuclei in the cat. J. Comp. Neurol., *102*, 607–632.

Larsell, O., 1937: The cerebellum. A.M.A. Arch. Neurol. Psychiat., *38*, 580–607.

Larsell, O., 1951: *Anatomy of the Nervous System*. Appleton-Century-Crofts, Inc., New York.

Larsell, O., 1967: *The Comparative Anatomy and Histology of the Cerebellum from Myxinoids Through Birds*. J. Jansen, Ed. University of Minnesota Press, Minneapolis.

Morin, F., and Haddad, B., 1953: Afferent projections to the cerebellum and the spinal pathways involved. Amer. J. Physiol., *172*, 497–510.

Morin, F., and Lindner, O., 1953: Pathways for conduction of tactile impulses to the paramedian lobule of the cerebellum of the cat. Amer. J. Physiol., *175*, 247–250.

Pompeiano, O., 1967: Functional organization of the cerebellar projections to the spinal cord. In *Progress in Brain Research*, Vol. 25, *The Cerebellum*. C. Fox and R. S. Snider, Eds., Elsevier, Amsterdam, pp. 282–331.

Snider, R. S., 1943: A fifth cranial nerve projection to the cerebellum. Fed. Proc., *2*, 46.

Snider, R. S., 1950: Recent contributions to the anatomy and physiology of the cerebellum. A.M.A. Arch. Neurol. Psychiat., *64*, 196–219.

Snider, R. S., 1952: Interrelations of cerebellum and brain stem. Res. Publ. Ass. Res. Nerv. Ment. Dis., *30*, 267–281.

Snider, R. S., and Stowell, A., 1944a: Receiving areas of the tactile, auditory and visual systems in the cerebellum. J. Neurophysiol., *7*, 331–357.

Snider, R. S., and Stowell, A., 1944b: Electroanatomical studies on a tactile system in the cerebellum of monkey (*Macaca mulatta*). Anat. Rec., *88*, 457.

Sprague, J. M., and Chambers, W. W., 1953: Regulation of posture in intact and decerebrate cat. I. Cerebellum, reticular formation, vestibular nuclei. J. Neurophysiol., *16*, 451–463.

Sprague, J. M., and Chambers, W. W., 1954: Control of posture by reticular formation and cerebellum in the intact, anesthetized and unanesthetized and in the decerebrated cat. Amer. J. Physiol., *176*, 52–64.

Tomasch, J., 1969: The numerical capacity of the human cortico-ponto-cerebellar system. Brain Res., *13*, 476–484.

Wiener, N., 1961: *Cybernetics or Control and Communication in the Animal and the Machine*. The M.I.T. Press and John Wiley & Sons, New York.

Yoss, R. E., 1953: Studies of the spinal cord. Part II. Topographic localization within the ventral spino-cerebellar tract in the *Macaque*. J. Comp. Neurol., *99*, 613–638.

Chapter 20

Cerebellar Dysfunction

The primary function of the cerebellum is the regulation or control of movement, posture, and tonus. It may be that it exerts some control on many other functions of the nervous system, since it has extensive fiber connections with other parts of the brain and with the spinal cord. In fact, there are indications from physiological studies as well as from observations of human cases that the cerebellum influences autonomic functions. It is appropriate to note, however, that extensive injuries to the cerebellum produce no apparent sensory disturbances.

The **flocculonodular lobe** is concerned with the maintenance of equilibrium or balance. It has been demonstrated that monkeys in which this lobe was removed had gross disturbances of equilibrium without impairment in volitional movements or changes in reflexes. An animal thus impaired by operation is unable to stand or walk without swaying or falling, but uses his hands effectively in feeding without tremor. Tumors (medulloblastomas) of the flocculonodular lobe, which occur not uncommonly in children, cause symptoms comparable to those produced by the isolated ablations in monkeys. The patient is very unsteady on his feet, walks on a wide base, sways from side to side, and may be unable to maintain an upright position. The individual movements of the limbs are not impaired when lying in bed and there are no reflex changes.

The flocculonodular lobe, therefore, appears to be exclusively concerned with the maintenance of equilibrium, as might be expected, since most of its afferent and efferent connections are with the vestibular nerves and nuclei (Chap. 19).

Recent experimental studies support the morphological observations that, as indicated above, emphasize the importance of the concept of cerebellar organization in terms of longitudinal corticonuclear zones for the corpus cerebelli. Ablation and stimulation experiments have defined three bilaterally symmetrical zones in the cerebellum of cats. Each medial zone (vermal cortex and fastigial nucleus) regulates tone, posture, locomotion, and equilibrium of the entire body. Each intermediate zone (paravermal cortex and nucleus interpositus) is concerned with the regulation of spatially organized and skilled movements as well as with the tone and posture associated with these movements of the ipsilateral limbs. Each lateral zone (cortex and dentate nucleus) is also concerned with the regulation of skilled and spatially organized movements of the ipsilateral limbs but with no apparent role in the regulation of posture and tone. This analysis shows that vestibular function is not limited to the flocculonodular lobe, and that the anterior lobe is not a functional unit as implied by the more conventional division of the cerebellum into lobes by the transverse fissures.

The studies show that the paravermal and lateral zones of the cerebellum particularly are concerned with the control of volitional movements. The development of the lateral zone especially may be correlated with the development of manual dexterity in primates. Thus, particularly in man, pronounced symptoms are produced by disease processes that disturb neocerebellar mechanisms.

With lesions that involve the lateral and intermediate zones of the cerebellum or the cerebellocerebral circuit, movements tend to become *ataxic* (jerky and intermittent) and *dysmetric* (overshoot their objectives). The direction of movements is inaccurate (*pastpointing*) and rapidly alternating movements such as pronation and supination of the hands or flexion and extension of the fingers are not well performed; the latter deficiency is termed *adiadochokinesis. Rebound phenomena* and *decomposition of movement* are also likely to be present. In the former condition the patient tries to maintain flexion of the elbow against traction applied by the examiner; sudden cessation of traction results in abrupt and uncontrolled flexion of the elbow. By decomposition of movement is meant the breaking down of a complex movement, which is normally accomplished by simultaneous movements of several joints, into a succession of movements that involve only one joint at a time. (It will be recalled that the lateral and intermediate zones are essentially comparable to neocerebellum.)

Neocerebellar lesions in man may also cause *hypotonia* (diminished resistance to passive movement) and *tremor.* Cerebellar tremors increase toward the end of a given movement and are associated with dysmetria. Lesions confined to the cerebellar cortex do not result in enduring and pronounced tremors; when such tremors are produced by cerebellar le-

sions it indicates that the central nuclei have been damaged.

Nystagmus, as a manifestation of damage to the internal ear, vestibular nerve, or vestibular nuclei, is discussed in Chapter 9. That the cerebellum is superimposed on the vestibuloocular pathways is indicated by the fact that nystagmus is very likely to be a symptom of cerebellar lesions in man. It is probable that the cerebellum exerts its influence on the extrinsic muscles of the eyes through the cerebellovestibular connections described in the preceding chapter and through connections from cerebellar nuclei to the central gray matter surrounding the cerebral aqueduct in the midbrain, and to the posterior commissural nuclei that send fibers caudally through the medial longitudinal fasciculi. The motor nuclei of the nerves to the muscles of the eye may receive impulses from either central gray matter or posterior commissural nuclei. Nystagmus may appear in patients with lesions in any part of the cerebellum, except the posterior midline portions.

Asynergia, or lack of coordination of the many muscles involved in *speech,* results from cerebellar lesions. Consequently, the speech of individuals with such lesions tends to be thick and monotonous in character. *Speech coordination* has been variously localized in the lingula, lobulus simplex (declive monticuli and posterior part of the quadrangular lobule), uvula, and nodule. As has been suggested, it would seem more logical to believe that speech was integrated by the newer parts of the cerebellum, since speech is one of the latest capacities to develop in evolutionary history. There is no evidence of dominance of one side of the cerebellum in relation to speech such as exists in the cerebral cortex.

The influence of the cerebellum is exerted ipsilaterally; ataxia, tremor, hypotonia, dysmetria, and other signs of cerebellar deficit localized to one or the other side of the body indicate a lesion in the ipsilateral half of the cerebellum. Furthermore, the signs of cerebellar deficit are qualitatively the same whether the cerebellum itself, its afferent pathways, or its efferent pathways are damaged.

Localization of function in the cerebellum, so far as the control of specific parts of the body is concerned, is indefinite. In general, the cerebellar hemispheres control the ipsilateral extremities and the vermis controls the trunk. In cases of involvement of one hemisphere the subject staggers to that side and there is likely to be irregular overstepping and overabduction of the ipsilateral lower extremity; there may be slight inward deviation of the foot (pes varus). The upper extremity may swing less freely than is normal when walking, and the slight flexion normally present in the elbow and fingers may be lost. The trunk is often concave toward the involved side, and the head may be inclined toward that side. Lesions of the anterior part of the vermis in man cause the subject to stagger forward, and disease of the posterior vermis may result in a tendency to fall backward.

Tabes dorsalis, sometimes known as locomotor ataxia, is referred to in Chapter 5. In the tabetic type of ataxia there is loss or diminution of conscious perception of all types of sensibility carried by the posterior funiculi, and loss or marked diminution of deep reflexes. In cerebellar ataxia there is no interference with the conscious perception of posterior column sensibility and there is only slight diminution of the deep reflexes; in addition, there may be nystagmus and postural deviations. There may be a pendular type of knee jerk in cerebellar ataxia, disturbances in equilibrium, and speech abnormalities. The sensory loss in tabes and the preservation of all types of sensory perception in cerebellar lesions are the most important considerations in differentiating the two conditions.

In the hereditary condition known as *Friedreich's ataxia* the spinocerebellar tracts in the spinal cord, the posterior

funiculi, and the lateral corticospinal tracts are all more or less degenerated. The subject is ataxic in all skilled movements, and there is hypotonia of the muscles of the extremities. The symptoms are due to the involvement of the spinocerebellar tracts and illustrate the fact that such involvement may give rise to the same syndrome as lesions in the cerebellum itself. Friedreich's ataxia is further characterized by defective joint and muscle sensibility, loss of vibratory sensibility, and diminution in tactile discriminative ability. The symptoms are due to degeneration of the posterior funiculi. The abdominal reflexes are usually absent bilaterally, and there are bilateral Babinski signs as a result of lateral corticospinal tract involvement.

Cerebellopontile angle tumors (acoustic neurinomas) are discussed in Chapter 9. Reference was made to the fact that the biventral lobule of the cerebellum is likely to be involved by them. This results in the development of symptoms of neocerebellar deficit such as have been described, in addition to the sensory and motor loss attributed to involvement of the eighth, fifth, ninth, seventh, sixth, and tenth cranial nerves, all of which enter or emerge from the brain stem in the region of the cerebellopontile angle. Eighth nerve neurinomas were mentioned previously as the type of tumor most commonly encountered in this location. However, tumors arising in the cerebellum and expanding downward into the angle may produce the same combination of symptoms.

BIBLIOGRAPHY

Brodal, A., and Jansen, J., 1946: The pontocerebellar projection in the rabbit and cat. Experimental investigations. J. Comp. Neurol., *84,* 31–118.

Carpenter, M. B., and Correll, J. W., 1961: Spinal pathways mediating cerebellar dyskinesia in the rhesus monkey. J. Neurophysiol., *24,* 534–551.

Chambers, W. W., and Sprague, J. M., 1955a: Functional localization in the cerebellum. I.

Organization in longitudinal corticonuclear zones and their contribution to the control of posture, both extrapyramidal and pyramidal. J. Comp. Neurol., *103,* 105–129.

Chambers, W. W., and Sprague, J. M., 1955b: Functional localization in the cerebellum. II. Somatotopic organization in cortex and nuclei. A.M.A. Arch. Neurol. Psychiat., *74,* 653–680.

Dow, R. S., 1936: The fiber connections of the posterior parts of the cerebellum in the rat and cat. J. Comp. Neurol., *63,* 527–548.

Dow, R. S., 1938a: Effect of lesions in the vestibular part of the cerebellum in primates. A.M.A. Arch. Neurol. Psychiat., *40,* 500–520.

Dow, R. S., 1938b: Efferent connections of the flocculonodular lobe in *Macaca mulatta.* J. Comp. Neurol., *68,* 297–305.

Dow, R. S., 1969: Cerebellar syndromes including vermis and hemispheric syndromes. In *Handbook of Clinical Neurology.* P. J. Vinken and G. W. Bruyn, Eds., Vol. 2. North-Holland Publishing Co., Amsterdam.

Dow, R. S., and G. Moruzzi, 1958: *The Physiology and Pathology of the Cerebellum.* University of Minnesota Press, Minneapolis.

Fulton, J. F., 1949: *Physiology of the Nervous System.* Oxford University Press, New York.

Growdon, J. H., Chambers, W. W., and Liu, C. N., 1967: An experimental study of cerebellar dyskinesia in the rhesus monkey. Brain, *90,* 603–632.

Jansen, J., and Brodal, A., 1954: *Aspects of Cerebellar Anatomy.* J. Jansen and A. Brodal, Eds. Gunderson, Oslo.

Parker, H. L., and Kernohan, J. W., 1933: Parenchymatous cortical cerebellar atrophy (chronic atrophy of Purkinje's cells). Brain, *56,* 191–212.

Rand, R. W., 1954: An anatomical and experimental study of the cerebellar nuclei and their efferent pathways in the monkey. J. Comp. Neurol., *101,* 167–223.

Chapter 21

The Diencephalon

The diencephalon (Fig. 196) is the rostral-most portion of the brain stem. Recall that in the developing neural tube (Chap. 2) the primitive cephalic vesicle, the prosencephalon, differentiates into the diencephalon and telencephalon as the outpocketing cerebral hemispheres are formed. The diencephalon retains its proximity to the third ventricle and in the adult is traditionally divided into *epithalamus; dorsal thalamus,* more commonly referred to as thalamus proper; *hypothalamus;* and *subthalamus.*

In a general way, the diencephalon can be thought of as a station that is interposed between cortex and lower levels of the brain stem and as such is intimately related to motor and sensory functions in both the somatic and visceral spheres. The classical sensory pathways and extralemniscal (reticular arousal) system are interrupted at this level before they

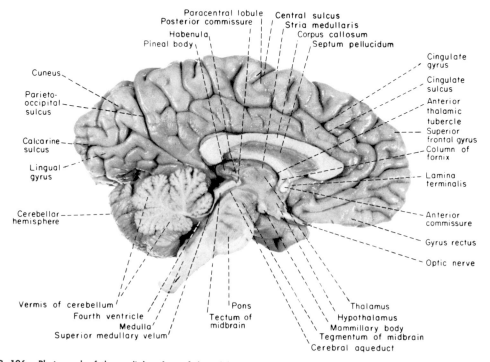

FIG. 196. Photograph of the medial surface of the adult brain cut in sagittal section.

222

project information to cortex. In addition, parts of the extrapyramidal system as well as visceral motor and visceral sensory systems are importantly linked with diencephalic structures. Because of its unique position, the diencephalon is sometimes referred to as the interbrain or between brain.

EPITHALAMUS

The epithalamus is superiorly, caudally, and medially placed with respect to the other divisions of the diencephalon. It is continuous caudally with the pretectum of the mesencephalon (Figs. 197, 199). The structures that constitute the epithalamus are the *pineal body,* the *habenula,* the *habenular commissure,* and the *striae medullares* (Figs. 197, 199, 200).

The *pineal body,* or epiphysis, is a small projection of tissue from the dorsal diencephalic roof at the caudal margin of the habenular trigones in the region of the posterior commissure. Its dorsocaudal extension is in relation to the superior

colliculi. Most of the cells within the epiphysis are of glial types. In addition, there are parenchymal cells (pineocytes) which probably have a secretory role. Photoreceptor cells, which are characteristic of lower vertebrate pineal systems, have not been described for birds and mammals. Little is known about the function of the epiphysis in man and other mammals. An input of fibers from the striae medullares and habenular ganglia has been described.

The habenula receives terminals from the stria medullaris and is the origin of the habenulopeduncular tract (Chap. 24).

THALAMUS

The dorsal thalamus (thalamus proper) is a receiving station for sensory information from receptors throughout the body and, in fact, except for primary olfactory stimuli, serves as a relay station for all incoming sensory information that is destined for the cerebral cortex. It also serves to distribute impulses to other regions of

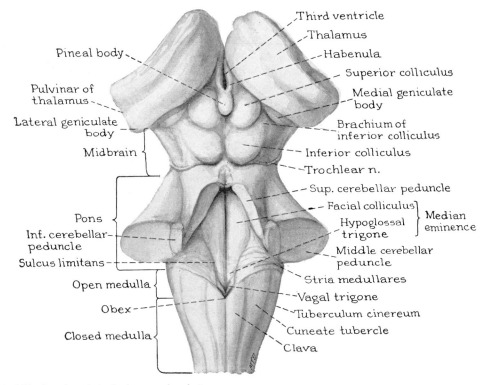

FIG. 197. Drawing of the brain stem, dorsal view.

the brain, and there is good evidence that the thalamus integrates much of the information received. As mentioned earlier, it would appear that pain and perhaps other sensory modalities are appreciated at thalamic level. In addition to the incoming sensory information, the thalamus receives impulses from the cerebral cortex, basal ganglia, and cerebellum. Although a brief orientation to the thalamus, together with an account of certain nuclei including their afferent and efferent connections, is given in preceding chapters, it seems desirable to present a more organized account of all the major thalamic nuclei and related fiber systems in this section.

The thalamus lies in direct contact with the third ventricle medially and forms a part of the floor of the lateral ventricle dorsally. Laterally it is bounded by the *external medullary lamina* and beyond that, just outside the reticular nucleus, by the internal capsule. The internal configuration of the thalamus is very complex, though different categories have been made which simplify its organization into nuclear groups. The category used here divides the thalamus into five major nuclear groups, *anterior, midline, medial,*

lateral, and *posterior* (Figs. 198–203). This division, which is based on the monkey thalamus, has been shown to be applicable for man and is generally used for all primates.

A thin band of myelinated fibers, called the *internal medullary lamina,* separates the thalamus into medial and lateral nuclear groups (Figs. 200, 203). Rostrally, this lamina splits to enclose an anterior group. Midline and posterior groups are located in the positions their respective names indicate. Each of these groups is dealt with separately, though not all of the described nuclei are included here since our knowledge of their connections and functions is incomplete. It should also be noted that where precise thalamocortical projections are described, corticothalamic connections generally exist also. In considering thalamic "functions" it is therefore difficult to separate out those that do not also involve some portion of the cortex.

Anterior Nuclei (anteromedial, anterodorsal, and anteroventral)

The anterior nuclei (Figs. 201–203) are enclosed by the diverging limbs of the internal medullary lamina at the rostral

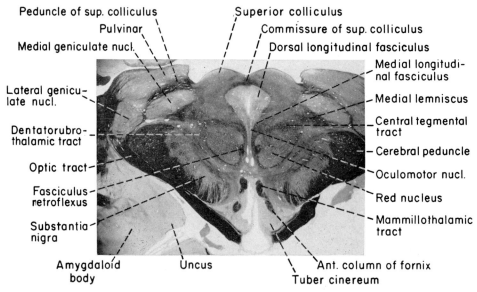

Peduncle of sup. colliculus
Pulvinar
Medial geniculate nucl.
Superior colliculus
Commissure of sup. colliculus
Dorsal longitudinal fasciculus
Medial longitudinal fasciculus
Lateral geniculate nucl.
Medial lemniscus
Dentatorubrothalamic tract
Central tegmental tract
Optic tract
Cerebral peduncle
Fasciculus retroflexus
Oculomotor nucl.
Substantia nigra
Red nucleus
Mammillothalamic tract
Amygdaloid body
Uncus
Ant. column of fornix
Tuber cinereum

FIG. 198. Photomicrograph of a transverse section through the rostral part of the superior collicular level of the midbrain which passes through the posterior thalamic nuclei. Weil stain.

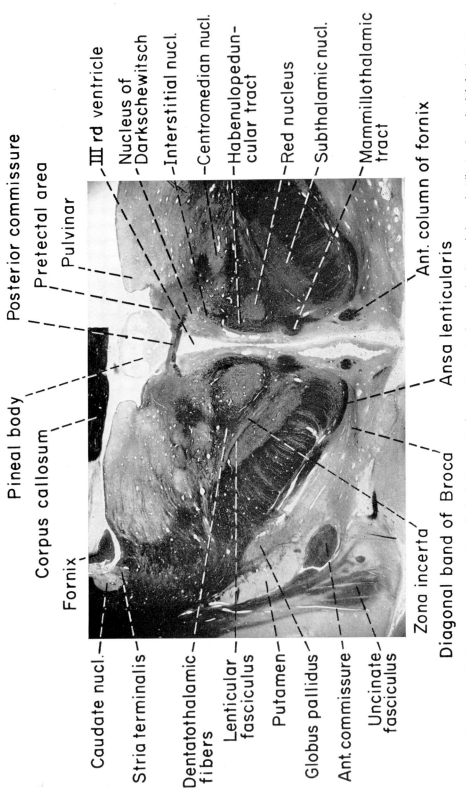

FIG. 199. Photomicrograph of a transverse section through the brain stem in the transition region between the diencephalon and midbrain. Several subthalamic structures are shown in addition to thalamic nuclei. Weil stain.

end of the thalamus. They can be observed grossly as a prominent protuberance that bulges into the lateral ventricle. Of the three described nuclei in this group, the anteroventral is the best developed in man (Fig. 201). These nuclei receive connections from the hypothalamus via the *mammillothalamic tract* and project to the cingulate gyrus (Fig. 199), especially to areas 23 and 24 of Brodmann (Fig. 134).

Midline Nuclei

The midline nuclei include groups of cells adjacent to the wall of the third ventricle as well as cells in the interthalamic adhesion (massa intermedia) (Figs. 200, 207). The latter body is absent in about 25 percent of human brains. The midline nuclei receive fibers from the major ascending sensory tracts (spinotha-

lamic, trigeminothalamic, and medial lemniscus), from the reticular formation, and from other thalamic nuclei. Midline nuclei have efferent projections to the hypothalamus, to the cortex of the anterior rhinencephalon, and probably to the basal ganglia. Efferent connections are also made with other thalamic nuclei. Whereas a complex group of midline nuclei have been described in several species, they are very poorly developed in man where they serve no known function.

Medial Nuclei (dorsomedial, centromedian)

The medial nuclear mass is situated between the internal medullary lamina and the midline nuclei. It is very prominent in man and is composed of two major nuclei, dorsomedial and centromedian (Figs. 202, 203). The dorsomedial nucleus receives

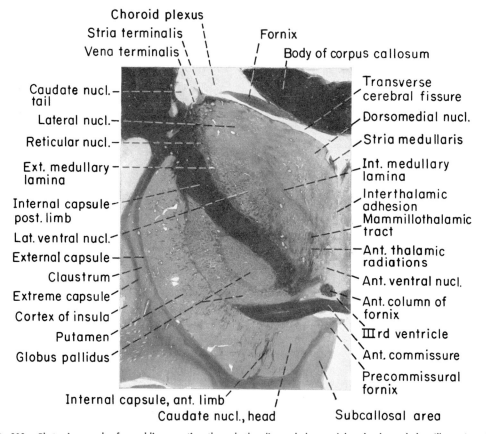

FIG. 200. Photomicrograph of an oblique section through the diencephalon and basal telencephalon illustrating the thalamus and basal ganglia. The section passes through the middle third of the thalamus. Weil stain.

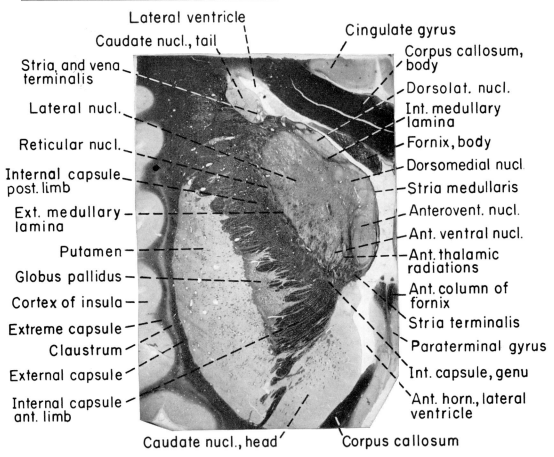

Lateral ventricle

Caudate nucl., tail

Stria, and vena terminalis

Lateral nucl.

Reticular nucl.

Internal capsule post. limb

Ext. medullary lamina

Putamen

Globus pallidus

Cortex of insula

Extreme capsule

Claustrum

External capsule

Internal capsule ant. limb

Cingulate gyrus

Corpus callosum, body

Dorsolat. nucl.

Int. medullary lamina

Fornix, body

Dorsomedial nucl.

Stria medullaris

Anterovent. nucl.

Ant. ventral nucl.

Ant. thalamic radiations

Ant. column of fornix

Stria terminalis

Paraterminal gyrus

Int. capsule, genu

Ant. horn., lateral ventricle

Caudate nucl., head

Corpus callosum

FIG. 201. Photomicrograph of an oblique section through the rostral third of the thalamus showing the relation of the thalamus to the internal capsule, lentiform nucleus, and head of caudate.

afferents from other nearby thalamic nuclei, prefrontal cortex, septal (subcallosal) areas, and basal ganglia. Its major projections are to prefrontal cortex. Interconnections with the hypothalamus have been described but the evidence is not conclusive. Since this nucleus receives fibers from many of the surrounding nuclei, it probably serves to integrate much of the visceral and somatic information coming into the thalamus and then projects it to the frontal lobe.

The centromedian nucleus is large and easily recognized since it is partially surrounded by fibers of the internal medullary lamina. Little is known about the connections of this nucleus in man, although connections to other thalamic nuclei and to the putamen and caudate nucleus have been described. In the monkey, considerable retrograde degeneration in the centromedian nucleus occurs after lesions of the caudate and putamen. In addition, it receives a massive projection from the globus pallidus. Although the literature relative to the connections of nucleus centromedian is quite controversial, generally it is agreed that it does not project to the cortex. Functionally, emphasis is placed on its interrelations with the basal ganglia and on possible intrathalamic correlations. Because the centromedian nucleus is almost entirely surrounded by the internal medullary lamina, it is sometimes referred to as one of the intralaminar nuclei. These nuclei are gen-

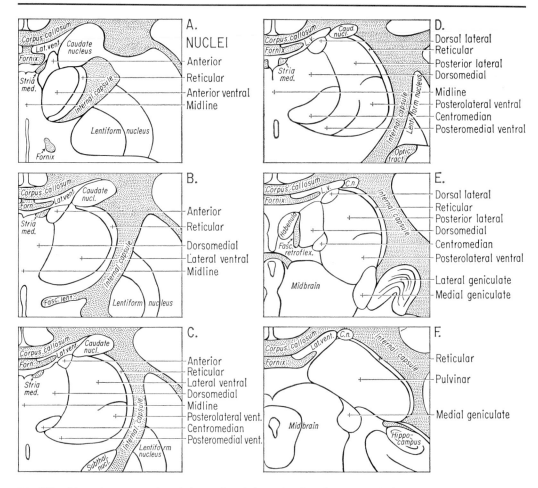

FIG. 202. Schematic representation of the monkey thalamus in aligned rostrocaudal planes of frontal sections (A–F) showing major nuclear groupings and divisions within each group.

erally considered to be a part of the *non-specific* or *diffuse thalamocortical system* that is discussed on page 232.

Lateral Nuclei (anterior ventral, lateral ventral, posterolateral ventral, posteromedial ventral, dorsal lateral, posterior lateral, and reticular)

The lateral nuclei are a large group of nuclei located between the internal and external medullary laminae extending to the *pulvinar* posteriorly (Figs. 200–203). The group also includes the reticular nucleus which is outside the external medullary lamina. The anatomical position of these nuclei is made clearer by considering the whole group as being divided into "lateral" and "ventral" portions. Thus the

"lateral" portion (posterior lateral and dorsal lateral nuclei) are found only posteriorly, just rostral to the pulvinar. The "ventral" division, containing the remaining nuclei, extends throughout the thalamus and occupies a true ventral position posteriorly (posteromedial ventral and posterolateral ventral nuclei), but fills the entire lateral thalamus (lateral ventral and anterior ventral nuclei) in more anterior planes of section (Figs. 200, 203).

Anterior Ventral and Lateral Ventral Nuclei. The anterior ventral nucleus is located at the rostral end of the complex lateral thalamic group of nuclei. It receives fibers from the globus pallidus through the thalamic fasciculus and sends

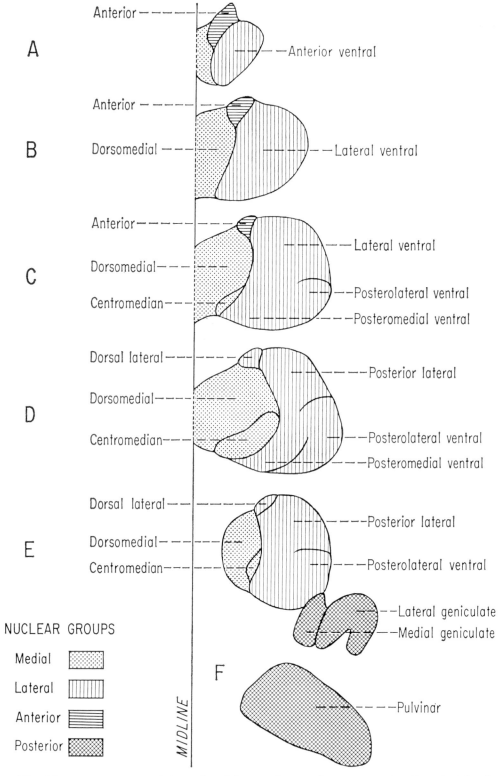

FIG. 203. Schematic representation of the monkey thalamus and surrounding structures. A to F are frontal sections serially arranged in a rostrocaudal order. Major thalamic nuclei are labeled.

fibers to the corpus striatum (see Chap. 17). Connections of the anterior ventral nucleus with frontal lobe cortex seem to be certain, though details of its specific projections have not been resolved.

The lateral ventral nucleus receives fibers from the cerebellum through the superior cerebellar peduncle (Fig. 195) and from the globus pallidus via the thalamic fasciculus (Fig. 169). The efferent fibers course through the posterior limb of the internal capsule to the motor and premotor areas of the cerebral cortex (Fig. 195). In monkeys, fibers from the premotor cortex to the lateral ventral nucleus have been described.

The anterior ventral and lateral ventral nuclei are considered as part of the complex circuitry involved in motor systems (Chap. 17). This is readily apparent from their connections with the cerebellum, basal ganglia, and motor cortex. The anterior ventral nucleus has also been considered one of the nonspecific nuclei (see p. 233).

Posterolateral Ventral and Posteromedial Ventral Nuclei. These nuclei fill the posterior ventral part of the lateral thalamus at the level of the centromedian nucleus and extend to the pulvinar (Figs. 202, 203). The two nuclei are readily distinguishable by the semilunar or arcuate appearance of the posteromedial ventral nucleus in myelin preparations. These nuclei are of major importance since they form the thalamic sensory relay station for somesthetic afferents.

The posterolateral ventral nucleus is the terminus of the spinothalamic tracts and of the medial lemniscus (Chaps. 5 and 6). Fibers from the cervical segments end medially and those from more caudal segments end more laterally in the nucleus (Fig. 204). The posteromedial ventral nucleus is the terminus of the secondary trigeminal fibers and of the secondary taste fibers. These two nuclei send their fibers through the posterior limb of the internal capsule (Fig. 205) to cortical areas 3, 1, and 2 of the postcentral gyrus where the topographical pattern is inverted (Fig. 204). Thus, the medial to lateral representation of head, arm, and leg in the thalamus is reflected on the cor-

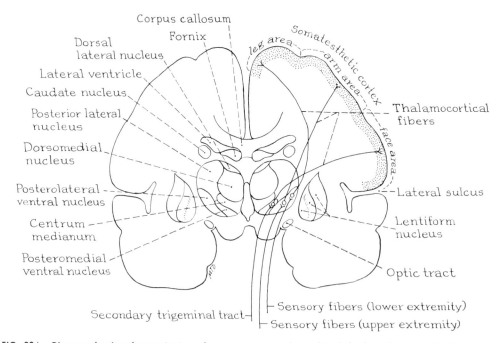

FIG. 204. Diagram showing the termination of sensory tracts in the nuclei of the lateral part of the thalamus, and the projection of these nuclei on the somesthetic cortex by way of the internal capsule (modified from Ranson).

tex with the leg area placed dorsomedially, the face area most laterally, and the arm area in between. This projected topographical pattern is sometimes difficult to appreciate in two dimensional drawings because the sensory radiations in the internal capsule do not actually intermix with each other, but rather maintain their orderly pattern while turning in three dimensions. In the internal capsule, the fibers from the posteromedial ventral nucleus pass somewhat anterior and ventral to those from the posterolateral ventral nucleus which project in a more posterior and dorsal direction.

Dorsal Lateral and Posterior Lateral Nuclei. The posterior lateral nucleus extends through the lateral nuclear mass from the pulvinar posteriorly to the lateral ventral nucleus anteriorly (Figs. 202, 203). Its posterior portion lies immediately dorsal to the posterolateral ventral and posteromedial ventral nuclei just described. The dorsal lateral nucleus is much smaller than the posterior lateral nucleus. It lies along the dorsomedial edge of the posterior lateral nucleus and is actually separated from it to some extent by the internal medullary lamina. The dorsal lateral and the posterior lateral nuclei receive fibers from other thalamic nuclei and project to parietal lobe cortex. Fibers from the parietal lobe to these nuclei have also been described. Some authors emphasize the projection of the lateral dorsal nucleus to posterior cingulate cortex and prefer to include it as a part of the anterior nuclear group.

Reticular Nucleus. The reticular nucleus forms a thin band of cells between the internal medullary lamina and the internal capsule (Figs. 200–202). It stretches from the most anterior to the most posterior part of the thalamus and ventrally blends with the zona incerta. Afferents to it from the *entire cerebral cortex,* midline, medial and intralaminar nuclei of the thalamus, and the brain stem reticular formation have been described. It is also grouped with the nonspecific nuclei, though considerable controversy exists regarding its anatomical projection sites and functional roles. Retrograde degeneration studies have indicated that the reticular nucleus has a wide projection to cortical areas that are organized in a rostrocaudal direction. On the basis of Golgi preparations of normal material, it has been argued that the great majority of axons from the reticular nucleus are projected to other thalamic nuclei and that many course as far caudally as the

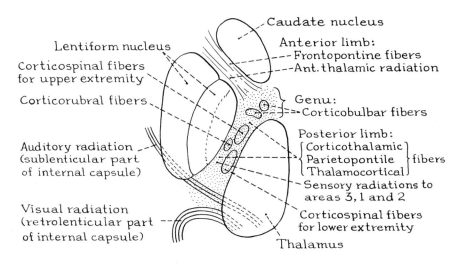

FIG. 205. Diagram illustrating the parts of the internal capsule and the various fiber systems in the respective parts as seen in horizontal section.

16

midbrain tegmentum, thus possibly representing a centrifugal system rather than a cortically directed one.

Posterior Nuclei (pulvinar and medial and lateral geniculate nuclei)

Pulvinar. The posterior nuclei are at the most caudal part of the thalamus, lateral and dorsal to the transition area (pretectum) between the diencephalon and midbrain. The pulvinar (Figs. 198, 199, 202, 203) comprises the largest part of the posterior thalamic mass and to some extent overhangs the superior colliculus dorsolaterally. It is generally considered to receive fibers from adjacent nuclei, the lateral group in particular, and from the medial and lateral geniculate nuclei. The pulvinar projects to the cortex of the parietal, temporal, and occipital lobes and probably receives fibers from these cortical areas.

Medial Geniculate Nucleus. In transverse section, the medial geniculate nucleus forms an outcropping on the lateral side of the midbrain at superior collicular levels between the cerebral peduncle and the lateral geniculate nucleus (Figs. 198, 202, 203). It receives auditory information through the brachium of the inferior colliculus and projects to the auditory cortex through the acoustic radiations that course in the sublenticular part of the internal capsule (Fig. 205). Recall that in contrast to other sensory systems, auditory information is bilaterally represented throughout the central nervous auditory pathways (see Chap. 9).

Lateral Geniculate Nucleus. The lateral geniculate nucleus (Figs. 198, 202, 203) is situated lateral to the medial geniculate nucleus immediately ventral to the pulvinar. It is a laminated structure composed of six major layers that receive the optic tract fibers. Each lateral geniculate receives visual information from both eyes, crossed fibers synapsing in layers 1, 4, and 6, and uncrossed fibers in layers 2, 3, and 5. In turn, the geniculates project to their respective ipsilateral

striate cortex along the calcarine fissure in the occipital lobe (Brodmann area 17) via the retrolenticular part of the internal capsule (Fig. 205). The medial part of the lateral geniculate nucleus receives fibers from the upper retinal quadrants and projects to the upper lip of the calcarine cortex. The lateral part of the nucleus receives fibers from the lower retinal quadrants and projects to the lower lip of the calcarine cortex. Macular fibers end in the caudal part of the geniculate nucleus which projects to the posterior part of the visual cortex. Representation of the more peripheral fields is on the anterior part of the visual cortex (see Chap. 9).

Specific Thalamic Nuclei. More general nomenclatures for thalamic nuclei have been used by different authors which are based on known connections and/or functional characteristics evidenced by electrophysiological methods. *Specific* thalamocortical projection nuclei are those that receive well-defined afferents and send efferents to well-defined cortical areas. Within this group are the *cortical relay nuclei,* which include the major sensory relay nuclei described above as receiving specific sensory tracts and projecting to circumscribed cortical receiving areas, that is, the posteromedial ventral, posterolateral ventral, medial geniculate, and lateral geniculate. Other cortical relay nuclei are the lateral ventral and the anterior ventral, included because of their known inputs from cerebellum and basal ganglia and outputs to motor cortex. Another group of nuclei, the *association* nuclei, are also considered as part of the specific category, though their connections form a somewhat less specific pattern, and their functions are only poorly understood. The association nuclei (dorsomedial, dorsolateral, posterior lateral, and pulvinar) receive inputs primarily from other thalamic nuclei and project to wider areas of cerebral cortex, the so-called association areas.

Nonspecific Thalamic Nuclei. The nuclei most frequently considered as comprising a nonspecific nuclear group are the *intralaminar, midline, centromedian, reticular,* and *anterior ventral.* The intralaminar nuclei are formed by neurons irregularly clustered in relation to the internal medullary lamina. Whereas several of these have been defined, their connections are poorly understood. There is evidence that they are interconnected with adjacent thalamic nuclei and receive afferents from the brain stem reticular formation. The other nonspecific nuclei are described previously in the above text. Most of the nonspecific nuclei are also considered as a *subcortical* group because they either do not project directly to cortex or their cortical projection is in dispute. They are the centromedian, midline, and reticular nuclei, and posterior parts of the intralaminar group.

Repetitive electrical stimulation of the nonspecific group of thalamic nuclei leads to cortical potentials that increase and then decrease in amplitude in a periodic waxing and waning fashion ("recruiting response"). The waves can be recorded over areas of cortex that are more widespread ("diffuse") than those assigned to specific sensory or motor functions, however, their distribution is restricted to more circumscribed areas depending on such factors as which nucleus is stimulated and the general level of arousal in the animal. The neurophysiological concept of such a diffuse thalamocortical system with multisynaptic connections among nonspecific thalamic nuclei still remains somewhat of an enigma regarding its precise functional and anatomical properties. The difficulty in assigning specific functions to thalamic nuclei that

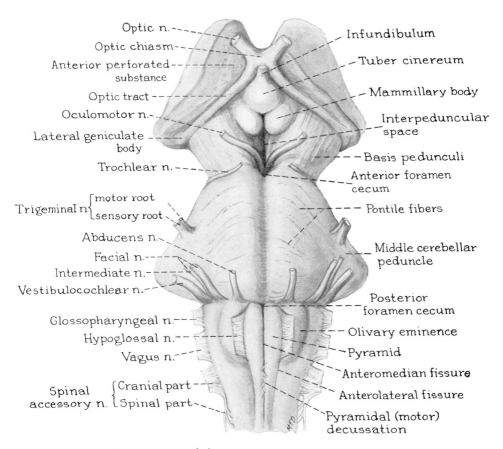

FIG. 206. Drawing of the brain stem, ventral view.

are grouped together because of their "nonspecific" effects can be readily appreciated.

The nonspecific nuclei are often considered to be the cephalic component of the brain stem reticular formation, part of which is considered an "ascending activating system" concerned with maintenance of consciousness. There has been considerable controversy over the role played by the reticular formation and nonspecific thalamic nuclei on such generalized higher nervous functions as alterations in levels of consciousness, focusing of attention, discriminations, and perceptions. A major unresolved problem is the anatomical route by which information projected to the thalamus from the reticular formation, or cortical effects elicited by stimulation of nonspecific thalamic nuclei, finally reaches the cortex. Several indirect pathways have been proposed via the striatum, anterior ventral nuclei, or other basal telencephalic structures, though the mechanisms by which reticular formation, thalamus, and cortex are interrelated are by no means clear.

HYPOTHALAMUS

The hypothalamus is the most ventral part of the diencephalon. Its rostral and caudal boundaries are marked on the ventral surface by the *optic chiasm* and the *mammillary bodies* respectively, and the region between these is the *tuber cinereum* (Fig. 206). Internally, the hypothalamus is divided into halves by the third ventricle, and it is continuous rostrally with the telencephalic *preoptic area* and caudally with the midbrain tegmentum. Dorsally, the hypothalamic sulcus marks the boundary between the thalamus and hypothalamus (Figs. 196, 207).

Each half of the hypothalamus can be divided arbitrarily into three longitudinal zones: a *periventricular region* adjacent to the third ventricle; a *medial region* just lateral to the periventricular region, which contains several nuclear groups; and a *lateral region,* or area, roughly separated

from the medial region by the path of the *fornix* (Fig. 207). The lateral hypothalamic area contains fewer cells than the medial, but has many thinly myelinated fibers which run longitudinally. The nuclei of the ventral thalamus (subthalamus) form the lateral boundary of the hypothalamus (Fig. 199). The hypothalamus can also be subdivided, for purposes of localizing the nuclear groups, into three rostrocaudal parts: a *supraoptic area* at the level of the optic chiasm; a *middle* or *tuberal area;* and a *mammillary area* at the level of the mammillary bodies (Fig. 207A, B, C).

The nuclei in the medial part of the supraoptic area (Fig. 207A) include the anterior *hypothalamic, paraventricular,* and *supraoptic.* In man the anterior hypothalamic nucleus is composed of an irregular mass of small cells and is more appropriately called *anterior hypothalamic area.* The paraventricular nucleus is an elongated group of cells along the sides of the third ventricle, and the supraoptic nucleus overlies the optic tract. The paraventricular and supraoptic nuclei contain neurosecretory material and send their axons into the neurohypophysis (Fig. 208). Although the anterior hypothalamic area and the lateral hypothalamic area cannot be distinguished histologically from the preoptic area, it is customary to limit the supraoptic portion of the hypothalamus by a transverse plane rostral to the optic chiasm.

Nuclei in the tuberal region of the hypothalamus (Fig. 207B) include the *arcuate nucleus* within the ventral part of the periventricular gray, the *ventromedial* and *dorsomedial nuclei* of the medial region, and the *lateral tuberal nuclei,* which are located ventrally in the lateral region. The dorsomedial nucleus is not well defined in man.

The nuclei of each mammillary body, a large medial and a small lateral nucleus, are considered in this text without subdivision (Fig. 207C).

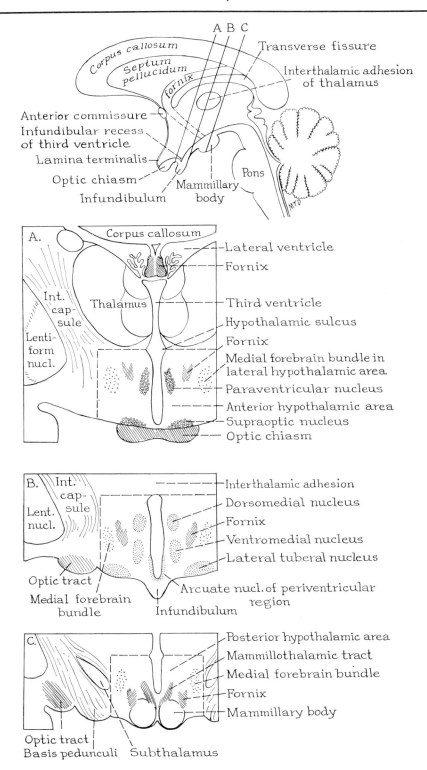

FIG. 207. The upper schematic drawing is a sagittal section of the brain stem showing the relations of the hypothalamus to surrounding brain structures. The lines, A, B, and C, correspond to the levels at which the three lower drawings were made. Section A is through the supraoptic area, B is through the tuberal area, and C is through the mammillary area of the hypothalamus.

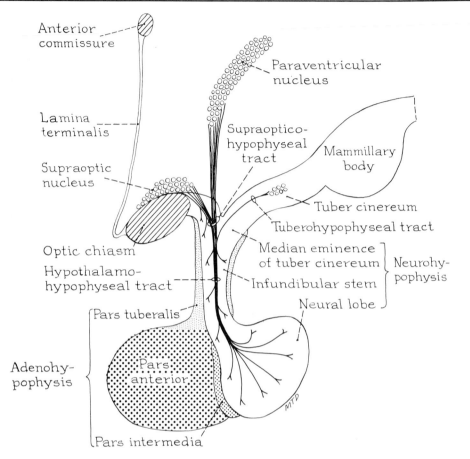

FIG. 208. Sagittal section through the hypothalamus and hypophysis demonstrating the origin and distribution of the hypothalamohypophyseal tract.

Hypophysis

The hypophysis, or pituitary gland, is attached to the hypothalamus at the rostral part of the tuber cinereum, the region known as the median eminence (Fig. 208). The hypophysis is comprised of two major divisions, *neurohypophysis* and *adenohypophysis,* that have separate embryonic origins. The neurohypophysis arises from the embryonic infundibular process of the diencephalic floor and in the adult includes the *neural lobe, infundibular stem,* and *median eminence.* The adenohypophysis differentiates from a diverticulum of the stomodeal roof (Rathke's pouch) and in the adult is composed of the *pars anterior, pars intermedia,* and *pars tuberalis* (Fig. 208).

Fiber Systems

Of numerous fiber systems that interconnect the hypothalamus with other areas of the brain, only the major systems will be described. One of the systems discussed in connection with the rhinencephalon (Chap. 24), is the *medial forebrain bundle* (Figs. 199, 207). This bundle includes both ascending and descending fibers that connect the septal or medial olfactory area with the preoptic and hypothalamic areas and with the tegmental areas of the midbrain. Several hypothalamic nuclei, particularly the ventromedial nucleus, are believed to have connections with the medial forebrain bundle.

The *mammillary peduncle,* described

as taking origin from the medial lemniscus at midbrain levels, ends in the mammillary body. A number of fibers from the tegmental gray are believed to be incorporated in the mammillary peduncle. It is probable that this system includes descending as well as ascending fibers.

The *fornix* is the most prominent fiber system of the hypothalamus. In the main, it arises in the hippocampus (Fig. 194) and terminates in the mammillary body (Figs. 196, 207). It is considered in relation to the rhinencephalon (Chap. 24). As the fornix approaches the anterior commissure, it divides into a small precommissural and a large postcommissural division. The precommissural fornix connects with the preoptic and anterior hypothalamic areas (Fig. 199). The postcommissural fornix terminates in the anterior hypothalamic area, mammillary nuclei, and possibly other hypothalamic nuclei. There is evidence that fibers of the fornix arise in the septal area and conduct to the cortex of the temporal pole via the hippocampus.

The *stria terminalis* arises from the amygdaloid body and connects with the preoptic and anterior hypothalamic areas and ventromedial nucleus.

Adjacent to the ventricle throughout the diencephalon is a system of finely medullated and nonmedullated fibers known as the *periventricular fiber system*. Many of the fibers are arranged obliquely; others course in a rostrocaudal direction. The rostral part of the system connects the preoptic and anterior hypothalamic areas with the dorsomedial and midline nuclei of the thalamus. The caudally directed fibers have connections with essentially all areas of the hypothalamic gray and extend to the tegmental gray of the midbrain and reticular areas of more caudal levels. The dorsal longitudinal fasciculus, a fairly discrete grouping of fibers in the periaqueductal region of the midbrain, is generally considered to be part of the periventricular system (Figs. 169, 199). There is evidence of

projections from this system coursing to the dorsomedial thalamic nuclei, thus providing a link between the hypothalamus and frontal cortex. In addition to these indirect connections, direct fibers from the preoptic and anterior hypothalamic areas to the orbitofrontal areas have been described. However, it should be noted that hypothalamoneocortical interconnections are somewhat in dispute.

The *mammillothalamic tract* is a conspicuous bundle of fibers that projects from the mammillary nuclei to the anterior thalamic nuclei (Figs. 200, 207). The *mammillotegmental tract* arises from the mammillothalamic tract and courses dorsocaudally to the dorsal tegmental nucleus (Figs. 196, 199).

The *hypothalamohypophyseal tract,* which is composed of two parts, relates the hypothalamus with the neurohypophysis (Fig. 208). The larger component, the *supraopticohypophyseal tract,* arises from the supraoptic and paraventricular nuclei. The lesser component, the *tuberohypophyseal tract,* is thought to arise from the basal tuberal regions of the hypothalamus. The two tracts join to form the hypothalamohypophyseal tract, which courses centrally in the pituitary stalk to the neurohypophysis (Fig. 208). The fibers probably terminate in relation to blood vessels. Fibers of the tuberohypophyseal tract actually end in the median eminence and proximal part of the stalk. The major portion of the supraopticohypophyseal tract ends in the neural lobe.

Hypothalamic Functions: General

It has been established that the hypothalamus plays an important role in the regulation of metabolic activities and in the control of the functions of the autonomic nervous system. Related to the control of autonomic functions is the involvement of the hypothalamus in the behavioral responses to emotional states. Other functions under hypothalamic influence include the regulation of pituitary hormone output, control of body temper-

ature, drinking, eating, sleep, and wakefulness.

The many hypothalamic regulatory
mechanisms are mediated primarily
through the neuronal connections described above. In the case of the hypophysis, humoral factors as well as nerve
fibers are involved (see below). Through
its hormones the adenohypophysis controls most of the endocrine glands and
thus has a widespread influence over re-
productive, metabolic, and related processes.

Hypothalamic Control of Pituitary Gland

There is good evidence that venous
connections from the median eminence
to the adenohypophysis (hypophyseal
portal system) provide the functional relationship between the hypothalamus and
adenohypophysis. If the pituitary stalk is
transected the adenohypophysis must re-
establish a vascular relationship with the
hypothalamus before normal gonadotropic, adrenocorticotropic, and thyrotropic functions are restored. It now
seems likely that neurohumoral trans-
mitters, *releasing factors,* are present in
the median eminence region that are secreted into the hypophyseal portal vessels, thus forming the important chemical
link between hypothalamus and anterior
pituitary gland. Although the final definition of these is not yet established, it
appears that separate factors exist for
each of the anterior lobe hormones.

It is well established that the release of
adrenocorticotropic, thyrotropic, and
gonadotropic hormones of the adenohypophysis is regulated by the hypothalamus.
Although it has not always been possible
to outline precisely the specific hypothalamic nuclei controlling the release of
each pituitary tropin, it is generally accepted that overlapping pituitary regulat-
ing "centers" exist in the more ventral
portions of the hypothalamus throughout
its rostrocaudal extent.

The neurohypophysis liberates an *anti-
diuretic* hormone (vasopressin), which

mediates the resorption of water in the
renal tubules, and *oxytocin,* which causes
uterine contractions and the ejection of
milk from lactating mammary glands.
The supraoptic and paraventricular neurons of the hypothalamus form these two
neurohypophyseal hormones that are
transported by the supraopticohypophyseal tract to the neurohypophysis
where they are stored. Injury to the supraopticohypophyseal system produces *dia-
betes insipidus* in which large volumes of
dilute urine are formed (polyuria). The
excessive loss of water in the urine causes
pronounced thirst and excessive intake of
water (polydipsia).

The reader interested in additional
background material in the area of hypothalamic control of the pituitary gland is
directed to the bibliography which contains several recent comprehensive re-
views of the rapidly expanding field of
Neuroendocrinology.

Autonomic Functions

With respect to hypothalamic control
of the autonomic nervous system, descending nervous pathways, probably
mainly multisynaptic, provide for the relay of information from hypothalamic
integrative regions to motor centers of
the brain stem and spinal cord. Autonomic functions in which the hypothalamus has an integrative or regulative role
include both sympathetic and parasympathetic phenomena. Sympathetic responses that have been obtained by electrically stimulating the hypothalamus include cardiac acceleration, increased
blood pressure, pilo-erection, pupillary
dilatation, sweating, hyperglycemia, and
cessation of gastrointestinal movement.
Parasympathetic responses that have been
elicited, particularly from stimulating the
more anterior hypothalamic regions, include cardiac depression, vasodilatation,
bladder contraction, and increased gastrointestinal movement. These responses
following anterior hypothalamic stimulation suggest that separate areas are con-

cerned with sympathetic and parasympathetic regulation. There is, however, considerable intermingling of the elements responsible for these responses throughout the hypothalamus. Furthermore, the responses are generally more easily elicited from the lateral hypothalamic area, which contains many fibers and few neurons. Generally, the responses are not isolated effects, but are a part of more complex behavioral alterations.

Regulation of Temperature

Animals with lesions of the anterior hypothalamus dorsal to the optic chiasm and infundibulum (including the preoptic region) are unable to avoid extreme rises in body temperature when in a warm environment. Heating this region with electrodes has long been known to activate heat loss mechanisms such as panting and sweating. Local cooling of the region induces various effects which result in heat production and/or preservation. They include shivering, vasoconstriction, and the activation of the thyroid and adrenal glands. Lesions in the caudal hypothalamus, dorsolateral to the mammillary bodies, render animals incapable of maintaining normal body temperature in either a warm or cold environment. It is believed that the dorsomedial portion of the posterior hypothalamus is responsible, in part, for cold-induced shivering, and that a more dorsolateral region of the posterior hypothalamus is involved in other motor responses to cold. It seems likely that the changes in thermoregulatory responses that follow posterior hypothalamic lesions may be due to the interruption of traversing fibers as well as to the destruction of cells therein.

A number of studies support the view that the preoptic-anterior hypothalamic regions contain thermosensitive elements that are involved in the regulation of body temperature. The specific nerve cells which may act as temperature "receptors" have not been identified by direct anatomical methods, though there is increasing evidence that changes in single unit activity of neurons in this region occur during small displacements of hypothalamic temperature.

Food and Water Intake

It is well established that neural mechanisms reside in the hypothalamus which regulate food and water intake, although specific functions cannot easily be ascribed to any one isolated nuclear group. Rather, it appears that separate but interconnected widespread regions control the many aspects of eating and drinking behavior. Stimulation of the region between the columns of the fornix and mammillothalamic tract produces polydipsia and pronounced over-hydration, and lesions in this general region cause temporary adipsia; however, impairment of drinking has also been obtained by lateral hypothalamic lesions. With regard to the regulation of food intake, a variety of experiments have indicated that the lateral hypothalamic area is a feeding "center" and the medial hypothalamic region a satiety "center." Hyperphagia and resultant obesity ensue from lesions of the ventromedial nucleus, whereas lesions of the lateral hypothalamus result in aphagia and eventual starvation unless the animals are force fed. Correspondingly, food intake is decreased by electrical stimulation of the medial hypothalamus and increased by stimulating the lateral hypothalamus.

It can readily be seen that many parts of the hypothalamus enter into the regulation of food and water intake. Although it seems justifiable to call the ventromedial nucleus a satiety center, the lateral hypothalamus does not have the character of a center due to its scarcity of neurons. It has been suggested that ascending tracts in the lateral zone may transmit the urges to eat and drink to higher centers, and that the medial forebrain bundle may play a role in the neural organization of feeding areas. It has been further stressed that motivational factors

Sleep

Bilateral lesions in the hypothalamus of monkeys have produced somnolence, and it has been suggested that, in the rat, there is a cephalic hypothalamic sleep center and a more caudal waking center. Additionally, sleep has been produced in cats by diencephalic stimulation. Although these and a number of other studies have suggested the presence of an active sleep center in the hypothalamus, sleep itself cannot be considered without direct attention to wakefulness since sleep is, at least in part, the condition that occurs in the absence of wakefulness. Studies on the reticular activating system provide substantial support for the view that sleep ensues from the decreased flow of afferent impulses to the cerebral cortex. However, it has been reported that stimulation of the basal forebrain in cats produces behavioral and electroencephalographic manifestations of sleep. Moreover, it has been suggested that in addition to the activating system there are deactivating structures in the brain stem, primarily medulla and pons, which are responsible for deep sleep without EEG synchronization.

Emotional Expression

It is readily appreciated that the hypothalamus is involved in the expression of emotional states since it serves as a regulatory center for both parasympathetic and sympathetic divisions of the autonomic nervous system. Stimulation or the placement of lesions in localized regions of the hypothalamus has produced responses not unlike those produced by comparable procedures applied to rhinencephalic and related cortical areas. For example, lesions of the ventromedial nuclei of the hypothalamus elicit rage and savageness in animals and "sham" rage has been produced by ablating the orbital cortex. A variety of responses may, in fact, be elicited from stimulating the hypothalamus in unanesthetized animals which mimic normal defense reactions. It is probable, however, that the role of the hypothalamus is that of integrating the activity from cortical centers, thus controlling the expressive or motor aspects of emotion.

SUBTHALAMUS

The subthalamus, often called the ventral thalamus, is functionally interrelated with the extrapyramidal system and is described in Chapter 17.

BIBLIOGRAPHY

The Thalamus

Brodal, A., 1969: The reticular formation. In *Neurological Anatomy*. Oxford University Press, Inc., New York. Chap. 6.

Chow, K. L., and Pribram, K. H., 1956: Cortical projection of the thalamic ventrolateral nuclear group in monkeys. J. Comp. Neurol., *104,* 57–75.

Krupp, P., and Monnier, D., 1966: The unspecific intralaminary modulating system of the thalamus. Int. Rev. Neurobiol., *9,* 45–94.

Magoun, H. W., 1963: *The Waking Brain.* Charles C Thomas, Springfield, Ill.

Nauta, W. J. H., and Kuypers, H. G. J. M., 1957: Some ascending pathways in the brain stem reticular formation. In *Reticular Formation of the Brain.* H. H. Jasper et al., Eds., Henry Ford Hosp. Intern. Symposium, Little, Brown & Co., Boston, pp. 3–30.

Nauta, W. J. H., and Mehler, W. R., 1966: Projections of the lentiform nucleus in the monkey. Brain Res., *1,* 3–42.

Purpura, D. P., and Yahr, M. D., 1966: *The Thalamus.* Columbia University Press, New York.

Scheibel, M. E., and Scheibel, A. B., 1966: The organization of the nucleus reticularis thalami: a Golgi study. Brain Res., *1,* 43–62.

Sheps, J. G., 1945: The nuclear configuration and cortical connections of the human thalamus. J. Comp. Neurol., *83,* 1–56.

Toncray, J. E., and Krieg, W. J. S., 1946: The nuclei of the human thalamus. A comparative approach. J. Comp. Neurol., *85,* 421–459.

Walker, A. E., 1966: *The Primate Thalamus.* University of Chicago Press, Chicago.

must be considered when studying alterations in eating and drinking behavior due to hypothalamic interference.

Walker, A. E., 1959: Normal and pathological physiology of the thalamus. In *Introduction to Stereotaxis with an Atlas of the Human Brain*. I. G. Schaltenbrand and P. Bailey, Eds. Thieme, Stuttgart, pp. 291–330.

The Hypothalamus

Anand, B. K., 1961: Nervous regulation of food intake. Physiol. Rev., *41*, 677–708.

Andersson, B., Ekman, L., Gale, C. C., and Sundsten, J. W., 1963: Control of thyrotrophic hormone (TSH) secretion by the "heat loss center." Acta Physiol. Scand., *59*, 12–33.

Benzinger, T. H., 1962: The thermostatic regulation of human heat production and heat loss. Proc. XXII Intern. Congr. Physiologic Sci., Leiden, Vol. I, pp. 415–438.

Bligh, J., 1966: The thermosensitivity of the hypothalamus and thermoregulation in mammals. Biol. Rev., *41*, 317–367.

Brobeck, J. R., 1960: Regulation of feeding and drinking. In *Handbook of Physiology*, Vol. II, Section I., *Neurophysiology*. John Field, Ed.-in-Chief. Williams & Wilkins Co., Baltimore, Chap. 47, pp. 1197–1206.

Eisenman, J. S., and Jackson, D. C., 1967: Thermal response patterns of septal and preoptic neurons in cats. Exp. Neurol., *19*, 33–45.

Ganong, W. F., and L. Martini, 1969: *Frontiers in Neuroendocrinology*. Oxford University Press, Inc., New York.

Hardy, J. D., 1961: Physiology of temperature regulation. Physiol. Rev., *41*, 521–606.

Harris, G. W., and Donovan, B. T., 1966: *The Pituitary Gland*. Vols. 1–3. Butterworths, London.

Hellon, R. F., 1967: Thermal stimulation of hypothalamic neurones in unanesthetized rabbits. J. Physiol., *193*, 381–395.

Ingram, W. R., 1960: Central autonomic mechanisms. In *Handbook of Physiology*, Vol. II, Section I, *Neurophysiology*. John Field, Ed.-in-Chief. Williams & Wilkins Co., Baltimore, Chap. 37, pp. 951–978.

Martini, L., and Ganong, W. F., 1967: *Neuroendocrinology*. Vols. 1–2, Academic Press, New York.

Morgane, P. J., 1969: Neural regulation of food and water intake. N.Y. Acad. Sci., *157*, 531–1216.

Ortmann, R., 1960: Neurosecretion. In *Handbook of Physiology*, Vol. II, Section I, *Neurophysiology*. John Field, Ed.-in-Chief. Williams & Wilkins Co., Baltimore, Chap. 40, pp. 1039–1065.

von Euler, C., 1961: Physiology and pharmacology of temperature regulation. Pharmacol. Rev., *13*, 361–398.

The Epithalamus

Kelly, D. E., 1962: Pineal organs: photoreception, secretion and development. Amer. Sci. *50*, 597–625.

Kitay, J. I., 1966: Possible functions of the pineal gland. In *Neuroendocrinology*, Vol. II, L. Martini and W. F. Ganong, Eds. Academic Press, New York.

Chapter 22

The Autonomic Nervous System

The autonomic (visceral) nervous system is comprised of the nerve cells and fibers that are distributed to smooth muscle, cardiac muscle, and glands, and thus it is concerned with the regulation of visceral activities. These activities are usually not under voluntary influence.

It has been traditional to include in the autonomic nervous system only the visceral efferent (motor) components that supply visceral structures in accordance with the original definition by Langley. It is recognized, however, that most visceral efferent fibers are accompanied by sensory fibers, and it is the more common practice to include both visceral efferent and visceral afferent fibers as components of the autonomic nervous system. Moreover, the original connotation that the autonomic system included only peripheral elements, i.e., excluding central neural structures, is no longer tenable.

Visceral afferent neurons, like those with somatic afferent functions, have their cell bodies in the sensory ganglia of spinal and cranial nerves; specific locations, distribution of peripheral processes, and termination of central processes of these neurons have been discussed.

The *visceral efferent system* is divided, on the basis of function and outflow from the central nervous system, into *thoracolumbar* and *craniosacral* portions. The former division is also classified as *sympathetic system* and the latter as *para-*

sympathetic (Fig. 209). It is pointed out in Chapter 21 that both sympathetic and parasympathetic divisions are influenced by nervous impulses from the hypothalamus through the medium of descending hypothalamic pathways. Direct and indirect corticohypothalamic connections have been described, and the role of the hypothalamus in integrating activity from cortical centers and thus controlling motor aspects of emotion has been indicated.

Both divisions of the visceral efferent system (sympathetic and parasympathetic) employ two neurons for the transmission of impulses from the central nervous system to the structures innervated. The first or *preganglionic neuron* is located in the spinal cord or brain stem; the second or *ganglionic neuron* has its cell body in a sympathetic trunk or collateral ganglion. Examples of *collateral ganglia* are the ciliary, otic, submandibular, and sphenopalatine in the head region, and the celiac, aorticorenal, and superior and inferior mesenteric in the abdominal cavity. *Intrinsic ganglia,* situated in the walls of the visceral organs, may be included in the collateral classification. Nerve cells in the adrenal medulla, which are derived from the neural crest, may be included also since preganglionic fibers from the spinal cord reach them by way of the splanchnic nerves.

The sympathetic trunk ganglia com-

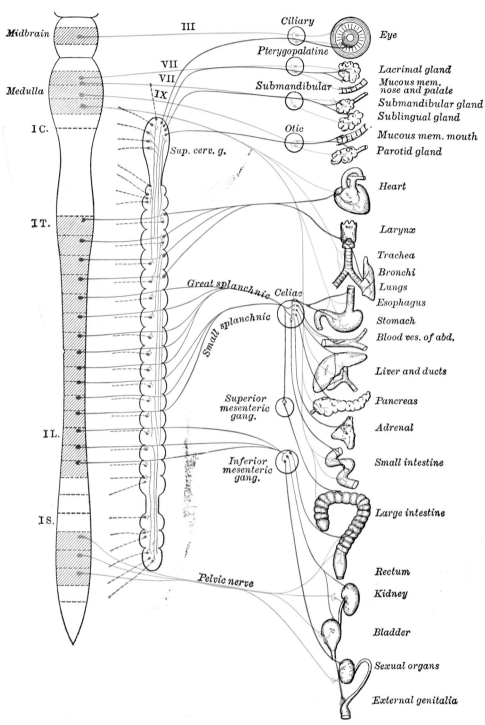

FIG. 209. Diagram of efferent autonomic nervous system. *Blue,* cranial and sacral outflow, parasympathetic. *Red,* thoracolumbar outflow, sympathetic. - - - - - -, postganglionic fibers to spinal and cranial nerves to supply vaso-motors to head, trunk, and limbs; motor fibers to smooth muscles of skin and fibers to sweat glands. (Modified after Meyer and Gottlieb.) This is only a diagram and does not accurately portray all the details of distribution. (From Gray's Anatomy, 28th ed., Charles Mayo Goss, Ed., Lea & Febiger, Philadelphia.)

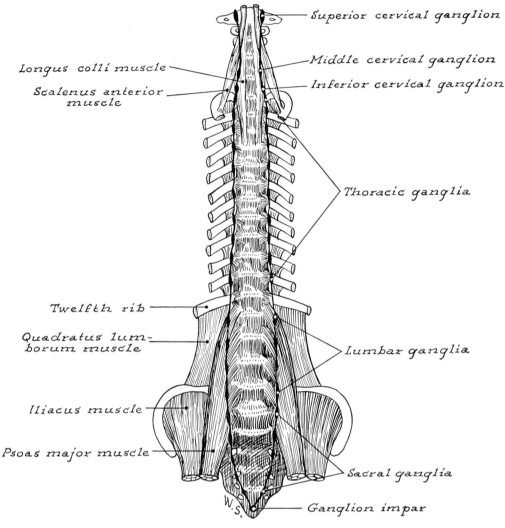

Longus colli muscle

Scalenus anterior
muscle

Superior cervical ganglion

Middle cervical ganglion

Inferior cervical ganglion

Thoracic ganglia

Twelfth rib

Quadratus lum-
borum muscle

Lumbar ganglia

Iliacus muscle

Psoas major muscle

Sacral ganglia

W. S.

Ganglion impar

FIG. 210. The ganglionated trunks of the sympathetic division of the autonomic system.

prise paired ganglionated trunks located lateral to the vertebral column; they extend from the base of the skull to the coccyx where the two trunks fuse in the ganglion impar (Fig. 210).

Preganglionic fibers (axons of centrally located neurons) proceed to the peripheral ganglia by way of spinal or cranial nerves and synapse on the ganglionic cells whose axons are then distributed as *postganglionic fibers* to the visceral structures (Fig. 209). Preganglionic fibers in spinal nerves reach the sympathetic ganglia via white rami communicantes (Fig. 5). Postganglionic fibers traverse the gray

rami communicantes from sympathetic ganglia to the spinal nerves with which they are distributed.

Most visceral organs have a dual innervation, i.e., they receive both sympathetic and parasympathetic impulses. It is still not definitely known whether the peripheral blood vessels have a dual innervation, although it is well established that all of them receive fibers from the sympathetic division of the autonomic system.

Pupillary constriction is produced by parasympathetic nerve impulses. The preganglionic neurons have their cell bodies in the *Edinger-Westphal nucleus* in the mesencephalon (Fig. 70). The nucleus is dorsolateral to the rostral half of the oculomotor nucleus and extends forward to a level slightly beyond the rostral limit of the latter nucleus. *Preganglionic fibers* reach the *ciliary ganglion* by way of the oculomotor nerve and synapse on ganglionic cells whose axons are distributed, as postganglionic fibers, through the short ciliary nerves to the sphincter muscle of the pupil and to the ciliary body (Fig. 209).

Dilatation of the pupil is effected by sympathetic impulses. The preganglionic neurons are located in the *intermediate gray column* of the upper two thoracic segments of the spinal cord; preganglionic fibers emerge from the cord over the anterior roots of the corresponding spinal nerves, proceed to the sympathetic trunk by way of the *white rami communicantes,* and then course upward in the trunk to finally synapse on cells in the *superior cervical ganglion* (Fig. 211). Postganglionic fibers from this ganglion reach the dilator pupillae muscle by way of the sympathetic plexus surrounding the internal carotid artery; they enter the orbit

through the superior orbital fissure and pass through or near the ciliary ganglion without interruption therein. Sympathetic fibers complete their course to the iris and ciliary body by way of the short ciliary nerves.

It has been demonstrated conclusively, in the monkey, that pupillary dilatation elicited by electrical stimulation of area 8 is a sympathetic response that is mediated by indirect corticohypothalamic and hypothalamicospinal connections. The response was abolished by section of the cervical sympathetic chain.

The **submandibular** and **sublingual glands** receive their *parasympathetic* innervation by way of a two-neuron pathway that begins with preganglionic cells in the *superior salivary nucleus* in the pontile tegmentum. Preganglionic fibers pass to the *submandibular ganglion* through the *nervus intermedius* and *chorda tympani*. Postganglionic fibers, axons of cells in the ganglion, are distributed to the glands (Fig. 209).

The **lacrimal gland** and the **glands of the nose and palate** also receive *parasympathetic* impulses from the *superior salivary nucleus*. Preganglionic fibers

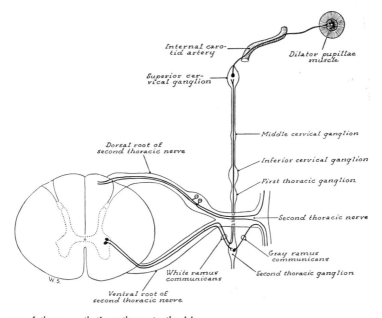

FIG. 211. Diagram of the sympathetic pathway to the iris.

from the nucleus traverse the *nervus intermedius* and *major petrosal* nerve to reach the *pterygopalatine ganglion* in the pterygopalatine fossa. Postganglionic fibers from the ganglion are distributed to the glands.

The **parotid gland** is innervated by preganglionic parasympathetic fibers that originate in the *inferior salivary nucleus,* in the reticular formation of the medulla; they reach the *otic ganglion* by way of the *glossopharyngeal nerve.* Postganglionic fibers from the otic ganglion are distributed to the gland through the *auriculotemporal nerve* (Fig. 209).

Direct parasympathetic innervation of secretory cells in parotid and submandibular glands (from otic and submandibular ganglia) has been demonstrated anatomically to satisfactorily explain the copious secretory effects produced by parasympathetic stimulation. The sympathetic nerves supplying these glands are distributed predominantly or exclusively to the intraglandular blood vessels, which implies that salivary secretion in response to sympathetic stimulation is the result of vasomotor activity. This concept coincides with the observation that occlusion of arteries supplying the glands prevents secretion due to sympathetic stimulation.

The **salivary nuclei** are not distinguishable in sections through the brain stem, but their approximate locations have been determined through stimulation experiments. The superior salivary nucleus has been found to be dorsolaterally placed in the caudal end of the pontile tegmentum with the inferior nucleus directly caudal to it in the reticular formation of the medulla.

The **sympathetic supply to all the salivary glands** and to other glands in the head region comes from preganglionic cells in the upper two thoracic segments of the spinal cord. Preganglionic fibers pass through the first and second thoracic nerves, the white rami communicantes, and the sympathetic trunk to the *superior cervical ganglion* (Fig. 211). Postgan-

glionic fibers from the ganglion are distributed to the glands by way of the plexuses that accompany the internal and external carotid arteries (Fig. 209).

The **upper extremity** derives its *sympathetic supply* from preganglionic cells located in the *intermediate gray column* of the upper seven or eight thoracic segments of the spinal cord. Axons of these cells reach the sympathetic trunk in the usual manner, and, after ascending in the trunk, synapse on cells in the middle and inferior cervical and upper two thoracic ganglia. Postganglionic fibers, through the gray rami communicantes, join the lower four cervical and first thoracic nerves and are distributed to the vascular and glandular structures and arrector pili muscles of the upper extremity by way of the brachial plexus and its branches (Fig. 212). Sweating, pilo-erection, and vasoconstriction are produced by impulses traversing these fibers. If there are vasodilator fibers to the blood vessels of the extremities they have still to be conclusively demonstrated.

A *sympathetic vasodilator outflow* from the motor cortex to skeletal muscles by way of the hypothalamus has been demonstrated in the dog. Such a pathway probably exists in the cat as well, but is said to be lacking in rabbits and monkeys and its existence in man is doubtful. The sympathetic vasodilator fibers are cholinergic rather than adrenergic, and it has been suggested that they are capable of increasing blood flow to skeletal (and possibly to cardiac) muscle in situations of emergency or other conditions requiring sudden muscular effort. In connection with humoral mediation between autonomic nerves and effector mechanisms, it should be noted that the sympathetic fibers to sweat glands are also cholinergic. As a general rule sympathetics are adrenergic and parasympathetics are cholinergic. Within peripheral ganglia, however, transmission from preganglionic fiber to ganglionic neuron is facilitated by acetylcholine regardless of whether that neuron

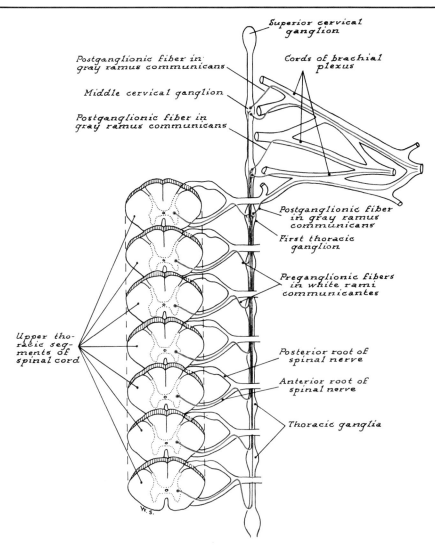

FIG. 212. Diagram of the sympathetic innervation of the upper extremity by way of the brachial plexus.

depends on norepinephrine or acetylcholine for its functional contact with an effector.

The **lower extremity** receives its sympathetic supply from preganglionic cells in the intermediate gray column of the lower five thoracic and the upper two lumbar segments of the spinal cord. After reaching the sympathetic trunk by way of white rami communicantes, the preganglionic fibers course downward within the trunk and synapse on ganglion cells in the lower lumbar and sacral ganglia (Fig. 215). Postganglionic fibers from these ganglia join the lumbar and sacral nerves as gray rami communicantes and, through the branches of the lumbar and sacral plexuses, are distributed to the blood vessels, arrector pili muscles, and sweat glands of the lower extremity.

The **thoracic viscera** are innervated by *sympathetic preganglionic neurons* in the intermediate gray columns of the upper five thoracic segments of the spinal cord. Preganglionic fibers enter and course upward in the sympathetic trunk where they synapse on cells in the superior, middle, and inferior cervical ganglia. Postganglionic fibers enter the thorax by way of the *superior, middle,* and *inferior cardiac nerves* and are distributed to the heart and lungs through the *cardiac* and *pulmonary plexuses* (Fig. 213). Some postganglionic fibers reach the pulmonary plexuses by passing directly forward from the third, fourth, and fifth thoracic ganglia. All cardiac nerves contain both efferent and afferent fibers with the exception of the superior one (derived from the superior cervical ganglion), which has only efferent fibers. This is important in operations devised for the relief of cardiac pain.

The **sympathetic supply to the abdomi-** **nal viscera** comes from preganglionic neurons with cell bodies in the lower six thoracic segments of the spinal cord. Their axons reach the sympathetic trunk over the corresponding ventral roots and white rami communicantes. They pass through the trunk ganglia without synapsing therein and form the splanchic nerves (greater, lesser, and least). The *splanchnic nerves* (Fig. 213) pierce the diaphragm and their component fibers (preganglionic) synapse on ganglionic cells in the *celiac, aorticorenal, superior mesenteric,* and *inferior mesenteric ganglia.* Postganglionic fibers from the ganglia are distributed with the branches of

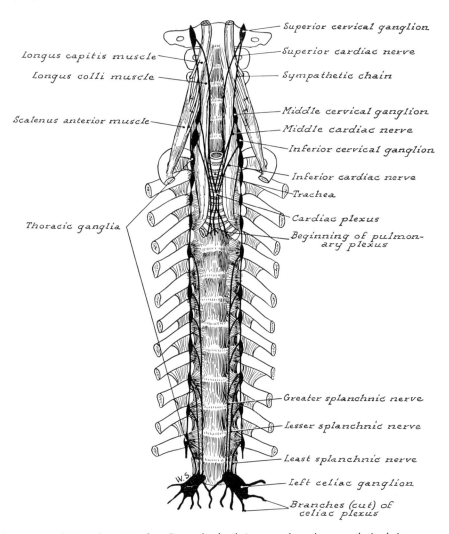

FIG. 213. Diagram showing the origin of cardiac and splanchnic nerves from the sympathetic chains.

the aorta to smooth muscle in the abdominal and pelvic organs and in the blood vessels that supply the organs.

The **parasympathetic supply to the thoracic and abdominal viscera,** including the digestive tract as far down as the transverse colon, originates in the *dorsal motor nucleus* of the *vagus nerve.* The nucleus is located in the medulla, just beneath the floor of the fourth ventricle and immediately lateral to the hypoglossal nucleus. The area of the rhomboid fossa overlying it is called the *vagal trigone* (Fig. 214). Preganglionic fibers

are distributed by way of the vagus nerve and the cardiac, pulmonary, celiac, and hypogastric plexuses to intrinsic ganglia, which have been previously described as being within the walls of the visceral structures (Fig. 209).

The **descending colon,** the **pelvic viscera** (pelvic colon, rectum, bladder, and uterus), and the **external genitalia** receive parasympathetic fibers from the intermediate (parasympathetic) gray column of the middle sacral segments of the spinal cord. Preganglionic fibers emerge from the cord through the anterior roots

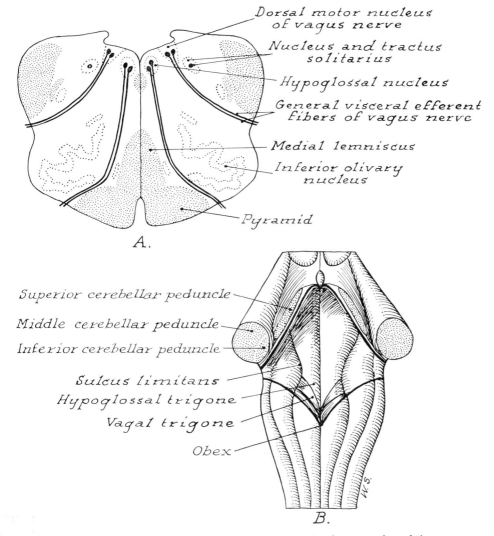

FIG. 214. A, Section of the medulla demonstrating the position of the dorsal motor nucleus of the vagus nerve. B, Diagram showing the position of the vagal trigone in the floor of the fourth ventricle (rhomboid fossa).

of the corresponding sacral nerves and, without passing through the sympathetic trunk, unite to form the *pelvic nerve* (*nervus erigens*), which is distributed through the *pelvic* (*inferior hypogastric*) *plexuses,* to the intrinsic ganglia in the pelvic viscera and external genitalia (Fig. 209).

Operative procedures on the visceral nervous system are carried out for the relief of pain, to correct circulatory disorders that appear to be due to abnormal vasomotor stimuli, and to adjust apparent motor imbalances in the smooth musculature of the colon and uterus. Pain is frequently associated with muscular spasm due to excessive autonomic impulses.

Cervicothoracic ganglionectomy has been performed for the relief of vascular spasm of such degree in the upper extremity as to interfere seriously with oxygenation of the tissues. The inferior cervical and upper two thoracic ganglia are excised; the preganglionic fibers from the upper two thoracic segments and the postganglionic fibers from these ganglia to the brachial plexus are thus severed, together with the removal of a large number of ganglionic cells (Fig. 212). The procedure promotes vasodilatation by decreasing the vasoconstrictor impulses to the extremity.

Horner's syndrome is an unavoidable sequel to cervicothoracic ganglionectomy since all preganglionic sympathetic fibers to the head region course upward through the part of the sympathetic chain that is excised. The syndrome is characterized by ipsilateral miosis, ptosis, enophthalmos, anhidrosis, and blushing of the face. *Miosis* (constriction of the pupil) occurs as the result of having interrupted the nerve supply to the dilator pupillae muscle. *Ptosis* of slight, but noticeable, degree results from paralysis of the smooth muscle (of Horner), which is associated with the levator palpebrae superioris in the upper eyelid. *Enophthalmos* may be due to paralysis of Mueller's muscle,

which bridges the inferior orbital fissure but has been termed an optical illusion due to narrowing of the palpebral fissure. *Anhidrosis* (absence or diminution of sweating) is due to interruption of the sympathetic nerves to the sweat glands, and *blushing* results from vasodilatation of peripheral vessels whose sympathetic innervation has been interrupted.

The oculopupillary features of Horner's syndrome can be avoided if, instead of performing cervicothoracic ganglionectomy, only the second or second and third thoracic ganglia are removed. Preganglionic sympathetic fibers to the upper extremity have been shown to come from the intermediate gray column of the first thoracic segment of the spinal cord in only about 10 percent of individuals. A theoretical advantage of second thoracic ganglionectomy, so far as sympathectomy of the upper extremity is concerned, is that the procedure is essentially a preganglionic resection with respect to the ganglion cells in the lower two cervical and first thoracic ganglia whose cells actually distribute postganglionic fibers to the upper extremity. Sensitization to circulating epinephrine, which has been supposed to be responsible for unsatisfactory results when the cervicothoracic ganglion cells are removed, is thus reduced or eliminated.

Lumbar ganglionectomy is performed for the relief of disorders of the circulation in the lower extremities and is particularly applicable to cases of thromboangiitis obliterans that are not too far advanced. The second and third and, frequently, the fourth lumbar ganglia are removed and this, in addition to removing some ganglionic cells, interrupts all the preganglionic fibers from the lower thoracic and upper lumbar segments of the cord that have to do with the sympathetic innervation of the lower extremity (Fig. 215). The relief of the excruciating pain usually associated with thromboangiitis obliterans, by lumbar ganglionectomy, may be due to the inter-

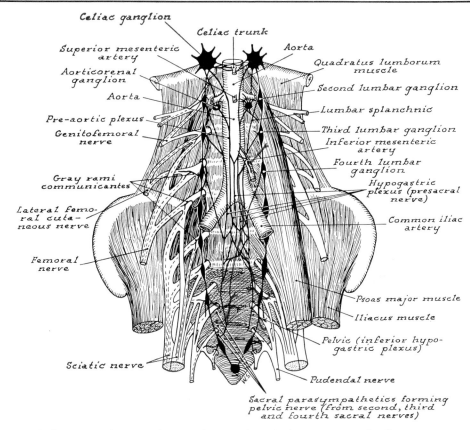

FIG. 215. The hypogastric plexus and the sympathetic supply to the lower extremity. The fibers diagrammed in red are parasympathetic, some of which course as far cephalad as the inferior mesenteric artery and are distributed with its branches (in part after Gask and Ross).

ruption of visceral afferent fibers, to the increased blood supply to the extremity, or to a combination of both factors.

It has been generally believed that bilateral removal of the upper lumbar ganglia in the male would result in sterility because of the location in the lumbar cord of the ejaculatory center, responsible for the sympathetic innervation of the ejaculatory mechanism (seminiferous tubules, vas deferens, and ejaculatory ducts). A study of 30 cases, however, following bilateral lumbar ganglionectomy in which the first, second, and third ganglia were removed, showed that only three individuals were sterile. On the contrary, seven of eight cases of hypertension, in whom the sympathetic chain from ninth thoracic to third lumbar was removed, had complete absence of ejac-

ulation. These observations were explained by the assumption that *postganglionic* ejaculatory innervation arises in the twelfth thoracic ganglion and reaches the pelvis via the least splanchnic and *presacral nerves* (Fig. 215).

The **hypogastric plexus (presacral nerve),** through which the distal part of the colon, rectum, bladder, and uterus receive their sympathetic supply, is formed by three roots (Fig. 215). The central root descends over the bifurcation of the aorta from the pre-aortic plexus and is joined on each side by a lateral root. The lateral roots are formed by the union, on both sides, of the lumbar splanchnics that arise from the upper lumbar segments of the spinal cord. The *lumbar splanchnics* pass through the sympathetic trunks without synapsing on ganglionic cells and eventually synapse on cells in ganglia scattered among the fibers of the pelvic plexuses. The hypogastric plexus is located between the common iliac arteries, anterior to the fifth lumbar vertebra and the sacral promontory. It continues into the pelvis and divides into right and left *pelvic (inferior hypogastric) plexuses,* which course downward on both sides of the rectum. The pelvic nerves, or sacral parasympathetics, also enter into the pelvic plexuses.

Hirschsprung's disease or **congenital megacolon** was formerly thought to be due to an autonomic imbalance, i.e., the sympathetic impulses to the colon were supposed to be in excess of the parasympathetic. Since the sympathetics have been shown to inhibit peristalsis and the parasympathetics to increase it, the imbalance would result in stasis of intestinal content with the tremendous dilatation of the colon which is characteristic of the condition.

More recently it has been demonstrated that there is, in most cases of congenital megacolon, an absence of ganglion cells in the myenteric (Auerbach's) plexuses of the distal colon. It appears that the aganglionic portion of the colon is tonically contracted and that there is absence, in this segment, of propulsive peristaltic activity, leading to accumulation of intestinal content in the proximal colon; this results in thinning out of the muscular layers and, eventually, loss of propulsive activity with stasis in this segment.

Dysmenorrhea (painful menstruation) has been successfully treated by *presacral neurectomy* (excision of the hypogastric plexus). The relief of pain may be dependent on the division of visceral afferent fibers, but it is probable that the division of efferent fibers, necessarily a part of the procedure, may be a potent factor through lessening of the severe smooth muscle spasm which accounts for the pain.

The musculature of the urinary bladder is innervated by parasympathetic fibers that arise from sacral segments 2, 3, and 4. These fibers course to the bladder through the pelvic nerve and end in relation to neurons of the vesical ganglia. The postganglionic fibers induce contraction of the bladder musculature (detrusor). The sympathetic fibers to the bladder are apparently restricted to the musculature of the vesical trigone in relation to the openings of the ureters and urethra and thus have no motor function in micturition. (The trigonal muscles contract during ejaculation and prevent the entry of seminal fluid into the bladder.) The external sphincter of the bladder, which is under voluntary control, is innervated by somatic motor fibers of the pelvic nerve which arise from sacral segments 2, 3, and 4.

Sensory fibers from the bladder, which mediate sensations of fullness as well as pain, course in the hypogastric nerves and sympathetic trunk to reach the lower thoracic and upper lumbar segments of the spinal cord.

BIBLIOGRAPHY

Cannon, W. B., and Rosenblueth, A., 1937: *Autonomic Neuro-effector Systems.* The Macmillan Company, New York.

Cheatham, M. L., and Matzke, H. A., 1966: Descending hypothalamic medullary pathways in the cat. J. Comp. Neurol., *127,* 369–380.

Craig, J. D., and Fuller, R. C., 1948: Cervical sympathetic paralysis. Brit. Med. J., *1,* 1182–1184.

Emmelin, N., 1967: Nervous control of salivary glands. In *Handbook of Physiology,* Section 6, Vol. II, *Secretion.* C. F. Code, Ed. American Physiological Society, Washington, D.C., Chap. 37, pp. 595–632.

Kuntz, A., 1953: *The Autonomic Nervous System,* Lea & Febiger, Philadelphia.

Langley, J. N., 1921: *The Autonomic Nervous System,* Vol. 1. W. Heffer and Sons, Cambridge.

Langworthy, O. R., 1943: General principles of autonomic innervation. A.M.A. Arch. Neurol. Psychiat., *50,* 590–602.

Magoun, H. W., and Beaton, L. E., 1942: The salivatory motor nuclei in the monkey. Amer. J. Physiol., *136,* 720–725.

Mitchell, G. A. G., 1953: The innervation of the heart. Brit. Heart J., *15,* 159–171.

Naquin, H. A., 1954: Argyll Robertson pupil following herpes zoster ophthalmicus: with remarks on the efferent pupillary pathways. Amer. J. Ophthalmol., *38*, 23–33.

Norberg, K. A., 1967: Transmitter histochemistry of the sympathetic nervous system. Brain Res., *5*, 125–170.

Nyberg-Hansen, R., 1966: Innervation and nervous control of the urinary bladder. Acta Neurol. Scand., *42, Suppl. 20*, 7–24.

Ray, B. S., 1953: Sympathectomy of the upper extremity. Evaluation of surgical methods. J. Neurosurg., *10*, 624–633.

Richins, C. A., and Kuntz, A., 1953: Role of sympathetic nerves in the regulation of salivary secretion. Amer. J. Physiol., *173*, 417–473.

Rose, S. S., 1953: An investigation into sterility after lumbar ganglionectomy. Brit. Med. J., *1*, 247–250.

Smith, O. A., Jr., and Clarke, N. P., 1964: Central autonomic pathways. A study in functional neuroanatomy. J. Comp. Neurol., *122*, 399–406.

Uvnäs, B., 1954: Sympathetic vasodilator outflow. Physiol. Rev., *34*, 608–618.

van Duzen, R. E., and Duncan, C. G., 1953: Anatomy and nerve supply of urinary bladder. J.A.M.A., *153*, 1345–1347.

von Euler, U. S., 1959: Autonomic neuroeffector transmission. In *Handbook of Physiology,* Section I, Vol. I, *Neurophysiology.* J. Field, H. W. Magoun, and V. E. Hall, Eds. American Physiological Society, Washington, D.C., pp. 215–237.

Wang, S. C., 1943: Localization of the salivatory center in the medulla of the cat. J. Neurophysiol., *6*, 195–202.

Ward, A. A., and Reed, H. L., 1946: Mechanism of pupillary dilatation elicited by cortical stimulation. J. Neurophysiol., *9*, 329–335.

Warwick, R., 1954: The ocular parasympathetic nerve supply and its mesencephalic sources. J. Anat., *88*, 71–93.

White, J. C., Smithwick, R. H., and Simeone, F. A., 1952: *The Autonomic Nervous System.* Macmillan, New York.

Chapter 23

Visceral Reflex Arcs

Visceral reflex arcs, including *viscerovisceral, viscerosomatic,* and *somatovisceral,* facilitate automatic adjustments of the entire organism to its internal and external environments. When food is ingested the visceral blood supply is increased at the expense of that to the periphery in order to promote digestion. When muscular activity results in increased demand for oxygen, respiration is correspondingly increased in rate and depth. In a cold environment the peripheral vessels are constricted to prevent loss of heat from the body surface.

Many visceral reflex arcs are centered in the spinal cord; others have their centers in the medulla oblongata. In many instances, the afferent limb of the arc includes the thalamus, which may send impulses to the hypothalamus or to the cerebral cortex; thus, visceral reflexes may be centered at diencephalic or cortical levels. That the cortex functions in visceral reflex arcs is indicated by the fact that there are several cortical areas that give rise to visceral responses when stimulated electrically.

The **carotid sinus reflex** (Fig. 216) is an important example of the viscerovisceral type. The *carotid sinus* is a slight dilatation of the common carotid artery at its level of bifurcation into internal and external divisions or of the proximal portion of the internal carotid artery. Its walls contain specialized receptors that are stimulated by increases in intrasinus pressure. Peripheral processes of nerve cells in the inferior petrosal ganglion of the glossopharyngeal nerve are distributed to the receptors by way of the *carotid sinus nerve.*

When the pressure within the carotid sinus is increased as the result of a general rise in blood pressure the nerve impulses thus initiated are conducted to the nucleus solitarius in the medulla. Direct or indirect connections from the nucleus solitarius to the dorsal motor nucleus of the vagus nerve complete a reflex arc through which a reduction in heart rate is produced. Other reflex connections from the nucleus solitarius to the vasomotor center in the reticular formation of the medulla inhibit the activity of the center, and thus allow dilatation of the circulatory system to occur. The combined effect resulting from decreased heart rate and dilatation of the vascular system is reduction in blood pressure.

When the blood pressure is low the number of nerve impulses reaching the vasomotor center from the receptors in the carotid sinus is correspondingly reduced; thus, the inhibitory effect on the center is lessened and vasoconstriction occurs with a resultant increase in blood pressure.

Sympathetic impulses emanating from the vasomotor center may also increase the cardiac rate and thereby contribute

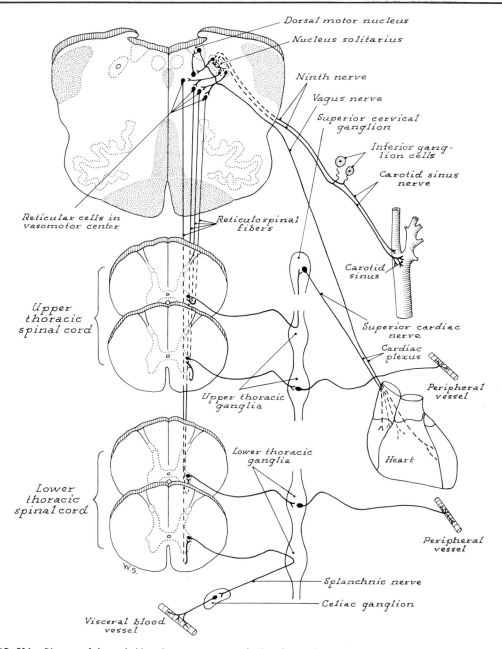

FIG. 216. Diagram of the probable reflex connections involved in the regulation of blood pressure by the carotid sinus.

to an increase in blood pressure. Vaso-constrictor and cardioaccelerator impulses from the vasomotor center are conducted to the proper cells in the intermediate gray columns of the spinal cord by way of reticulospinal fibers originating from cells within the center (Fig. 216). Evidence has been presented that large retic-

ular cells situated in the ventromedial area of the reticular formation of the medulla, immediately dorsal to the inferior olivary nucleus, regulate circulation. Damage to these cells invariably produces clinical symptoms of vasomotor disturbance, such as irregular feeble pulse, low pulse pressure, irregularities of blood pressure, and terminal shock. Based on detailed studies of the pons from individuals having bulbar poliomyelitis, the vasomotor center has been described as having its rostral half within large reticular cells in the caudal part of the pons. Involvement of this area resulted in circulatory collapse.

The **depressor nerve,** a branch of the vagus, functions as the afferent limb of another reflex arc through the nucleus solitarius, vasomotor center, and dorsal motor nucleus which effects lowering of blood pressure. The depressor nerve consists of peripheral processes of inferior ganglion cells and is distributed to the proximal portion of the aortic arch. It is not as well defined in man as in some of the lower animals (cat, rabbit, dog). Currently, there is evidence that afferent connections from almost all divisions of the vascular system affect the vasomotor center and contribute to regulation of blood pressure.

Chemoreceptors in the carotid sinus and carotid body are stimulated by increases in carbon dioxide tension and decreases in oxygen tension of the blood. Impulses arising from stimulation of these special receptors serve to stimulate the respiratory center when it might otherwise fail to maintain respiration because of abnormal conditions such as deep anesthesia. It has been shown that the chemically induced part of the carotid sinus reflex is transmitted principally by nerves other than the glossopharyngeal (vagus, sympathetic).

The **respiratory reflex** functions through a viscerosomatic arc (Fig. 217) since the muscles responsible for respiration originate from mesodermal somites. Peripheral processes of cells in the inferior ganglion of the vagus are distributed, by way of the vagus nerve and pulmonary plexuses, to special receptors in the lungs. Special receptors are found throughout the bronchial tree and as far distally as the atria. Impulses originating in these receptors reach the nucleus soli-

tarius from which they are conducted to the respiratory center in the reticular formation of the medulla; the impulses initiated by inflation of the lungs inhibit, and those resulting from deflation excite, inspiration. Many reticulospinal fibers from the respiratory center terminate in relation to anterior gray column cells in the third, fourth, and fifth cervical segments of the spinal cord and thus serve, through the phrenic nerve, to activate the diaphragm; others terminate in relation to anterior gray column cells in the thoracic levels of the cord whose axons are distributed to the intercostal muscles through the intercostal nerves.

The **respiratory center** consists of a diffusely arranged group of reticular cells extending from the rostral part of the medulla to the level of the obex (Fig. 217). The cells in the more dorsal and rostral parts of the medullary reticular formation have been shown to be concerned with the expiratory phase of respiration and those in the ventral part with the inspiratory phase. Afferent impulses from the lungs by way of the vagus nerve and from the carotid sinus by way of the glossopharyngeal do not constitute the only sources of activation of the respiratory center; slight increases in the carbon dioxide tension of the blood circulating through the center augment its activity. The function of the vagi in limiting inspiration and permitting the inception of expiration may be shared to some extent by the so-called pneumotaxic center.

A **pneumotaxic center** and its location in the rostral pons or mesencephalon have been postulated from experiments in which the vagus nerves were sectioned bilaterally in association with transection of the brain stem at various levels. After section of both vagi, breathing continues although it is deep and slow. If, however, section of the vagi is combined with transection of the brain stem at a level slightly rostral to the middle cerebellar peduncles, respiration ceases in a state of deep inspiration. Section of the brain stem at the same level without section of the vagi results in the same type of respiration as produced by vagal section alone. Apneustic breathing has not been produced in vagotomized cats, decerebrated at the midcollicular level after separate or seriatim ablation of inferior colliculi, central gray matter, and tegmentum at the inferior collicular level, pontile

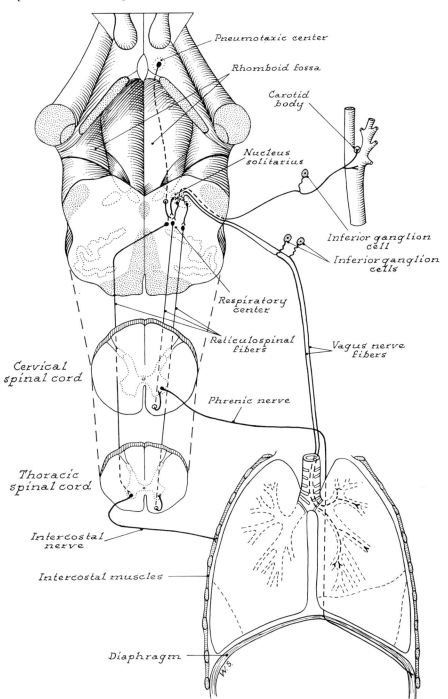

FIG. 217. The respiratory reflex arc.

central gray matter, and central part of the anterior pontile tegmentum. However, small bilateral lesions in the extreme dorsolateral part of the anterior pontile tegmentum consistently produced apneustic breathing, indicating that this is the location of the pneumotaxic center.

On the basis of studies of the entire medulla from each of eighty cases of bulbar poliomyelitis, it has been concluded that small reticular cells in the ventrolateral area of the reticular formation of the medulla, just dorsal to the inferior olivary nucleus, regulate respiratory function. Involvement of these cells by the virus resulted in irregularity of respiratory rhythm and depth, periods of apnea, and, finally, cessation of respiration.

The **light reflex** is dependent on a somatovisceral arc (Fig. 218). The receptors are the rods and cones of the retina. The course of the afferent impulses from the rod and cone cells through bipolar and ganglion cells, optic nerve, optic tract, and superior quadrigeminal brachium was described in Chapter 9. On reaching

the pretectum by way of the quadrigeminal brachium, the impulses are relayed to the Edinger-Westphal nuclei, ciliary ganglion, and constrictor pupillae muscle as described in Chapter 22.

The **accommodation reflex** differs from the light reflex in that the cerebral cortex is included in its arc and in that both smooth and striated muscles are included in its effector mechanism. The reflex consists of the adjustments of the eyes that occur when they are rather suddenly focused on a near object after an interval of staring at a distant wall or landscape. Clinically, the elicitation of the reflex is accomplished by asking the patient to look at the farthest wall of the examining room or out of the window; when his eyes are well adjusted to distant vision, a pencil, pen, or other small object is quickly placed in front of his eyes at a distance of 12 to 14 inches and he is asked to focus on it. Two important adjustments, reflex in character, occur when this procedure is carried out: the eyes converge to some extent (through con-

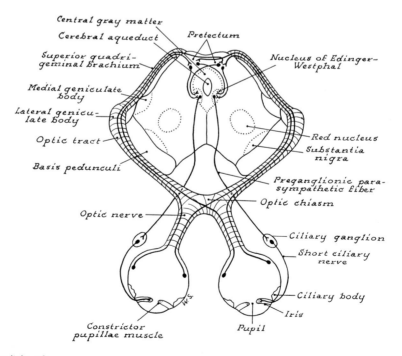

FIG. 218. The light reflex arc.

traction of the internal recti), and the lenses are thickened through contraction of the ciliary muscles. These adjustments serve to focus properly the near object on the retinae of the two eyes. Convergence and thickening of the lenses are accompanied by bilateral pupillary constriction, which may or may not be essential to accommodation; it should serve to reduce the amount of light entering the eyes and thus produce more clearly defined images as is the case when the aperture in the

diaphragm of a camera or microscope is reduced in diameter. Pupillary constriction in accommodation has sometimes been attributed to a failure of functional separation of the impulses from the Edinger-Westphal nuclei to ciliary and pupilloconstrictor muscles; it may be secondary to the convergence of the eyes and thus be dependent on a separate reflex arc beginning with proprioceptors in the extrinsic muscles of the eye.

Convergence of the eyes and constric-

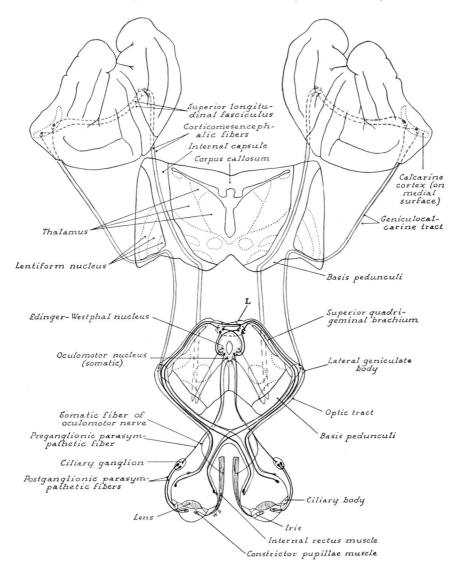

FIG. 219. Diagram demonstrating the reflex connections responsible for the light reflex and connections that may be involved in the accommodation reflex. The Argyll Robertson pupil, in which there is loss of the light reflex with preservation of accommodation, would be explained by a lesion (L) within the circle.

tion of the pupils constitute the observable reactions in the accommodation reflex. The arc traversed by the impulses responsible for the reflex has not been as definitely determined as has that for the light reflex. The receptors are the rods and cones from which impulses are conducted through the cell layers of the retina, the optic nerve, and the optic tract. Since the reflex depends on the conscious perception of an object or objects within the visual fields, it seems logical to assume that the afferent impulses are relayed from the lateral geniculate body to the visual cortex by way of the geniculocalcarine tract. It is possible, and highly probable, that intracortical connections from the visual cortex to the frontal eye fields by way of the superior longitudinal fasciculus and between the visual cortex and area 19 by way of short association fibers account for the inclusion of these areas in the accommodation reflex arc. Descending fibers from the various extrapyramidal areas of the cerebral cortex have been traced through the internal capsule to various subcortical centers (Chap. 17); those having to do with pupillary constriction and convergence as they occur in the accommodation reflex may enter the basis pedunculi of the mesencephalon and be distributed from it to the Edinger-Westphal and oculomotor nuclei (Fig. 219). It will be recalled, in this connection, that corticomesencephalic fibers from the frontal cortex have been traced to the oculomotor nuclei. The efferent pathways from the oculomotor nuclei to the internal recti and from the Edinger-Westphal nuclei to the ciliary and constrictor pupillae muscles have been previously described.

The **Argyll Robertson pupil** is one in which there is no constriction of the pupil in response to light, but normal constriction occurs in association with the accommodation reflex. It is obvious, since both reflexes have the same efferent pathway from the Edinger-Westphal nucleus to the constrictor pupillae muscle and since

both have the same afferent pathway from retina to the lateral geniculate body, that the interruption in the light reflex arc must occur at some point between the lateral geniculate body and the Edinger-Westphal nucleus (Fig. 219). If pupillary constriction in accommodation is effected by cortical projection fibers that reach the Edinger-Westphal nucleus by way of the basis pedunculi and mesencephalic tegmentum, the loss of the light reflex with preservation of accommodation is easily explained on the basis of a lesion in the rostrodorsal part of the mesencephalon (Fig. 219). Such a lesion would destroy the fibers from the pretectum to the Edinger-Westphal nucleus without damaging those from the basis pedunculi to the same nucleus.

The **pupillary-skin reflex arc** is of the somatovisceral type (Fig. 220). It consists of pupillary dilatation in response to scratching or pinching the skin of the cheek or chin. The reflex arc begins with receptors in the skin to which peripheral processes of trigeminal ganglion cells are distributed. Central processes of the ganglion cells terminate in the spinal nucleus of the trigeminal nerves, and axons of cells in that nucleus synapse on reticular cells whose axons course caudally through the spinal cord to synapse on intermediate gray column cells in the upper two thoracic segments. Preganglionic fibers from the intermediate column cells enter the sympathetic trunk by way of the ventral roots and white rami communicantes of the first and second thoracic nerves, course upward in the trunk, and end in relation to ganglionic cells in the superior cervical ganglion. Postganglionic fibers reach the dilator pupillae muscle by way of the internal carotid plexus and the ciliary nerves.

Reflex pupillodilatation has been attributed to inhibition of the nucleus of Edinger-Westphal and thus is due to inhibition of the parasympathetic innervation. This is the same mechanism responsible for the dilatation that occurs during ex-

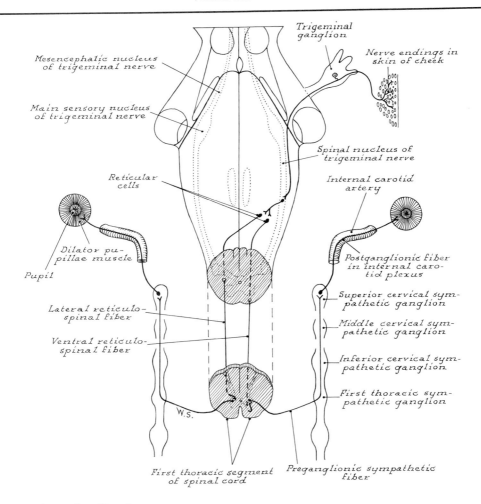

FIG. 220.   The pupillary-skin reflex.

citement. There is, nevertheless, no doubt that sympathetic stimulation produces pupillary dilatation.

Moreover, in lesions of the cervical cord in which stimuli from above could not reach the sympathetic outflow in the spinal cord, studies have shown that pupillary dilatation was absent, as observed in the ciliospinal (pupillary-skin) reflex, when the face was stimulated. However, when the chest below the level of the lesion was similarly stimulated, pupillary dilatation did occur and could be mediated only through pathways causing sympathetic excitation.

The **vomiting reflex** (Fig. 221) begins with receptors in the mucosa of the stomach, gallbladder, or duodenum. Irritative substances stimulate the receptors and the nerve impulses thus produced are carried by peripheral and central processes of the vagus nerve to the nucleus solitarius. From the nucleus the impulses are conducted to reticular cells whose axons course downward to anterior horn cells in the cervical and thoracic segments of the spinal cord; the axons of these cells innervate the diaphragm and the anterior abdominal muscles. A *vomiting center* has been located in the reticular formation of the medulla; it is in the vicinity of the dorsal motor nucleus of the vagus nerve and close to the respiratory center. Some of the descending (reticulospinal) fibers from the vomiting center terminate in the intermediate gray columns of the lower thoracic segments; impulses traversing these fibers are relayed to the stomach by way of the splanchnic nerves, celiac ganglion, and celiac plexus. Connections from the vomiting center to the dorsal motor nucleus of the vagus nerve account for vagal impulses to the stomach. Contraction of the pyloric sphincter and antrum of the stomach are produced by the vagal (parasympathetic) impulses, and inhibition of the cardiac sphincter and fundus by the splanchnic (sympathetic) impulses.

The **cough reflex** traverses an arc which is very similar to that for the vomiting reflex. Peripheral processes of cells in the inferior ganglion of the vagus are distributed to receptors in the mucosa of the larynx by way of the superior laryngeal nerve. Irritation of the mucosa gives ori-

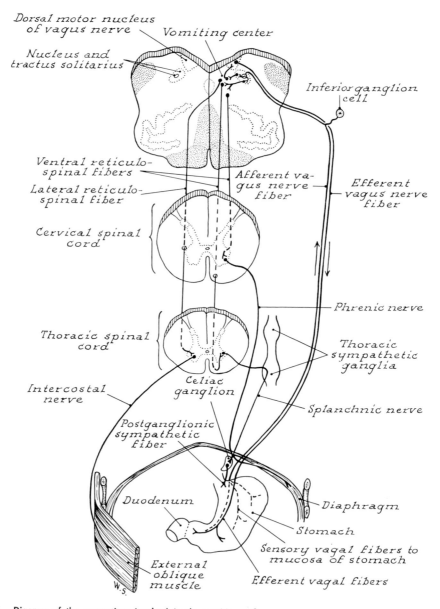

FIG. 221. Diagram of the connections involved in the vomiting reflex.

gin to nerve impulses that reach the nucleus solitarius and are then relayed to anterior horn cells through the medium of reticular cells and reticulospinal fibers. The diaphragm and abdominal muscles are thus activated. The closure of the glottis and inhibition of respiration which immediately precede the explosive phase of the reflex are no doubt effected by indirect connections from the nucleus solitarius to the nucleus ambiguus and respiratory center. The simultaneous closure of the glottis and contraction of the abdominal muscles produce the explosive pressure within the bronchial tree which is released in the form of a cough.

BIBLIOGRAPHY

Arieff, A. J., and Pyzik, S. W., 1953: The ciliospinal reflex in injuries of the cervical spinal cord in man. A.M.A. Arch. Neurol. Psychiat., 70, 621–629.

Baker, A. B., Matzke, H. A., and Brown, J. R., 1950: Poliomyelitis. III. Bulbar poliomyelitis: a study of medullary function. A.M.A. Arch. Neurol. Psychiat., 63, 257–281.

Borison, H. L., and Wang, S. C., 1953: Physiology and pharmacology of vomiting. Pharmacol. Rev., 5, 193–230.

Bouckaert, J. J., and Heymans, C., 1933: Carotid sinus reflexes: influence of central blood pressure and blood supply on respiratory and vasomotor centers. J. Physiol., 79, 49–66.

Harris, A. J., Hodes, M. C. R., and Magoun, H. W., 1944: The afferent path of the pupillodilator reflex in the cat. J. Neurophysiol., 7, 231–243.

Kuntz, A., 1953: *The Autonomic Nervous System,* 4th Ed. Lea & Febiger, Philadelphia.

Langworthy, O. R., 1943: General principles of autonomic innervation. A.M.A. Arch. Neurol. Psychiat., 50, 590–602.

Larsell, O., and Dow, R. S., 1933: The innervation of the human lung. Amer. J. Anat., 52, 125–146.

Matzke, H. A., and Baker, A. B., 1952: Poliomyelitis. V. The pons. A.M.A. Arch. Neurol. Psychiat., 68, 1–15.

Merritt, H. H., and Moore, M., 1933: The Argyll Robertson pupil; an anatomic physiologic explanation of the phenomenon, with a survey of its occurrence in neurosyphilis. A.M.A. Arch. Neurol. Psychiat., 30, 357–373.

Mettler, F. A., 1935: Corticofugal fiber connections of the cortex of *Macaca mulatta*: the frontal region. J. Comp. Neurol., 61, 509–542.

Pitts, R. F., Magoun, H. W., and Ranson, S. W., 1939a: Localization of the medullary respiratory centers in the cat. Amer. J. Physiol., 126, 673–688.

Pitts, R. F., Magoun, H. W., and Ranson, S. W., 1939b: The origin of respiratory rhythmicity. Amer. J. Physiol., 127, 654–670.

Ray, B. S., and Stewart, H. J., 1948: Role of glossopharyngeal nerve in the carotid sinus reflex in man, relief of carotid sinus syndrome by intracranial section of the glossopharyngeal nerve. Surgery, 23, 411–424.

Tang, P. C., 1953: Localization of the pneumotaxic center in the cat. Amer. J. Physiol., 172, 645–652.

Wilson, W. C., 1952: Analysis of cerebral control of reflex pupillary dilation in cat and monkey. A.M.A. Arch. Neurol. Psychiat., 68, 393–397.

Woldring, S., and Dirken, M. N. J., 1951: Site and extension of bulbar respiratory centre. J. Neurophysiol., 14, 227–241.

Chapter 24

The Rhinencephalon

The rhinencephalon (nose brain) includes, in addition to the pathways and cortical areas directly related to the sense of smell, many centers and projection pathways to other telencephalic areas that are necessary for visceral and somatic responses to smell but are not primarily concerned with olfaction. Thus, the components of the rhinencephalon can be arbitrarily grouped in two major divisions. One division includes the rostral parts related to primary reception of olfactory stimuli. The other includes a medial complex of cortex, subcortical nuclei, and fiber tracts, which developed phylogenetically along with the strictly olfactory system and are known as the *limbic lobe* or *limbic system* (Figs. 222, 223). The limbic system is of far more interest functionally than the strictly olfactory portion of the rhinencephalon and has received much attention in recent years. The intimate structural and functional interrelations of parts in these two divisions, which are listed below, will be evident from the discussion that follows.

A. Primary olfactory components
   olfactory nerve
   olfactory bulb
   olfactory tract
   lateral olfactory stria and gyrus
   anterior part of parahippocampal gyrus
   amygdaloid body (corticomedial portion)

B. Limbic components

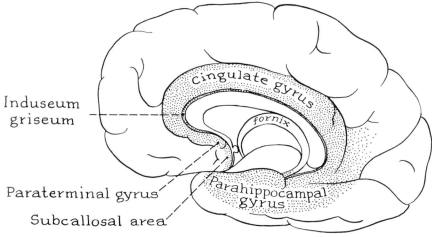

FIG. 222. Schematic drawing of the medial surface of the cerebral hemisphere illustrating the limbic lobe cortex (stippled areas).

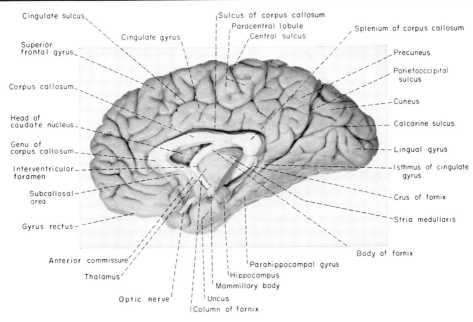

FIG. 223. Photograph of the medial surface of the adult brain cut in sagittal section and partially dissected to show the hippocampus and fornix.

1. Cortical areas
    medial olfactory area (septal area)
    hippocampal rudiment (induseum griseum)
    fornicate gyrus
        cingulate gyrus
        isthmus
        parahippocampal gyrus
    hippocampus
    amygdaloid body (a subcortical nuclear mass)
    posterior orbital and insular cortex
2. Pathways
    fornix
    mammillothalamic tract
    stria medullaris
    stria terminalis
    medial forebrain bundle
    cingulum
    anterior commissure

DEVELOPMENT

With respect to the phylogenetic and ontogenetic development of the cerebral cortex, the rhinencephalic components are more primitive. Accordingly, the terms *archipallium* (hippocampus and induseum griseum) and *paleopallium* (for the rostral part of the parahippocampal gyrus) are often applied to these older parts as opposed to the *neopallium,* which comprises the major part of the cerebral cortex in man. An additional term applicable to the cortex of the rhinencephalon is *allocortex* or *heterogenetic cortex,* which implies that it does not show six layers at some stage of ontogenetic development as is characteristic of neocortex which is *homogenetic. Mesopallium,* or *mesocortex,* is a term commonly used for the ring of cortex that is roughly equivalent to gyrus fornicatus (Fig. 222). Visceral responses may be elicited by electrical stimulation along the entire ring of limbic cortex.

SEPTAL AREA

The septal, or medial olfactory, area refers to the basal olfactory centers in the region of the anterior perforated substance (Figs. 222–224, 230). The area includes the subcallosal area and septal

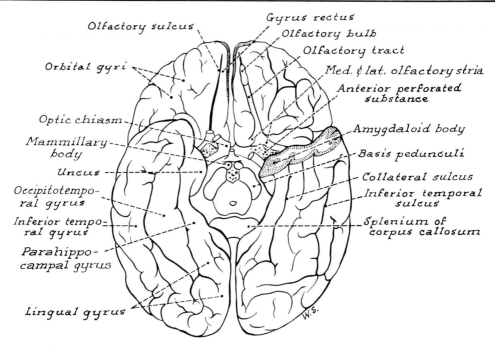

FIG. 224. The inferior surface of the cerebrum (after Toldt). The anterior part of the left temporal lobe, the brain stem caudal to the mesencephalic level, the right olfactory tract and bulb, and the left half of the optic chiasm have been removed.

nuclei that are in relation to the septum pellucidum and anterior commissure. Also included is the *hippocampal rudiment (induseum griseum)* that extends from the region of the medial olfactory stria to the hippocampus and encircles the corpus callosum (Figs. 222, 227); it contains the medial and lateral longitudinal striae. Olfactory fibers to the medial olfactory area course in the medial olfactory stria.

HIPPOCAMPAL FORMATION

The hippocampal formation is somewhat of an inclusive term commonly used in reference to the *dentate gyrus* and *hippocampus* proper and often for part of the immediately adjacent *parahippocampal gyrus*. The parahippocampal gyrus (Figs. 222–224), on the medial surface of the temporal lobe of the cerebral hemisphere, lies between the hippocampal and collateral fissures and turns back on itself at the anterior end of the hippocampal fissure as the *uncus*. The lateral olfactory stria, which contains axons of mitral cells in the olfactory bulb (Figs. 112, 113), courses posterolaterally from the olfactory tract and terminates in the lateral olfactory gyrus, rostral part of parahippocampal gyrus, uncus, and part of the underlying amygdaloid body (Figs. 224, 230). These areas comprise the *pyriform lobe*. The lateral olfactory gyrus is often called the prepyriform area, and the posterior part of the pyriform lobe is the entorhinal cortex, area 28 of Brodmann (Fig. 134). The latter does not receive direct fibers from the olfactory tract.

The **hippocampus** forms a long, curved elevation in the floor of the inferior horn of the lateral ventricle (Fig. 225). The presence of cortical gray matter in this location results from a complex expansion of temporal lobe cortex adjacent to the hippocampal fissure. In spite of convincing evidence that the hippocampus is not primarily an olfactory center, it is probable that it does function as an association center for olfactory *and other* im-

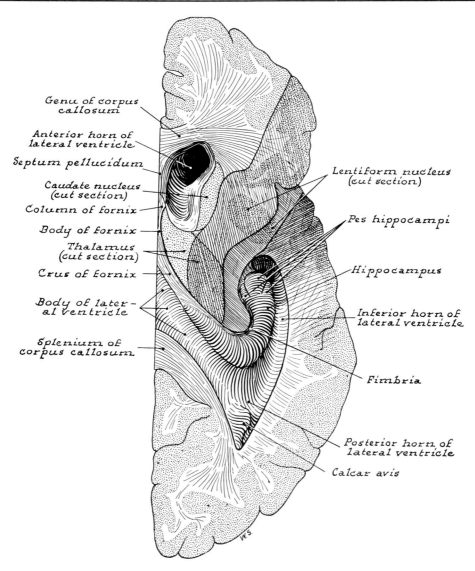

FIG. 225. The floor of the inferior horn of the lateral ventricle as seen from above.

pulses. Its relation to the hypothalamus is considered in Chapter 21. The definitive morphological and gross anatomical features of the hippocampus are considered under the heading of "Rhinencephalon" partly because of its associative olfactory function but mainly because it has become a matter of custom throughout neurological literature. Its other-than-olfactory roles include various possible involvements in memory and the behavioral, visceral, and endocrine spheres.

The structure and position of the hippocampus and **dentate gyrus** are best shown in frontal sections through appropriate sections of the temporal lobe of the cerebrum (Fig. 226). The temporal cortex immediately above the hippocampal fissure is designated the **dentate fascia** because its medial border presents numerous serrations. The dentate fascia is actually the surface of the *dentate gyrus,* which in turn is almost completely surrounded by hippocampal gray matter.

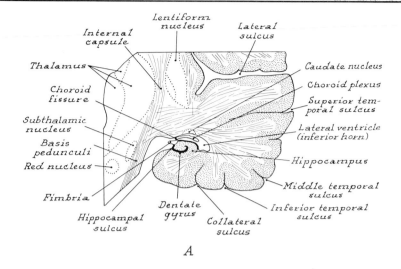

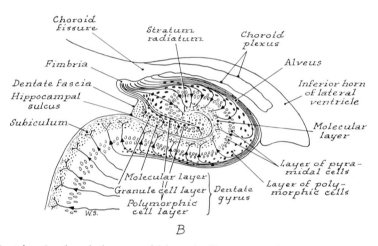

FIG. 226. A, Frontal section through the temporal lobe and adjacent areas of the right half of the brain to show the structure and relations of the hippocampus. B, Diagrammatic representation of the histological structure of the hippocampus.

It is evident that gray matter of the hippocampus has undergone more extensive development than the cortical cells of the dentate gyrus. The appearance of the hippocampus in cross-section (Fig. 226B) is responsible for its being called the *cornu ammonis* (ram's horn).

When examined microscopically, the dentate gyrus is found to consist of three layers (Fig. 226B): an outer *molecular layer,* an intermediate *granule cell layer* containing small ovoid or fusiform cells, and an inner *layer of polymorphic cells.* The hippocampus is similarly stratified

(Fig. 226B) but its intermediate layer contains medium-sized pyramidal cells and, therefore, is referred to as the *layer of pyramidal cells.* The apical dendrites of the pyramidal cells, as they course outward toward the molecular layer, form the *stratum radiatum.* The cortex of the parahippocampal gyrus adjacent to and continuous with the outer part of the hippocampus is known as the *subiculum* (Fig. 226).

Hippocampal stimulation evokes quick glancing or searching movements to the contralateral side and a facial expression indicating "attention" associated with possible bewilderment and anxiety; reaction to real external stimuli is decreased with fixation of attention on "something" in the environment. Such responses are referred to as "arrest" or "orienting" reactions. There is clinical and experimental evidence that the hippocampus is involved in processes such as learning and remembering, but there is no proof that these functions are specific to the hippocampus.

AMYGDALOID BODY

The amygdaloid body (Fig. 230) is a complex nuclear mass underlying the rostral part of the parahippocampal gyrus in the temporal lobe. It can be roughly divided into corticomedial and basolateral portions, though it has even more subdivisions. Stimulation of the phylogenetically old corticomedial part of the amyg-

daloid body elicits a variety of isolated patterns of somatomotor activity such as tonic and clonic movements of the extremities, licking, sniffing, and chewing, as well as various visceromotor responses such as pupillary dilatation, salivation, micturition, defecation, and pilo-erection. Stimulation of the phylogenetically younger basolateral division produces behavioral changes consisting of searching movements to the opposite side associated with apparent anxiety and sometimes defensive or aggressive behavior. The admixture of visceral with somatic responses, resulting from stimulation of the amygdaloid body, seems to indicate a close relationship with the hypothalamus.

MAJOR PATHWAYS

There are many pathways that interconnect the various components of the olfactory and limbic systems with each

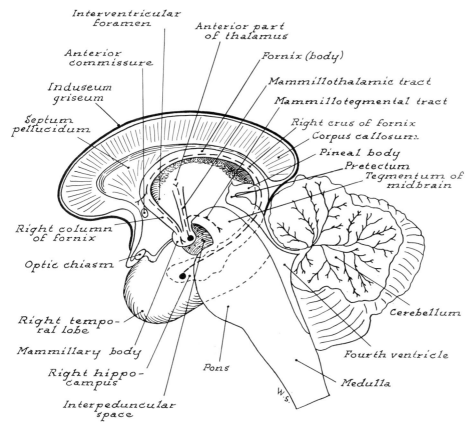

FIG. 227. Diagram demonstrating the origin, relations, and termination of the fornix.

other and with other parts of the forebrain and midbrain via projection, commissural, and association fibers. Most of
them are multisynaptic and reciprocally
connected. Only the major pathways are
considered here, and not all of their
known connections are given. Because of
such multiple interconnections, it has
been *particularly difficult to assign specific functions to individual structures in
this part of the forebrain.*

1. The fornix. The *alveus,* a thin layer
of white matter, covers the ventricular
surface of the hippocampus (Fig. 226).
The alveus consists of axons of neurons
in the hippocampus which enter the *fimbria* and then continue through the crus,
body, and anterior column of the *fornix*
to their termination in the mammillary
body (Fig. 227), and of commissural
axons from the hippocampus of the opposite side. Anterograde degeneration
studies have indicated that the hippo-
campal-fornix system projects to rather
wider areas including the septum, lateral
hypothalamus, thalamus, and as far caudally as the midbrain, and that different
hippocampal architectonic regions send
their axons to specific regions. The *commissure of the fornix* (hippocampal commissure), through which the two hippo-

campi are connected, consists of a band
of transversely coursing fibers between
the right and left crura of the fornix (Fig.
228). The fimbria is located on the medial side of the hippocampus (Fig. 226)
and is directly continuous with the crus
of the fornix (Fig. 228). The right and
left crura, after arching upward and forward around the posterior limits of the
thalami, unite to form the body of the
fornix. The columns of the fornix arch
downward and backward from the body
and enter the mammillary bodies (Fig.
227). The body and crura of the fornix
are attached to the undersurface of the
corpus callosum; the columns diverge
from the corpus callosum but are attached
to its body, genu, and rostrum by the
septum pellucidum. Several investigators
have suggested that the fornix contains
fibers coursing in both directions between
septal area and hippocampus. The fibers
from the septal region to the hippocampus
constitute the *dorsal fornix.* Stimulation
of the fimbria or hippocampus induces
motor fits and cortical electrical discharges similar to those of psychomotor
epilepsy.

2. The mammillothalamic tract. The
mammillothalamic tract (bundle of Vicq
d'Azyr) (Fig. 227) is a prominent bundle

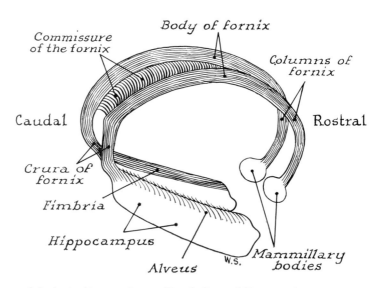

FIG. 228. Diagram of the fornix, hippocampi, mammillary bodies, and hippocampal commissure.

of fibers, demonstrable by gross dissection, that carries impulses from the mammillary body to the anterior nuclei of the thalamus. It may include some thalamomammillary fibers. The anterior nuclei of the thalamus projects mainly to areas 23 and 24 of the cingulate gyrus, as previously described (Chap. 21). Fibers that arise from the mammillary body in common with the mammillothalamic tract and are shunted to the tegmental nuclei of the midbrain comprise the *mammillotegmental tract*.

3. **The stria medullaris.** The stria medullaris thalami, originating in the medial olfactory area, provides a pathway through which impulses from the olfactory cortex may be projected caudally through the central nervous system; it arches upward anterior to the thalamus and then courses posteriorly along the dorsomedial border of the thalamus (Figs. 229, 230). The stria ends in the habenular nucleus, which is located in the *epithalamus*. The epithalamus, consisting of pineal body and habenular trigone, is located between the pretectum of the

mesencephalon and the tela choroidea of the third ventricle. The *habenular trigone* contains the right and left habenular nuclei and the habenular and posterior commissures. Efferent impulses from the medial olfactory area when reaching the habenular nucleus by way of the stria medullaris thalami (Figs. 229, 230) may be relayed to the interpeduncular nucleus through the *habenulopeduncular tract (fasciculus retroflexus of Meynert)*. As its name implies, the *interpeduncular nucleus* is located between the cerebral peduncles. Fibers from the interpeduncular nucleus course to the tegmental nuclei of the midbrain that, in turn, are connected with motor neurons through the dorsal longitudinal fasciculus and other descending pathways.

4. **Stria terminalis and anterior commissure.** The *stria terminalis* completes another complex pathway from "olfactory" cortex to the hypothalamus (Fig. 230). It is generally considered to arise from the corticomedial amygdala group of nuclei and follows a circuitous route along with (but *not* functionally related

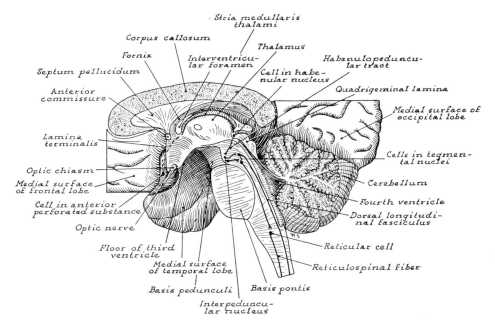

FIG. 229. Diagram of the olfactory projection through the stria medullaris thalami, habenular nucleus, and interpeduncular nucleus.

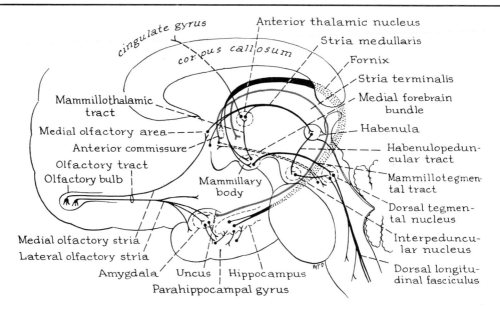

FIG. 230. Composite diagram illustrating the major components of the rhinencephalon, their relations, and their connections.

to) the tail of the caudate nucleus in close relation to the lateral ventricle until the *level* of the anterior commissure where many of its fibers then terminate in the preoptic and anterior hypothalamus. Some of the fibers continue to the ventromedial nucleus, and others join the anterior commissure and are distributed to the contralateral amygdaloid body. The *anterior commissure* itself has two major components. One component interconnects the olfactory bulbs, and the other interconnects the rostral portions of the temporal lobes including the amygdaloid body.

GENERAL CONCEPTS OF LIMBIC SYSTEM FUNCTIONS

Many olfactory projection pathways have been described, but, since the sense of smell does not play as important a part in the activities of man as it does in many of the other mammals, it is unnecessary to consider all their complex ramifications. It is of more significance that limbic system mechanisms represent an early neural development involved in affectively determined behavior.

For many years limbic structures, interconnected as they are with the hypothalamus and thalamus, have been thought to provide an anatomical substrate ("Papez circuit") for emotional responses. A number of stimulation and ablation experiments have provided support for this concept. Pronounced behavioral disturbances in monkeys are found subsequent to bitemporal lobectomies, which are collectively referred to as the Klüver-Bucy syndrome. They include visual agnosia, a compulsiveness to contact and examine objects, a strong oral tendency, an apparent loss of fear, and a marked increase in sexual behavior. Essentially the same behavioral disturbances are produced in cats and monkeys by removal of the amygdaloid bodies and adjacent cortex. Apparent contradictory results have been observed where ablations of the amygdaloid body along with some surrounding regions produce rage reactions. However, it is likely that savage behavior or rage reactions do not follow bilateral removal of the amygdaloid body and adjacent pyriform cortex unless there is damage to the hypothalamus. Removal of the pyriform cortex alone is thought to produce hypersexuality. Additional support for the role of rhinencephalic structures in emotional responses emerges from the results of implanting electrodes in the septal region and other parts of the limbic system. Following appropriate placement, the animals will stimulate themselves repeatedly, which suggests that the stimulation is related to motivation.

Another functional parameter of the rhinencephalon is suggested by the evidence that the hippocampus is related in some way to recent memory mechanisms. Additionally, it has been shown that the limbic cortex has important relationships with the reticular formation of the brain stem and probably plays a role in the alerting process. The limbic system is also implicated in the hypothalamic control of the pituitary gland, possibly acting as a regulator of different hypothalamic neuroendocrine "homeostats."

In spite of the many studies done on the limbic system, there still remains the problem of assigning its various components specific functional roles. This is perhaps not surprising in view of its many interconnections and its close relation to other parts of the brain.

Uncinate fits result from lesions of the temporal lobe that impinge on the uncus or the anterior part of the parahippocampal gyrus. They are characterized by olfactory hallucinations that usually consist of sensations of disagreeable odors. The attacks may be followed by a dreamy state of unreality and there may be associated sensations of taste. Motor phenomena, such as champing of jaws and smacking of lips, may appear. The stimulation experiments involving hippocampus and amygdaloid body suggest that they may be concerned in the phenomena that constitute uncinate fits.

The neurons in the hippocampus are very susceptible to damage from infectious, degenerative, or toxic processes. A marked loss of cells in the hippocampus is usually evident in the brains of indi-

viduals who die from carbon monoxide poisoning. A similar loss of cells is characteristic of the hippocampi in brains from neurosyphilitic and epileptic patients.

BIBLIOGRAPHY

Adey, W. R., and Tokizani, T., 1967: Structure and function of the limbic system. In *Progress in Brain Research*. Vol. 27. Elsevier, New York.

de Groot, J., 1966: Limbic and other neural pathways that regulate endocrine function. In *Neuroendocrinology*. L. Martini and W. F. Ganong, Eds. Vol. 1, Academic Press, New York, pp. 81–106.

Drachman, D. A., and Arbit, J., 1966: Memory and hippocampal complex. II. Is memory a multiple process? Arch. Neurol. (Chicago), *15,* 52–61.

Gloor, P., 1960: Amygdala. In *Handbook of Physiology,* Section I. *Neurophysiology,* Vol. 2. John Field, Ed.-in-Chief. Williams & Wilkins Co., Baltimore, pp. 1345–1372.

Green, J. D., 1957: The rhinencephalon: aspects of its relation to behavior and the reticular activating system. In *Reticular Formation of the Brain*. H. H. Jasper et al., Eds. Henry Ford Hosp. Intern. Symposium, Little, Brown & Co., Boston, pp. 607–619.

Green, J. D., 1964: The hippocampus. Physiol. Rev., *44,* 561–608.

Kaada, B. R., 1960: Cingulate, posterior orbital, anterior insular and temporal pole cortex. In *Handbook of Physiology,* Section I, *Neurophysiology,* Vol. II. John Field, Ed.-in-Chief. Williams & Wilkins Co., Baltimore, pp. 1395–1420.

Klüver, H., and Bucy, P. C., 1937: "Psychic blindness" and other symptoms, following bilateral temporal lobectomy in rhesus monkeys. Amer. J. Physiol., *119,* 352–353.

MacLean, P. D., 1958: The limbic system with respect to self-preservation and the preservation of the species. J. Nerv. Ment. Dis., *127,* 1–11.

Nauta, W. H. J., 1958: Hippocampal projections and related neural pathways to the midbrain in the cat. Brain, *81,* 319–340.

Nauta, W. H. J., 1963: Central nervous organization and the endocrine motor system. In *Advances in Neuroendocrinology*. A. V. Nalbandov, Ed. University of Illinois Press, Urbana, pp. 5–21.

Nilges, R. G., 1944: Arteries of mammalian cornu ammonis. J. Comp. Neurol., *80,* 177–190.

Olds, J., and Milner, P., 1954: Positive reinforcement produced by electrical stimulation of septal and other regions of the rat brain. J. Comp. Physiol. Psychol., *47*, 419–427.

Papez, J. W., 1937: A proposed mechanism of emotion. A.M.A. Arch. Neurol. Psychiat., *38*, 725–743.

Raisman, G., Cowan, W. M., and Powell, T. P. S., 1966: An experimental analysis of the efferent projection of the hippocampus. Brain, *89*, 83–108.

Schreiner, L., and Kling, A., 1953: Behavioral changes following rhinencephalic injury in cat. J. Neurophysiol., *16*, 643–659.

Summers, T. B., and Kaelber, W. W., 1962: Amygdalectomy: effects in cats and a survey of its present status. Amer. J. Physiol., *203*, 1117–1119.

Votaw, C. L., and Lauer, E., 1963: An afferent hippocampal fiber system in the fornix of the monkey. J. Comp. Neurol., *121*, 195–206.

Chapter 25

The Ventricles of the Brain

The ventricular system of the brain includes two lateral ventricles, the third ventricle, the cerebral aqueduct, and the fourth ventricle (Fig. 231). The lateral ventricles communicate with the third ventricle through the interventricular foramina. The cerebral aqueduct connects the third ventricle with the fourth; the fourth ventricle communicates with the subarachnoid space through the median foramen of Magendie and the lateral paired foramina of Luschka. The ventricular system is lined by a layer of ependymal cells.

The **lateral ventricles** are within the cerebral hemispheres; each consists of a body and anterior, posterior, and inferior horns (Fig. 232). The **body of the lateral ventricle** is bounded superiorly by the corpus callosum, inferiorly by the thalamus and caudate nucleus, and medially by the fornix. The corpus callosum and caudate nucleus approximate one another to form a narrow, lateral boundary (Fig. 233). The shallow, longitudinal groove between the dorsal convex surface of the caudate nucleus and that of the thalamus, in the floor of the body of the lateral ventricle, contains the stria and vena terminalis. The choroid plexus of the body of the lateral ventricle develops by evagination of the pia mater lining of the

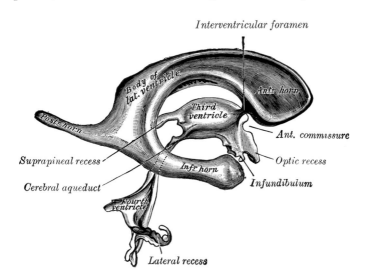

FIG. 231. Drawing of a cast of the ventricular system of the brain as seen from the side (Retzius in Gray's Anatomy).

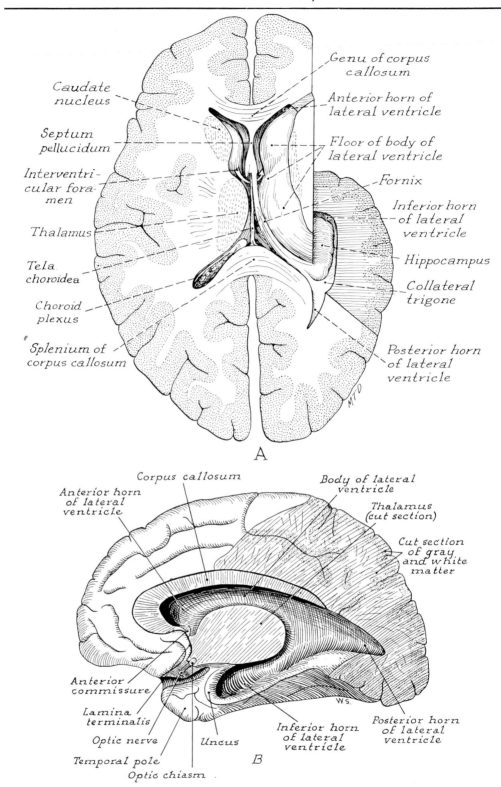

FIG. 232. A, Drawing showing the right lateral ventricle as seen from above. Note in the midline, the tela choroidea of the third ventricle, and on the left, the choroid plexus of the lateral ventricle. B, The right lateral ventricle exposed from its medial side.

cerebral fissure through the choroid fissure (Fig. 233). That portion of the ependymal lining of the ventricle which was originally reflected from the fornix to the dorsal surface of the thalamus across the choroid fissure is carried into the ventricle with the choroid plexus and thus comes to form its ependymal covering.

The **anterior horn of the lateral ventricle** extends forward and downward into the frontal lobe of the cerebral hemisphere. Its slanting floor is formed by the head of the caudate nucleus, and its roof by the corpus callosum (Figs. 232, 234). The anterior horn is limited anteriorly by the genu and rostrum of the corpus callosum; it is limited medially by the

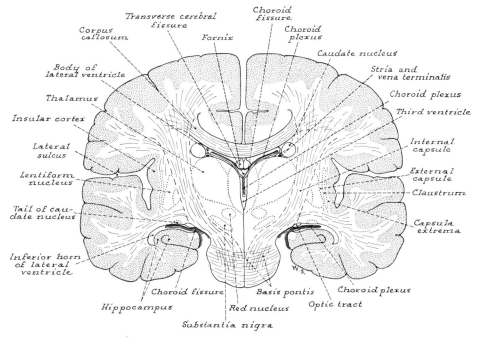

FIG. 233. Frontal section of the brain through the bodies of the lateral ventricles illustrating the relations of the cerebral fissure, choroid fissures, and ventricles to one another.

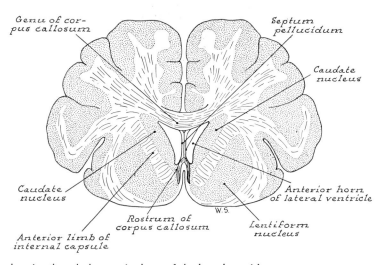

FIG. 234. Frontal section through the anterior horns of the lateral ventricles.

septum pellucidum, which also serves to separate it from its fellow of the opposite side. The *septum pellucidum* is a double-layered membranous structure extending from the corpus callosum to the columns of the fornix (Figs. 227, 234). The ventricular surface of each lamina is covered by the ependyma of the ventricle. A cavity, developed between the two layers of the septum and known as the *cavum pellucidum,* is sometimes referred to as the fifth ventricle, although it has no connection with the ventricular system. Fluid sometimes accumulates in the cavum pellucidum and results in marked dilatation, which may lead to severe pressure symptoms and require surgical intervention. The choroid plexus does not extend into the anterior horn of the lateral ventricle.

The **posterior horn of the lateral ventricle** extends into the central white matter of the occipital lobe (Figs. 232, 235). Its roof, lateral wall, and a considerable part of its medial wall are formed by radiations of the corpus callosum. The callosal fibers in its roof and lateral wall are distributed to the cortex of the temporal lobe; they constitute what has been termed the *tapetum* of the corpus callosum. The callosal fibers in the medial wall of the posterior horn contribute to the formation of the *forceps major* that connects the right and left occipital lobes (Fig. 236). The forceps major accounts for a longitudinal prominence in the medial wall of each posterior horn known as the *bulb of the posterior horn* (Fig. 235). A second longitudinal prominence immediately inferior to the bulb is produced by the rostral part of the calcarine fissure and is called the *calcar avis*. The choroid plexus does not extend into the posterior horn.

The **inferior horn of the lateral ventricle** begins at the junction of the body and posterior horn and curves inferiorly and anteriorly into the temporal lobe (Fig. 232). The triangular area developed between the diverging inferior and posterior horns is named the *collateral trigone* (Fig. 232*A*). The collateral eminence, formed by ingrowth of the collateral sulcus from the medial surface of the temporal lobe, begins at the collateral trigone and continues forward in the lateral part of the floor of the inferior horn. The *hippocampus,* which is described in Chapter 24, forms a prominent elevation in the medial part of the floor; it terminates rostrally in three or more digitations, which are responsible for the designation of *pes hippocampi* for this part of the hippocampus. The fimbria of

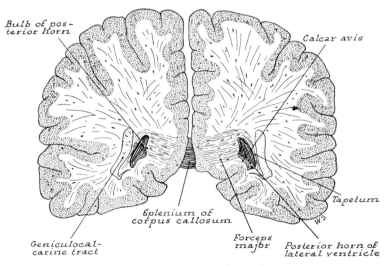

FIG. 235. Frontal section through the posterior horns of the lateral ventricles.

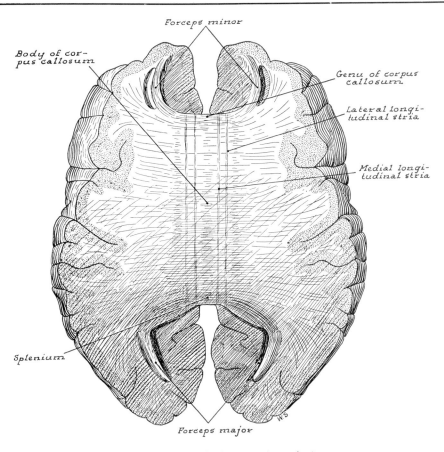

FIG. 236. Dissection of the corpus callosum showing the forceps major and minor.

the hippocampus lies along its medial side and, as has been noted, is continuous with the crus of the fornix. The roof of the inferior horn is formed by the central white matter of the temporal lobe (Fig. 237). The *stria terminalis,* which arises from the amygdaloid body, and the tail of the caudate nucleus are found in the medial part of the roof. The amygdaloid body is responsible for a slight bulge in the rostral part of the roof of the inferior horn known as the amygdaloid tubercle. The choroid plexus and the choroid fissure of the inferior horn are continuous with those of the body of the lateral ventricle (Fig. 238). The choroid fissure of the inferior horn is between the fimbria of the hippocampus and the basis cerebri. The plexus develops through ingrowth of pia mater through the fissure; it acquires an ependymal covering in the same manner as was described for the choroid plexus of the body of the ventricle.

The **interventricular foramen (of Monro)** is located between the column of the fornix and the anterior limit of the thalamus (Fig. 238). The column of the fornix, immediately below the point at which it forms the anterior boundary of the interventricular foramen, enters the substance of the hypothalamus through which it courses to the mammillary body. The choroid fissure of the lateral ventricle terminates anteriorly at the interventricular foramen while the choroid plexus is continuous through the foramen with the choroid plexus of the third ventricle.

The **third ventricle,** situated between the right and left thalami, is a narrow

19

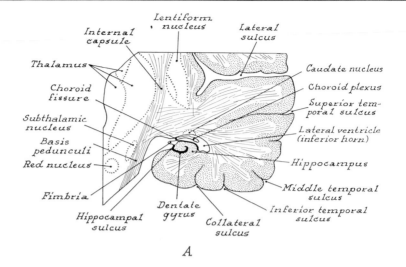

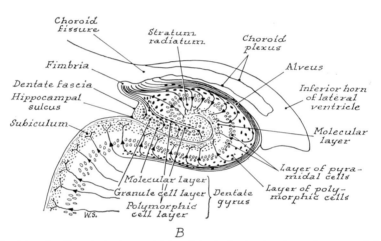

FIG. 237. A, Frontal section through the temporal lobe of the brain showing the conformation of the inferior horn of the lateral ventricle as it appears in cross-section. B, Enlarged drawing of the inferior horn and the microscopic structure of the hippocampus.

cavity whose floor is formed by the hypothalamus and, near its caudal limit, by the subthalamus (Fig. 239). The anterior boundary of the third ventricle is formed by the anterior commissure and the lamina terminalis (Fig. 229). The *lamina terminalis* extends from the anterior commissure to the optic chiasm. The *preoptic recess* of the third ventricle is in the angle formed between the lamina terminalis and optic chiasm (Fig. 240).

The ependymal roof of the third ventricle stretches between the dorsomedial borders of the thalami (Fig. 239). It is covered by a layer of pia mater known as the *tela choroidea*. The tela choroidea of the third ventricle is continuous with the pia mater lining the cerebral fissure. Vascular folds from the tela choroidea invaginate into the ventricle and form its choroid plexus. The ependymal membrane of the plexus is invaginated ahead of the vascular folds in the same manner as described in connection with the development of the choroid plexuses of the lateral ventricles. The tela choroidea, as such, ends posteriorly at the habenular trigone where it is continuous with pia mater covering that structure.

The **cerebral aqueduct** begins at the

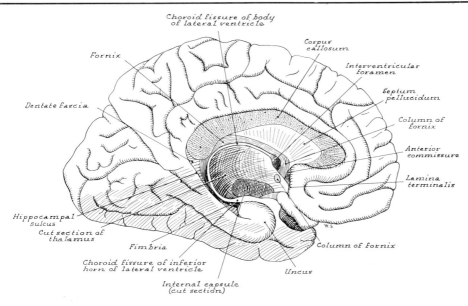

FIG. 238. Medial view of the left half of the brain showing the continuity of the choroid fissure of the body of the lateral ventricle with that of its inferior horn.

caudal limit of the third ventricle. It passes caudally through the midbrain, where it is surrounded by the central gray matter (aqueductal gray), and opens into the rostral end of the fourth ventricle (Fig. 240).

The **fourth ventricle** is bounded ventrally by the pons and medulla and dorsally by the cerebellum (Fig. 240). It is continuous caudally with the central canal of the spinal cord. The rostrolateral walls of the ventricle are formed by the superior and inferior cerebellar peduncles (Fig. 241). Caudally, the lateral boundaries consist of the clavae, cuneate tubercles, and inferior cerebellar peduncles. The latter contribute to the caudal and lateral boundaries before they turn upward to the cerebellum and to the rostrolateral boundaries as they course from the medulla to the cerebellum. The floor of the fourth ventricle, or *rhomboid fossa*, extends from the rostral limit of the pons to the junction of the open and closed portions of the medulla (Fig. 241). The rostal angle of the rhomboid fossa is between the right and left superior cerebellar peduncles; its caudal angle,

the *calamus scriptorius,* is found between the two clavae. The lateral angles are immediately caudal to the dorsally directed segments of the inferior cerebellar peduncles. The cavity of the fourth ventricle extends outward over the dorsal surfaces of the intramedullary portions of the inferior cerebellar peduncles to form the *lateral recesses* of the ventricle.

The **rhomboid fossa** is divided into right and left halves by the median sulcus, which extends from its rostral to its caudal angle. Each lateral half of the rhomboid fossa is subdivided into medial and lateral portions by the *sulcus limitans.* The area lateral to the sulcus limitans overlies the vestibular nuclei and is called the *area vestibularis.* The region medial to the sulcus, in the rostral half of the rhomboid fossa, overlies the abducens nucleus and the internal genu of the facial nerve; it is called *facial colliculus.* The medial area of the caudal half of the rhomboid fossa (medial to the sulcus limitans) is divided into a medial *hypoglossal trigone* and a lateral *vagal trigone* by a sulcus that begins at the inferior fovea and extends medially and caudally

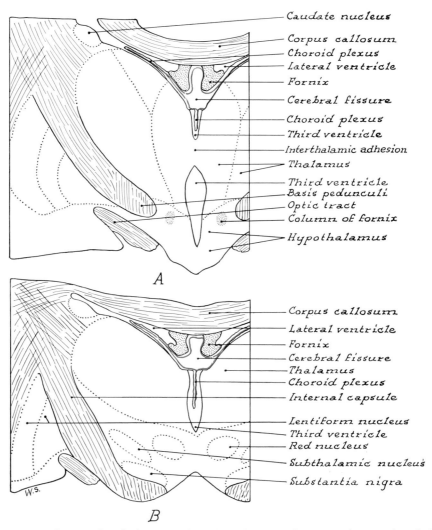

Caudate nucleus
Corpus callosum
Choroid plexus
Lateral ventricle
Fornix
Cerebral fissure
Choroid plexus
Third ventricle
Interthalamic adhesion
Thalamus
Third ventricle
Basis pedunculi
Optic tract
Column of fornix
Hypothalamus

A

Corpus callosum
Lateral ventricle
Fornix
Cerebral fissure
Thalamus
Choroid plexus
Internal capsule
Lentiform nucleus
Third ventricle
Red nucleus
Subthalamic nucleus
Substantia nigra

B

FIG. 239. A, Frontal section through the middle third of the third ventricle. B, Frontal section through the caudal part of the third ventricle.

to terminate at the median sulcus. The trigones overlie the hypoglossal nucleus and the dorsal motor nucleus of the vagus nerve. Because of its blue-gray color, the vagal trigone is also referred to as the *ala cinerea*. The *inferior fovea* is a depression in the sulcus limitans near the junction of the rostral and caudal halves of the rhomboid fossa. The *funiculus separans* is an obliquely placed ridge at the caudal limit of the vagal trigone. The

narrow area between the funiculus separans and the clava is termed the *area postrema*. Several narrow transverse ridges at the junction of the rostral and caudal halves of the rhomboid fossa are known as the *striae medullares;* the ridges are produced by transversely coursing fibers that originate in the arcuate nuclei and terminate in the cerebellum. A depression in the rostral part of the sulcus limitans is designated the *superior fovea*.

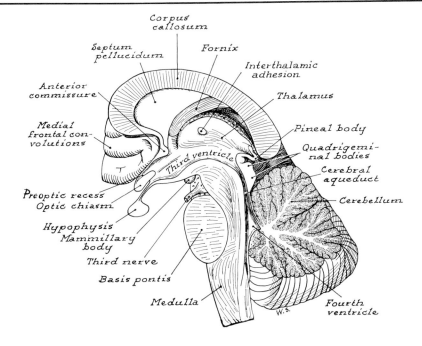

FIG. 240. Sagittal section of the brain stem (after Sobotta-McMurrich).

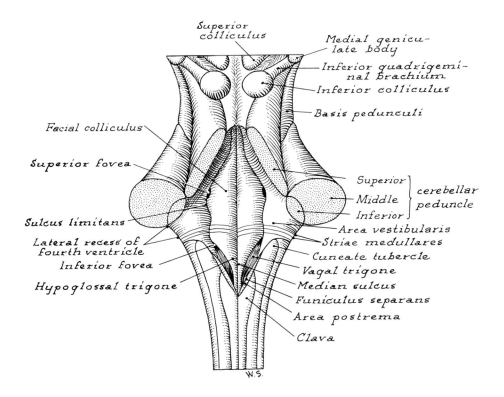

FIG. 241. Posterior view of a portion of the brain stem to show the boundaries and floor of the fourth ventricle.

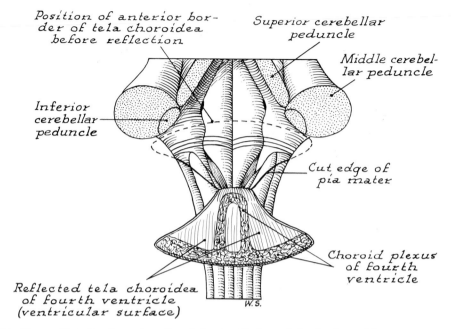

Position of anterior bor-
der of tela choroidea
before reflection

Superior cerebellar
peduncle

Middle cerebel-
lar peduncle

Inferior
cerebellar
peduncle

Cut edge of
pia mater

Reflected tela choroidea
of fourth ventricle
(ventricular surface)

Choroid plexus
of fourth
ventricle

W.S.

FIG. 242. Diagram illustrating the conformation of the choroid plexus of the fourth ventricle.

The **roof of the fourth ventricle** is formed by the superior medullary velum, the central white matter of the cerebellum, and the tela choroidea of the fourth ventricle (Fig. 240). The superior medullary velum stretches between the superior borders of the superior cerebellar peduncles. The tela choroidea, as that of the third ventricle, invaginates into the ventricle to form its choroid plexus. The choroid plexus of the fourth ventricle develops along a transverse and two longitudinal lines (Fig. 242) so that its ultimate configuration is that of the letter "T." The transverse bar of the "T" ex-

tends from the lateral recess of one side to that of the other. A posterior median aperture in the tela choroidea is called the *foramen of Magendie*. The *foramina of Luschka* are continuous with the lateral recesses of the ventricle. All three foramina serve to connect the fourth ventricle with the subarachnoid space.

BIBLIOGRAPHY

Truex, R. C., and Kellner, C. E., 1948: *Detailed Atlas of the Head and Neck*. Oxford University Press, New York.
Wolf-Heidegger, G., 1962: *Atlas of Systematic Human Anatomy*. Hafner Publishing Company, Inc., New York.

Chapter 26

The Cerebrospinal Fluid

The brain and spinal cord are suspended in the **cerebrospinal fluid** (CSF) that occupies the compartments within the ventricles and subarachnoid space (Fig. 243). The fluid is clear and differs largely from plasma in having a much lower protein content. It has higher sodium, chloride, and magnesium concentrations than plasma and lower concentrations of potassium, calcium, urea, and glucose. The osmolarities of the two fluids do not differ significantly. The differences in concentrations of substances within CSF and plasma clearly indicate that CSF is a secretory product and cannot be considered as a simple filtrate of blood plasma. Most of the CSF is actively secreted by the choroid plexuses of the brain ventricles (Fig. 243). Small amounts are derived from the interstitial spaces of the brain through the ependyma and from the capillaries of the pia-arachnoid.

The total volume of CSF in man is approximately 140 ml, and it has been estimated that about 700 ml is produced daily. Thus, there is an appreciable turnover of the fluid.

From the lateral ventricles, the primary sites of CSF formation, the fluid passes through the interventricular foramina to the third ventricle where some fluid is contributed by the choroid plexus of the third ventricle. The fluid then passes through the cerebral aqueduct into the fourth ventricle where fluid is added by the choroid plexus of that ventricle. From the fourth ventricle the CSF passes through three openings in the roof to enter the subarachnoid space. Two lateral openings (foramina of Luschka) are at the lateral recesses of the fourth ventricle which extend over the inferior cerebellar peduncles. Each of the lateral foramina opens into the pontine cistern at the angle between the pons and medulla. The third opening (foramen of Magendie) is medially placed and communicates directly with the cerebellomedullary cistern.

The **cisterns** are expansions of the subarachnoid space. The *cerebellomedullary cistern* (cisterna magna) is in the angle formed between the posterior inferior surface of the cerebellum and the tela choroidea of the fourth ventricle (Fig. 243). The pia mater is closely attached to the inferior surface of the cerebellum, as it is to all the surfaces of the central nervous system, whereas the arachnoid mater is reflected from the posterior border of the cerebellum to the dorsal surface of the closed portion of the medulla. The *pontine cistern* is situated about the pons, especially in its basilar sulcus and in the transverse sulci, at its rostral and caudal border. It is continuous caudally with the subarachnoid cavity around the medulla and rostrally with the *interpeduncular cistern*. The latter communicates with the *chiasmatic cistern* which is in relation to the optic chiasm.

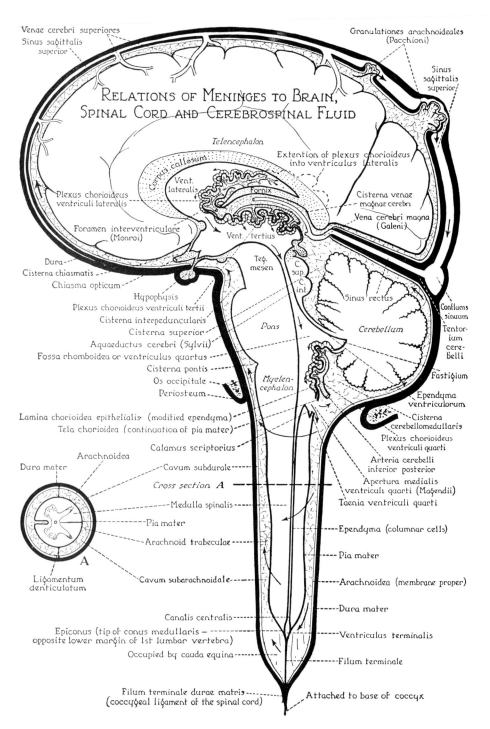

FIG. 243. The relations of the meninges to the brain, spinal cord, and cerebrospinal fluid. (From Rasmussen, The Principal Nervous Pathways, courtesy of the Macmillan Company.) (From Gray's Anatomy, 28th ed., Charles Mayo Goss, Ed., Lea & Febiger, Philadelphia.)

There is both clinical and experimental evidence which shows that obstruction of the foramina in the roof of the fourth ventricle causes a hydrocephalus that involves the entire ventricular system, whereas an occlusion of the cerebral aqueduct causes dilatation only of the third and lateral ventricles. Farther forward in the ventricular system, an obstruction of one interventricular foramen causes distention only of the corresponding lateral ventricle; if the choroid plexus of this ventricle is previously removed no distention results.

It has been shown that the fluid passes mainly upward around the brain from the cerebellomedullary cistern and basal areas and that it is absorbed into the venous system through arachnoid villi and arachnoidal granulations that project through the inner layer of dura into venous sinuses. The arachnoidal granulations, which are accumulations of numerous villi, are grossly visible and are most abundant along the superior longitudinal sinus. Arachnoid villi are also present in relation to other dural sinuses. Comparable structures have also been described in relation to veins of the spinal cord, spinal nerves, and certain of the cranial nerves.

It is generally considered that there are two forces that promote passage of CSF into the blood: the difference in the hydrostatic pressure of the CSF and the blood, and the colloid osmotic pressure of the blood owing to the higher concentration of proteins in plasma. It seems questionable, however, whether colloid osmotic pressure of the plasma proteins is a significant factor, since this would require that the cellular linings of the arachnoid villi be impermeable to plasma proteins or offer considerable restraint to their passage. In fact, it has been shown that large protein molecules pass from the CSF through the arachnoid villi at approximately the same rate as smaller molecules, such as inulin, which indicates the importance of bulk flow in the reabsorption of CSF. However, it may be pointed out that some solutes including iodide, thiocyanate, bromide, and perchlorate have been shown to be actively transported from the CSF by the choroid plexuses, more particularly the plexus of the fourth ventricle.

The **normal pressure of the cerebrospinal fluid** with the subject in the horizontal position varies from 70 to 180 mm of saline. The mean value, as measured in the lumbar sac from a large number of apparently normal individuals in the recumbent position, has been reported to be 148 mm saline and 397 mm in the sitting position. Since all of the CSF compartments are in communication, the pressures within different sites are related and influenced by such factors as body position, movement, and changes in blood volume and pressure. Thus, in the horizontal position the actual pressure is the same all along the subarachnoid space, and, when the pressure is increased at any point, it is instantaneously increased in all parts of the space. Recent studies have shown that insofar as CSF pressure is concerned, the determining factor is the altered volume of blood in the cranium owing to vasodilation or vasoconstriction. The pressure of the fluid is usually slightly higher than the venous pressure. It has been proposed that the effects of postural changes on cerebrospinal fluid pressure are due to altered gravitational pull on the fluid and to the relative levels of the venous pressure in the cerebral and lumbar regions; the effectiveness of the gravitational pull on the venous blood depends on the preexisting venous pressure in both regions, the amount of blood that flows from one region to the other during the postural change, and the associated reflex vascular adjustments. Because the pressure follows closely the intracranial venous pressure, it is easy to raise the pressure of the cerebrospinal fluid by obstructing the internal jugular veins in the neck; this obstruction results in intracranial venous congestion. When a tumor or other disease process has obstructed the subarachnoid space at some level above the level of spinal puncture (spinal block), the pressure in the cul-de-sac may rise very slowly or not at all when the jugular veins are compressed, thus confirming the presence of obstruction (Queckenstedt's test). When lateral sinus thrombosis is suspected, the response to jugular compression on the two sides should be compared. If thrombosis is present, increase in pressure is absent or delayed on the affected side.

The **volume and rate of the vascular circulation through the brain** depend on the caliber of the intracranial arterioles and capillaries and the difference between the arterial and venous blood pressures. The caliber of the intracranial arterioles is influenced by chemical substances in the blood stream, by vasomotor nerves, by variations of the venous pressure, and by *variations in the pressure of the cerebrospinal fluid*. The difference between the arterial and venous pressures is influenced by obstruction to the venous outflow from the cranial cavity by variations of the systemic arterial pressure, and by *variations in pressure of the spinal fluid*. Any increase in the pressure of the cerebrospinal fluid is immediately transmitted to the thin-walled veins, so that the pressure of the venous blood and of the cerebrospinal fluid becomes almost identical. The veins of the eyeball drain into the cranial cavity and because of this a general increase of intracranial pressure will interfere with their circulation. The result may be seen in the retina by examination with the ophthalmoscope. The veins become engorged and tortuous and the papilla of the optic nerve is edematous and swollen. The optic disc is said to be "choked." If the obstruction continues, hemorrhages occur and, finally, the optic nerve fibers atrophy.

The removal of cerebrospinal fluid from the dural cul-de-sac, caudal to the lower limit of the spinal cord, has been discussed. *Cisternal puncture* constitutes

another method of withdrawal of cerebrospinal fluid. In the procedure, a long needle is introduced into the cisterna magna penetrating the posterior midline structures of the neck and the atlanto-occipital membrane between the atlas and occipital bone. The needle enters the cranial cavity through the posterior limit of the foramen magnum and enters the cistern by piercing the arachnoid mater overlying it.

Withdrawal of cerebrospinal fluid is associated with a sudden fall in fluid pressure. Some observers have noted a more marked decrease in pressure after removal of a like amount from a subject in whom a cerebral tumor has impinged on the subarachnoid space and decreased the total amount of fluid. The difference was attributed to the fact that similar amounts of fluid removed in the tumor cases represented greater proportions of the total. The injection of saline solution or cerebrospinal fluid into the dural sac is accompanied by a steep rise in pressure that is followed by a rapid return to normal as the fluid is removed from the subarachnoid space.

BLOOD BRAIN BARRIER

The interrelations of the blood and tissues of the central nervous system, as reflected by a restricted passage of some substances from blood to the cells, are more complex than for other tissues. This restricted exchange, based originally on the observation that dyes injected into the blood stream did not stain the brain as they did other tissues, gave rise to the concept of a blood brain barrier. The view that the intercellular space in the brain is much smaller than in other tissues and that this related importantly to restricting the diffusion of substances into brain cells is no longer tenable, since recent studies have established that the space is similar to that of other tissues.

Although it has appropriately been pointed out that the phenomenon of a blood brain barrier probably cannot be explained by a single structure or mechanism, it appears that the basis for the barrier lies within the specific types of intercellular junctions of cells which are interposed between the fluid compartments and brain cells. For example, it is now established that intercellular tight junctions are characteristic of the endothelial cells of cerebral vessels, and these junctions form the basis for selectively excluding substance from spaces within the brain.

With respect to the choroidal vessels, the endothelium is fenestrated and studies have shown that peroxidase passes through them but is restricted in passing into the lumen by the tight junctions of the choroid epithelial cells.

Although it was earlier reported that tight junctions existed between astrocytic end-feet and the endothelium of vessels in the cerebral cortex, recent studies have established that these are gap junctions. Moreover, gap junctions have been described as joining ependymal cells and as the type of junction present between the glia and ependymal cells.

Since the gap junctions have been shown to be penetrated by peroxidase or lanthanum, it appears that they could have only a limited influence on intercellular passage. Thus the described endothelial and epithelial tight junctions are considered to serve as the structural basis for the blood brain and blood cerebrospinal fluid barriers.

BIBLIOGRAPHY

Adams, F. D., 1942: Cabot and Adams' *Physical Diagnosis*. 13th ed. Williams & Wilkins Co., Baltimore.

Ayala, G., 1925: Die Physiopathologie der Mechanik des Liquor cerebrospinalis und der Rachidial-quotient. Monatsschr. Psychiat. Neurol., *58*, 65–101.

Ayer, J. B., 1926: Cerebrospinal fluid pressure from the clinical point of view. Res. Publ. Ass. Res. Nerv. Ment. Dis., *4*, 159–171.

Bailey, P., 1948: *Intracranial Tumors*. Charles C Thomas, Springfield, Ill.

Barr, M. L., 1948: Observations on the foramen of Magendie in a series of human brains. Brain, *71*, 281–289.

Bondareff, W., and Pysh, J. J., 1968: Distribution of the extracellular space during postnatal maturation of rat cerebral cortex. Anat. Rec., *160*, 773–780.

Brightman, M. W., and Palay, S. L., 1963: The fine structure of ependyma in the brain of the rat. J. Cell Biol., *19*, 415–439.

Brightman, M. W., and Reese, T. S., 1969: Junctions between intimately apposed cell membranes in the vertebrate brain. J. Cell Biol., *40*, 648–677.

Broman, T., 1949: *Permeability of the Cerebrospinal Vessels in Normal and Pathological Conditions*. Munksgaard, Copenhagen.

Dandy, W. E., 1919: Experimental hydrocephalus. Ann. Surg., *70*, 129–142.

Davson, H., 1967: *Physiology of the Cerebrospinal Fluid*. Little, Brown & Company, Boston.

Masserman, J. H., 1934: Cerebrospinal hydrodynamics. IV. Clinical experimental studies. A.M.A. Arch. Neurol. Psychiat., *32*, 523–553.

Merritt, H. H., and Fremont-Smith, F., 1937: *The Cerebrospinal Fluid*. W. B. Saunders Co., Philadelphia.

Schaltenbrand, G., and Putnam, T. J., 1927: Untersuchungen zum Kreislauf des Liquor cerebrospinalis mit Hilfe intravenöser Fluorescineinspritzungen. Deutsche Ztschr. f. Nervenh., *96*, 123–132.

Walter, F. K., 1929: *Die Blut-Liquorschranke: eine physiologische und klinische Studie*. G. Thieme, Leipzig.

Weed, L. H., 1935: Certain anatomical and physiological aspects of the meninges and cerebrospinal fluid. Brain, *58*, 383–397.

Wolff, H. G., and Blumgart, H. L., 1929: The cerebral circulation: VI. The effect of normal and of increased intracranial cerebrospinal fluid pressure on the velocity of intracranial blood flow. A.M.A. Arch. Neurol. Psychiat., *21*, 795–804.

Chapter 27

The Blood Supply of the Central Nervous System

The brain derives its blood supply from the internal carotid and vertebral arteries. The former is a terminal branch of the common carotid artery; the latter is a branch of the subclavian artery. The internal carotid enters the cranial cavity through the carotid canal in the petrosa of the temporal bone. The vertebral artery, after coursing upward through the successive transverse foramina of the upper six cervical vertebrae, enters the cranial cavity through the foramen magnum.

The **internal carotid artery** courses forward through the cavernous sinus where it gives off small branches to the *trigeminal ganglion, pituitary body,* and the *tuberal area of the hypothalamus.* It turns upward and backward at the anterior limit of the cavernous sinus to the

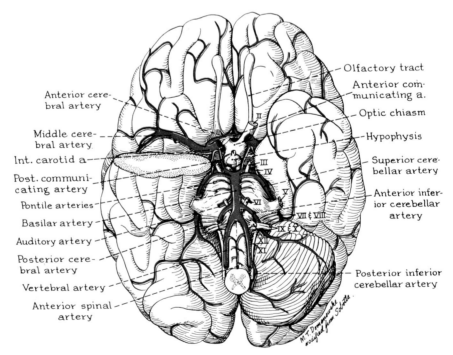

Anterior cerebral artery

Middle cerebral artery

Int. carotid a.

Post. communicating artery

Pontile arteries

Basilar artery

Auditory artery

Posterior cerebral artery

Vertebral artery

Anterior spinal artery

Olfactory tract

Anterior communicating a.

Optic chiasm

Hypophysis

Superior cerebellar artery

Anterior inferior cerebellar artery

Posterior inferior cerebellar artery

FIG. 244. The arteries of the base of the brain.

medial aspect of the anterior clinoid process, perforates the dura of the sinus roof, and then gives off the ophthalmic, posterior communicating, and anterior choroidal arteries. The internal carotid ends below the anterior perforated space by dividing into the anterior and middle cerebral arteries (Fig. 244). The **ophthalmic branch** enters the orbit through the optic foramen and is distributed to the structures therein, including the bulbus oculi.

The **posterior communicating artery** usually originates from the internal carotid (Figs. 244, 246), but it may arise from the middle cerebral artery. It courses backward over the optic tract and basis pedunculi, alongside the hippocampal gyrus, and joins the posterior cerebral, which is a terminal branch of the basilar artery. The posterior communicating artery gives off a *middle thalamic branch,* a branch to the *hippocampal gyrus,* and —particularly if the anterior choroidal artery is small—branches to the *optic tract.* The posterior communicating artery has also been found to distribute branches to the *lateral tuberal* and *lateral mammillary areas of the hypothalamus* and to the *genu of the internal capsule.* In about 8 percent of cases in which the posterior cerebral artery is a branch of the internal carotid, the posterior communicating artery connects the posterior, cerebral, and basilar arteries.

The **anterior choroidal artery** also passes backward on the optic tract and basis pedunculi (Figs. 246, 248); it enters the inferior horn of the lateral ventricle through the choroid fissure, supplies branches to the *hippocampus* and its *fimbria,* and ends in the *choroid plexus.* Branches are also distributed to the *globus pallidus, optic tract, amygdaloid body, tail of the caudate nucleus, uncus,* ventral part of the *posterior limb of the internal capsule, sublentiform part of the internal capsule,* and the anterior part of the *lateral geniculate body.* Branches of the anterior choroidal artery have been traced to the middle third of the *cerebral peduncle, red nucleus, lateral ventral nucleus of the thalamus,* and the *subthalamic nucleus.*

The **anterior cerebral artery** passes anteriorly and medially across the anterior perforated substance between the olfactory and optic nerves (Fig. 244). It enters the sagittal fissure between the frontal lobes of the brain and communicates with the corresponding artery of the opposite side through the anterior communicating artery. From this point it courses anteriorly and superiorly around the genu of the corpus callosum and then posteriorly along the upper surface of that commissural structure (Fig. 245). It gives off large branches to the cortex of the *medial surfaces of the frontal and parietal lobes,* branches to the *genu, body and splenium* of the *corpus callosum,* and eventually terminates by anastomosing with the posterior cerebral artery. The cortical branches terminate by crossing the superior border of the hemisphere and anastomosing with the cortical branches of the middle cerebral artery on the superior and lateral surfaces (Fig. 247). Branches of the anterior cerebral artery are also distributed to the olfactory bulb and to the medial part of the orbital surface of the frontal lobe.

A few small branches of the anterior cerebral artery are distributed to the basal ganglia through the anterior perforated substance; they are called *anterior striate branches* and they end in the anterior limit of the *head of the caudate nucleus,* in the same area of the *putamen,* and in the *medial part of the anterior limb of the internal capsule.* The so-called *central branches* of the anterior cerebral are given off in front of the optic chiasm and are distributed to the *supraoptic region of the hypothalamus, columns of the fornix, rostrum of the corpus callosum, lamina terminalis,* and *septum pellucidum.* The *recurrent artery (of Heubner)* arises from the anterior cerebral in the region of the anterior communicating artery (Fig. 246).

It divides into several branches that are distributed to the *external capsule,* antero-lateral aspect of the *lentiform nucleus,* head of the *caudate nucleus,* and *anterior limb of the internal capsule.* Two or three small branches of this artery penetrate the lentiform nucleus and continue to the *genu of the internal capsule;* the most posterior of these branches may extend into the anterior part of the posterior

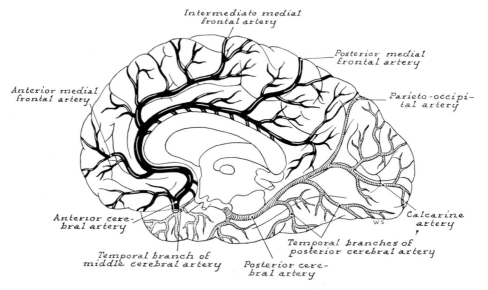

FIG. 245. Distribution of cerebral arteries on the medial and tertorial surfaces of the right cerebral hemisphere (redrawn from Gray's Anatomy).

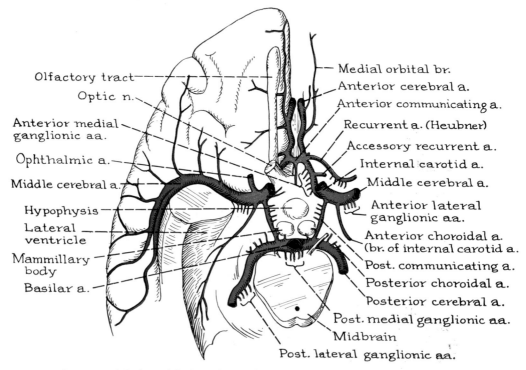

FIG. 246. The arteries of the base of the brain showing the origin of the recurrent artery (after Rubenstein, 1944).

limb of the internal capsule. The recurrent artery is also called *medial striate,* and it distributes mainly to the head of the caudate nucleus and the adjacent part of the internal capsule.

The **middle cerebral artery** is the larger of the two terminal branches of the internal carotid (Fig. 244). It passes laterally and obliquely upward into the lateral sulcus opposite the insula where it divides into several *cortical branches* that are distributed to the *dorsolateral surfaces of the frontal, parietal,* and *temporal lobes* of the hemisphere (Fig. 247). The cortical branches anastomose inferiorly and posteriorly with those of the posterior cerebral artery and superiorly with those of the anterior cerebral artery. The *central (striate) branches* of the middle cerebral artery enter the brain through the anterior perforated substance (Fig. 248); they are distributed to the *putamen* and *caudate nucleus* and to those parts of the *internal capsule* that are adjacent to these structures, i.e., the *anterior limb,* the *lateral portion of the genu,* and the *superior part of the posterior limb.* Injection studies have shown that the *external capsule* and the *claustrum* are also supplied by these branches. "Ganglionic twigs" from the middle cerebral artery are also distributed to the more lateral areas of the hypothalamus. Observations have shown that the more laterally placed of the striate branches of the middle cerebral artery (lateral striate arteries) in man tend to be considerably larger than the medial ones. Moreover, it has been reported that the concentration of arteries at the base of the external capsule is greater than in any other part of the brain, and explains why Charcot called this the site of election for cerebral hemorrhage, because chances of arterial rupture here are at least twice as great as anywhere else. Reference has been made to one or two larger lenticulostriate arteries in close relation to the internal capsule which correspond in position to Charcot's artery or arteries of cerebral hemorrhage.

The **intracranial portion of the vertebral artery** extends forward from the foramen magnum to the lower border of the pons where it unites with its fellow to form the basilar artery (Fig. 244). Its branches are: meningeal, posterior spinal, posterior inferior cerebellar, anterior spinal, and medullary. The *meningeal branch* is given off at the level of the

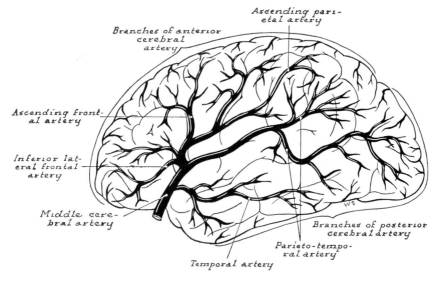

FIG. 247. Distribution of cerebral arteries on the dorsolateral surface of the cerebral hemisphere (redrawn from Gray's Anatomy).

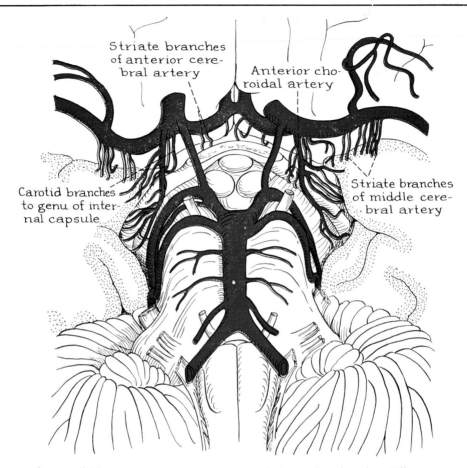

FIG. 248. The striopallidal arterial blood vessels at the base of the brain (after Alexander, 1942).

foramen magnum; it ramifies between the bone and dura mater in the posterior cranial fossa and supplies the *falx cerebelli*. The *posterior spinal artery* arises alongside the medulla and passes caudally into the spinal canal where it is in relation to the posterior roots of the spinal nerves.

The **posterior inferior cerebellar artery** is the largest branch of the vertebral artery. It is given off near the rostral limit of the medulla and winds dorsally around the medulla between the filaments of the hypoglossal nerve and then between those of the vagus and spinal accessory to be distributed to the posterior part of the *inferior surface of the cerebellum* (Fig. 244). It anastomoses with branches of the anterior inferior and supe-

rior cerebellar arteries and sends branches to the *choroid plexus of the fourth ventricle*. In its course over the medulla it distributes important *medullary branches* to the lateral areas of the medulla; these branches supply blood to the *lateral spinothalamic tract, nucleus ambiguus, spinal tract and nucleus of the fifth nerve*, and to the *ventral and dorsal spinocerebellar tracts*. Thrombosis of the posterior inferior cerebellar artery, which not infrequently occurs, results in symptoms referable to interference with the blood supply to these structures.

The **posterior inferior cerebellar artery syndrome** (of Wallenberg), due to thrombosis (Fig. 249), is characterized by loss of pain and thermal sensibility from the neck down on the side opposite the lesion

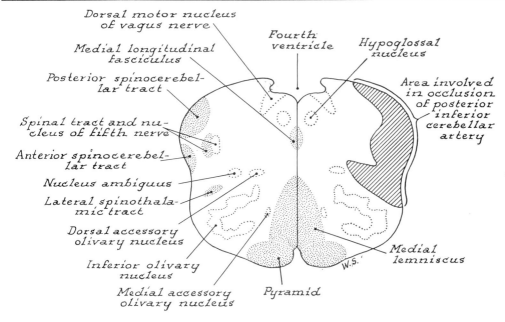

FIG. 249. Diagram showing the structures in the medulla that are damaged as the result of thrombosis of the posterior inferior cerebellar artery.

(lateral spinothalamic tract), loss of pain and thermal sensibility in the ipsilateral half of the face (spinal nucleus and tract of the trigeminal), ipsilateral paralysis of the soft palate, larynx, and pharynx (nucleus ambiguus), and ipsilateral ataxia (spinocerebellar tracts and cerebellum).

The **anterior spinal artery** arises from the vertebral artery near the point at which it joins its fellow to form the basilar artery (Fig. 244). It courses obliquely downward and inward and joins the corresponding artery of the opposite side. The combined vessel lies in the anteromedian fissure of the medulla and spinal cord and supplies branches to the anterior areas of each.

The **medullary branches** arise from the vertebral artery and its branches, and are distributed to the medulla. Those from the posterior inferior cerebellar branch, referred to above, are the most important.

The **basilar artery** is a single trunk formed by the junction of the two vertebral arteries; it extends from the lower to the upper border of the pons, lying in its median sulcus, and terminates by dividing into right and left posterior cerebral arteries (Fig. 244). The posterior cerebral artery may be a branch of the internal carotid, in which case its position is taken by the posterior communicating artery. (The posterior cerebral artery develops as a branch of the internal carotid.) In addition to its terminal branches the basilar artery gives off the following branches on each side: pontile, internal auditory, anterior inferior cerebellar, and superior cerebellar.

The **pontile arteries** pass transversely outward and curve around the lateral surfaces of the pons. They supply the *pons,* the *middle cerebellar peduncle,* and the *roots of the trigeminal nerve.*

The **internal auditory artery** traverses the internal auditory canal and is distributed to the *internal ear.*

The **anterior inferior cerebellar arteries** are given off about midway in the course of the basilar. They course posteriorly to be distributed to the inferior surface of the cerebellum where they anastomose with the posterior inferior cerebellar arteries.

The **superior cerebellar arteries** arise from the basilar artery near its termination. Each passes laterally around the basis pedunculi and reaches the tentorial surface of the cerebellum. A medial branch is distributed to the *superior vermis* and *anterior medullary velum;* a lateral branch supplies the superior surface of the cerebellar hemisphere and anastomoses posteriorly with the posterior inferior cerebellar artery.

The **posterior cerebral arteries** (Fig. 244), terminal divisions of the basilar, are separated from the superior cerebellar arteries by the third and fourth nerves. Each arches upward and backward between the basis pedunculi and the uncus and is distributed to the *medial and inferior surfaces of the temporal and occipital lobes* and to the *lateral surface of the occipital lobe* (Figs. 244, 245, 247). Anastomoses with the middle and anterior cerebral arteries have been mentioned in connection with those vessels. The *cortical branches* include *anterior and posterior temporal, calcarine, and parietooccipital.* The last two course along the sulci of the same name. The calcarine artery is of particular significance since it supplies the visual cortex. The *central branches* include three groups: posteromedial, posterolateral, and posterior choroid. The *posteromedial branches* enter the brain through the posterior perforated substance in the roof of the interpeduncular space; they supply the *mammillary bodies,* the *medial part of the thalamus* and the *tegmentum,* and *central gray matter of the midbrain.* The *posterolateral branches* are distributed to the *posterior part of the thalamus,* the *cerebral peduncles,* the *corpora quadrigemina,* the *geniculate bodies,* and the *posterior limb* and the *retro- and sublentiform* components of the *internal capsule.* The *posterior choroid branches* course forward through the transverse cerebral fissure and are distributed to the *telae choroideae* and *choroid plexuses* of the

third and lateral ventricles and to the *body* and *crura* of the *fornix.*

The **arterial circle (of Willis)**, at the base of the brain, is formed by the proximal portions of the two posterior cerebral arteries, the paired posterior communicating arteries, the internal carotids, the anterior cerebrals, and the anterior communicating artery. Free anastomosis between the two internal carotid and the two vertebral arteries through the arterial circle serves to equalize the flow of blood to the various parts of the brain. If one carotid or one vertebral is obstructed, the parts of the brain normally supplied by the vessel can still receive their blood supply through the remaining patent vessels by way of the circle. There is evidence from animal experiments to indicate that one vertebral artery is sufficient for the blood supply of the brain when there is a well-developed arterial circle.

The cortical branches of the cerebral arteries ramify and anastomose in the pia mater, giving off branches to the cortical substance; some of the branches extend through the cortex into the underlying white substance. The anastomosis between the various cortical arteries is not sufficient to provide adequate circulation in case a large branch is occluded. The central branches of the cerebral arteries, which ramify within the substance of the brain, are probably not end arteries as stated by some authors. It has been shown, in the brain of the cat, that there are anastomoses among the penetrating arteries, but such anastomoses ordinarily do not occur until the arteries reach precapillary size. The central anastomoses that have been demonstrated in mammalian brains are probably of considerable importance in preventing permanent damage to the brain from occlusion of small vessels, but they are not of sufficient caliber to assure an adequate blood supply to a given area when the main artery to that area has been occluded. Anatomically, then, the central arteries are not end arteries; functionally, however, the larger branches of the cortical arteries may be so considered.

The nervous mechanisms involved in the functioning of cerebral blood vessels have been studied in cat, monkey, and man. Summary observations for the monkey are as follows: most nerves are found along the arteries; they contain mostly small, unmyelinated axons; from nerve bundles found consistently along the larger pial arteries, nerve fibers are distributed less consistently to the smaller pial arteries and to arterioles in both pia and cortex; some cerebral arteries have a fine network of nervous tissue with a fibrillar or syncytial appearance and with nuclei typical of sheath cells; neurofibrils leave plexuses in the walls of small pial arteries and, after passing along the artery for a short distance, gradually disappear; the syncytial tissue is sometimes present along arterioles as they enter the cerebral cortex. Relative to the probable functions of the two types of nervous tissue around the pial and cerebral vessels, it seems that cerebral vasospasm may play an

important role in the phenomenon of thrombosis as it relates to apoplexy and that blocking the stellate ganglion in thrombotic apoplexy may be a justifiable procedure. This hypothesis assumes that the nervous tissue around pial and cerebral vessels is an extension of the internal carotid plexus which originates from the superior cervical sympathetic ganglion and enters the cranial cavity with the internal carotid artery.

The **blood supply of the spinal cord** comes from the anterior and posterior spinal arteries and from the spinal branches of the vertebral, intercostal, lumbar, and sacral arteries. The *anterior* and *posterior spinal arteries* originate from the vertebral arteries as they course on the anterolateral aspect of the medulla. The two anterior spinal branches unite anterior to the pyramid to form a single vessel (Fig. 244). As the spinal arteries course downward in the spinal canal they receive reinforcing branches from the segmental arteries. The posterior spinal arteries, as such, may terminate at any level of the cord by joining the ante-

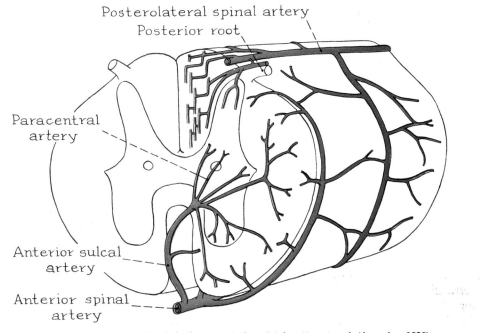

FIG. 250. Diagram of the arterial supply of the human spinal cord (after Herren and Alexander, 1939).

rior spinals. The three sets of arteries form an extensive *extramedullary plexus* around the spinal cord from which the intramedullary branches originate (Fig. 250).

A number of *anterior sulcal arteries* arise from the anterior spinal artery and enter the anterior median fissure of the cord (Fig. 250). They supply the *anterior* and *lateral horns,* the *central gray, part of the posterior horn,* and the *anterior* and *lateral funiculi.* Penetrating branches from the *posterior (posterolateral) spinal artery* supply the *posterior gray column* and the *posterior white column.* The *peripheral arteries* from the extramedullary plexus penetrate the *anterior, lateral,* and *posterior white columns;* their distribution is almost entirely limited to the white matter.

The **venous return from the brain** is facilitated by numerous veins, all of which are direct or indirect tributaries of the dural sinuses (Fig. 251*A*). The *superior* and *inferior sagittal sinuses* are found in the superior and inferior borders of the falx cerebri; the former drains into either right or left lateral sinus and the latter into the straight sinus. The *lateral sinuses* begin at the internal occipital protuberance and empty into the internal jugular veins; they consist of transverse portions within the posterior or attached border of the tentorium cerebelli and sigmoid portions which course downward in the angles formed between the petrous and mastoid parts of the temporal bones. The *straight sinus* is located at the junction of falx cerebri and tentorium cerebelli; it empties into either right or left lateral sinus. The *cavernous sinuses* are found on both sides of the body of the sphenoid; they receive the venous drainage from the eyes by way of the ophthalmic veins and empty into the superior and inferior petrosal sinuses. The *superior petrosal sinus* courses laterally along the superior border of the petrosa and empties into the lateral sinus. The *inferior petrosal sinus* is directed downward and

backward from the cavernous sinus, along the lateral margin of the basilar process of the occipital bone; it empties into the internal jugular vein. The *occipital sinus* is in the attached border of the falx cerebelli; it empties into one or the other of the lateral sinuses.

The **superior cerebral veins,** eight to twelve in number, drain the *superior, lateral and medial surfaces of the cerebrum* (Fig. 251*B*). Those from the superior and lateral surfaces are joined by those from the medial surface at the superior border of the hemisphere, and the combined vessels enter the superior sagittal sinus.

The **inferior cerebral veins** drain the blood from the *inferior surface of the cerebrum* and, to some extent, from the inferior part of the lateral surface (Fig. 253*A*). Veins from the inferior surfaces of the frontal lobes drain partly into the inferior sagittal sinus and partly into the cavernous sinuses. Veins from the inferior surfaces of the temporal lobes drain into the superior petrosal and transverse sinuses. A large vein from the occipital lobe empties into the great cerebral vein just before the latter enters the straight sinus.

The paired **internal cerebral veins,** formed in the transverse cerebral fissure, unite between the splenium of the corpus callosum and the tectum of the midbrain to form the great cerebral vein (Fig. 252). The main tributaries of each internal cerebral vein are the vena terminalis and the choroid vein, but they also receive direct tributaries from the *thalamus, corpus callosum, pineal body, corpora quadrigemina, cerebellum, occipital lobe* of the cerebrum, and the *choroid plexus* of the third ventricle.

The **vena terminalis,** formed by veins from the *thalamus* and *basal ganglia,* courses forward in the sulcus between the caudate nucleus and thalamus and joins the choroid vein in the region of the interventricular foramen. In addition to tributaries from the thalamus and basal

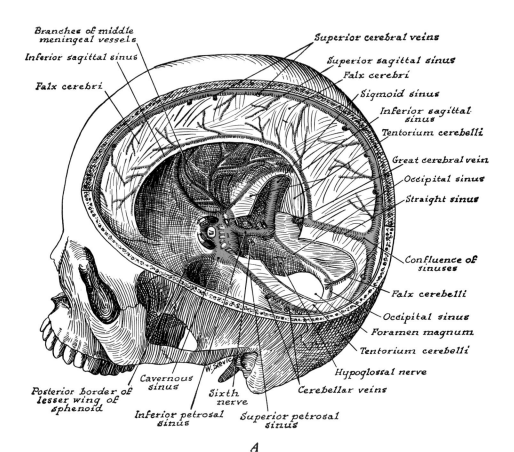

Branches of middle meningeal vessels

Inferior sagittal sinus

Falx cerebri

Superior cerebral veins

Superior sagittal sinus

Falx cerebri

Sigmoid sinus

Inferior sagittal sinus

Tentorium cerebelli

Great cerebral vein

Occipital sinus

Straight sinus

Confluence of sinuses

Falx cerebelli

Occipital sinus

Foramen magnum

Tentorium cerebelli

Hypoglossal nerve

Cerebellar veins

Posterior border of lesser wing of sphenoid

Cavernous sinus

Sixth nerve

Inferior petrosal sinus

Superior petrosal sinus

A

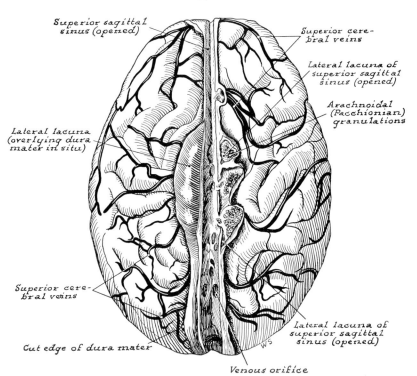

Superior sagittal sinus (opened)

Superior cerebral veins

Lateral lacuna of superior sagittal sinus (opened)

Arachnoidal (Pacchionian) granulations

Lateral lacuna (overlying dura mater in situ)

Superior cerebral veins

Cut edge of dura mater

Lateral lacuna of superior sagittal sinus (opened)

Venous orifice

B

FIG. 251.   A, The interior of the skull with brain removed and dural reflections shown. The dural sinuses are indicated (after Sobotta-McMurrich).   B, Veins of the dorsolateral surface of the hemisphere (redrawn from Toldt).

ganglia, the vena terminalis receives others from the *fornix* and *septum pellucidum.*

The **choroid vein** begins in the inferior horn of the lateral ventricle and ascends along the choroid plexus to the interventricular foramen. It receives tributaries from the *hippocampus, corpus callosum,* and *fornix.*

The **basal (basilar) veins** begin in the region of the anterior perforated substance (Fig. 253*A*) where they are formed by the junction of the deep middle cerebral (Sylvian) vein (from the insular region) and the anterior vein of the corpus callosum. They pass backward over the optic tract and basis pedunculi, curve dorsally around the midbrain, and empty into the great cerebral vein. The basal vein drains the *olfactory trigone, optic tract, tuber cinereum, mammillary bodies, posterior perforated substance, uncus,* and *cerebral peduncles.*

The **veins from the pons and medulla** terminate in the inferior petrosal and lateral sinuses.

The **superior cerebellar veins** ramify on the superior surface of the cerebellum; some cross the superior vermis and drain into the great cerebral vein and straight sinus; others run laterally to the transverse and superior petrosal sinuses.

The **inferior cerebellar veins** course forward and laterally to the inferior petrosal and transverse sinuses or directly backward to the occipital sinus.

The **venous drainage of the spinal cord** begins with the intramedullary veins which emerge from it and empty into anterior and posterior venous channels. Four longitudinal channels are usually present, the *anterior, anterolateral, posterior,* and *posterolateral* (Fig. 253*B*). The distribution of veins is similar to that of the arteries. In the cervical region the venous channels drain into the vertebral vein, in the thoracic region into the intercostal veins, and in the upper lumbar region into the lumbar and sacral veins.

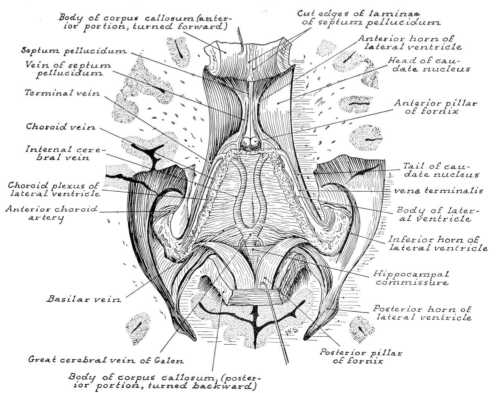

FIG. 252. **The internal cerebral and great cerebral veins (after Toldt).**

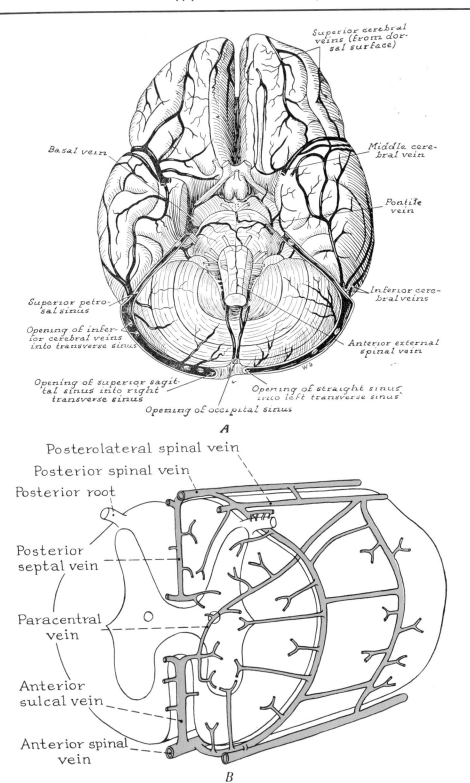

Superior cerebral veins (from dorsal surface)

Basal vein

Middle cerebral vein

Pontile vein

Inferior cerebral veins

Superior petrosal sinus

Opening of inferior cerebral veins into transverse sinus

Anterior external spinal vein

Opening of superior sagittal sinus into right transverse sinus

Opening of straight sinus into left transverse sinus

Opening of occipital sinus

A

Posterolateral spinal vein

Posterior spinal vein

Posterior root

Posterior septal vein

Paracentral vein

Anterior sulcal vein

Anterior spinal vein

B

FIG. 253. A, The veins on the base of the brain (redrawn from Toldt). B, Diagram of the veins of the spinal cord (after Herren and Alexander, 1939).

SUMMARY OF THE ARTERIAL DISTRIBUTION TO
THE CENTRAL NERVOUS SYSTEM

I. Cerebral Cortex

A. Frontal lobe
    Lateral surface—*middle cerebral artery*
    Medial surface—*anterior cerebral artery*
    Inferior surface—*middle cerebral artery* and *anterior cerebral artery*

B. Parietal lobe
    Lateral surface—*middle cerebral artery*
    Medial surface—*anterior cerebral artery*

C. Temporal lobe
    Lateral surface—*middle cerebral artery*
    Medial surface—*middle cerebral artery, posterior cerebral artery, anterior choroidal artery,* and *posterior communicating artery*
    Inferior surface—*posterior cerebral artery*

D. Occipital lobe
    Lateral surface—*posterior cerebral artery*
    Medial surface—*posterior cerebral artery*
    Inferior surface—*posterior cerebral artery*

II. Internal Capsule

A. Anterior limb—*striate branches of middle cerebral artery, striate branches of anterior cerebral artery,* and *recurrent branch of anterior cerebral artery*

B. Genu—*striate branches of middle cerebral artery, recurrent branch of anterior cerebral artery,* and *posterior communicating artery*

C. Posterior limb—*striate branches of middle cerebral artery, anterior choroidal artery,* and *posterolateral branches of posterior cerebral artery*

D. Sublentiform portion—*anterior choroidal artery* and *posterolateral branches of posterior cerebral artery*

E. Retrolentiform portion—*posterolateral branches of posterior cerebral artery*

III. Corpus Callosum

A. Rostrum—*central branches of anterior cerebral artery*

B. Genu, body, and splenium—*branches from the cortical trunk of anterior cerebral artery*

IV. Basal Ganglia

A. Caudate nucleus—*striate branches of middle cerebral artery, striate branches of anterior cerebral artery, anterior choroidal artery, recurrent branch of anterior cerebral artery,* and *posterolateral branches of posterior cerebral artery*

B. Putamen—*striate branches of middle cerebral artery, striate branches of anterior cerebral artery,* and *recurrent branch of anterior cerebral artery*

C. Globus pallidus—*anterior choroidal artery*
D. Amygdaloid body—*anterior choroidal artery*
E. Claustrum—*striate branches of middle cerebral artery*

V. Hippocampus—*anterior choroidal artery* and *posterior choroidal branches of posterior cerebral artery*

VI. Fornix

A. Anterior columns—*central branches of anterior cerebral artery*
B. Body and crura—*posterior choroidal branches of posterior cerebral artery*

VII. Thalamus—*anterior choroidal artery, posteromedial branches of posterior cerebral artery, posterolateral branches of posterior cerebral artery,* and *posterior communicating artery*

VIII. Hypothalamus

A. Lateral area—*striate branches of middle cerebral artery*
B. Supraoptic area—*central branches of anterior cerebral artery*
C. Tuberal area—*branches from internal carotid artery and posterior communicating artery*
D. Mammillary area (including mammillary bodies)—*posteromedial branches of posterior cerebral artery* and *posterior communicating artery*

IX. Subthalamus—*anterior choroidal artery* and *posteromedial branches of posterior cerebral artery*

X. Optic Tract—*anterior choroidal artery* and *posterior communicating artery*

XI. Geniculate Bodies

A. Lateral—*anterior choroidal artery* and *posterolateral branches of posterior cerebral artery*
B. Medial—*posterolateral branches of posterior cerebral artery*

XII. Olfactory Bulb—*anterior cerebral artery*

XIII. Lamina Terminalis—*central branches of anterior cerebral artery*

XIV. Septum Pellucidum—*central branches of anterior cerebral artery*

XV. External Capsule—*recurrent branch of anterior cerebral artery* and *striate branches of middle cerebral artery*

XVI. Pineal Body—*posterolateral branches of posterior cerebral artery*

XVII. Choroid Plexuses

A. Lateral ventricle—*anterior choroidal artery* and *posterior choroidal branches of posterior cerebral artery*

      B. Third ventricle—*posterior choroidal branches of posterior cerebral artery*

      C. Fourth ventricle—*posterior inferior cerebellar artery*

XVIII. Mesencephalon

      A. Basis pedunculi—*posterolateral branches of posterior cerebral artery* and *anterior choroidal artery*

      B. Tegmentum—*posteromedial branches of posterior cerebral artery* and *anterior choroidal artery*

      C. Central gray matter—*posteromedial branches of posterior cerebral artery*

      D. Corpora quadrigemina—*posterolateral branches of posterior cerebral artery*

XIX. Pons—*pontile branches of basilar artery*

XX. Medulla—*posterior inferior cerebellar artery, medullary branches of vertebral artery,* and *anterior spinal artery*

XXI. Cerebellum and Cerebellar Peduncles—*posterior inferior cerebellar artery, anterior inferior cerebellar artery, superior cerebellar artery,* and *pontile branches of basilar artery*

XXII. Spinal Cord—*anterior spinal artery, posterior spinal artery,* and *segmental branches of vertebral, intercostal, lumbar* and *sacral arteries*

BIBLIOGRAPHY

Abbie, A. A., 1934: The morphology of the forebrain arteries, with especial reference to the evolution of the basal ganglia. J. Anat., *68*, 433–470.

Alexander, L., 1942: The vascular supply of the striopallidum. In Diseases of the Basal Ganglia. Res. Publ. Ass. Res. Nerv. Ment. Dis., *21*, 77–132.

Carpenter, M. B., Noback, C. R., and Moss, M. L., 1954: The anterior choroidal artery. Its origins, course, distributions and variations. A.M.A. Arch. Neurol. Psychiat., *71*, 714–722.

Christensen, K., Lewis, E., and Stuesse, T., 1953: Innervation of cerebral blood vessels. XIX Intern. Physiol. Congr., Montreal, pp. 268-269.

Hassler, O., 1966: Deep cerebral venous system in man. A microangiographic study on its areas of drainage and its anastomoses with the superficial cerebral veins. Neurology, *16*, 505–511.

Hassler, O., 1967: Arterial pattern of human brain stem. Normal appearance and deformation in expanding supratentorial conditions. Neurology, *17*, 368–375.

Herren, R. Y., and Alexander, L., 1939: Sulcal and intrinsic blood vessels of human spinal cord. A.M.A. Arch. Neurol. Psychiat., *41*, 678–687.

Kaplan, H. A., and Ford, D. H., 1966: *The Brain Vascular System.* Elsevier, Amsterdam.

Kuhlenbeck, H., 1954: The human diencephalon. A summary of development, structure, function and pathology. Confin. Neurol., *14*, (*Suppl.*), 1–230.

Mettler, F. A., Liss, H. R., and Stevens, G. H., 1956: Blood supply of the primate striopallidum. J. Neuropath. Exp. Neurol., *15*, 377–383.

Rubinstein, H. S., 1944: Relation of circulus arteriosus to hypothalamus and internal capsule. A.M.A. Arch. Neurol. Psychiat., *52*, 526–536.

Scharrer, E., 1944: The blood vessels of the nervous tissue. Quart. Rev. Biol., *19*, 308–318.

Atlas of the Brain Stem and of the Whole Brain in Three Series of Sections

Figures A-1 through A-14—Transverse sections through the brain stem. These are the same as those which appear throughout the text section of the book.

Figures A-15 through A-24—Coronal sections of the whole brain.

Figures A-25 through A-44—Horizontal sections of the whole brain.

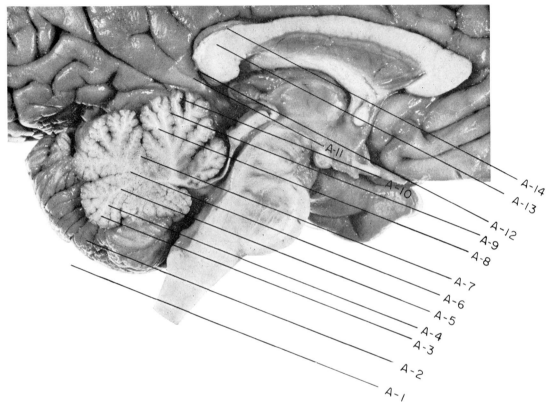

Medial view of brain stem showing the levels and planes of sections in Figures A-1 through A-14.

Fasciculus gracilis
Nucleus gracilis
Fasciculus cuneatus
Nucleus cuneatus
Spinal tract of Ⅴ
Nucleus of spinal tract Ⅴ
Post. spinocerebellar tract
Ant. spinocerebellar tract
Ant. horn
Pyramidal (motor) decussation
Anterior median fissure

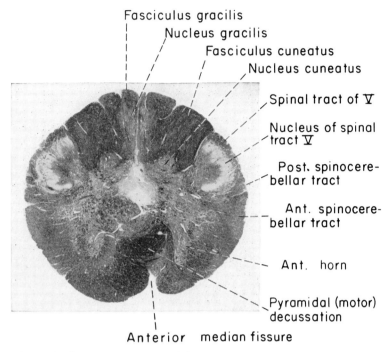

FIG. A-1. Photomicrograph of a transverse section of the neuraxis at the level of transition from spinal cord to medulla. Weil stain.

Posterior median sulcus
Fasciculus and nucleus gracilis
Fasciculus and nucleus cuneatus
Lateral cuneate nucleus
Central canal
Spinal tract and nucleus N. Ⅴ
Reticular substance
Sensory decussation
Medial lemniscus
Medial accessory olivary nucleus
Ventral arcuate nucleus
Pyramid

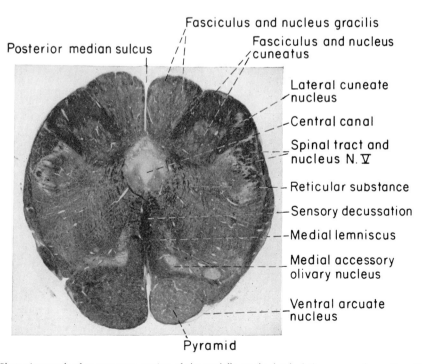

FIG. A-2. Photomicrograph of a transverse section of the medulla at the level of the sensory decussation. Weil stain.

Dorsal motor nucleus X
Hypoglossal nucleus
IV th ventricle
Fasciculus and nucleus solitarius
Fasciculus and nucleus gracilis
Fasciculus and nucleus cuneatus
Lateral cuneate nucleus
Inf. cerebellar peduncle
Post. spinocerebellar tract
Spinal tract and nucleus V
Anterior spinocerebellar tract
Spinothalamic tract
Medial accessory olive
Ventral superficial arcuate fibers
Medial longitudinal fasciculus
Medial lemniscus
Nucl. ambiguus
Lateral reticular nucleus
Olivocerebellar and cerebello-olivary fibers
Inferior olive
Interolivary fibers
Pyramid
N XII

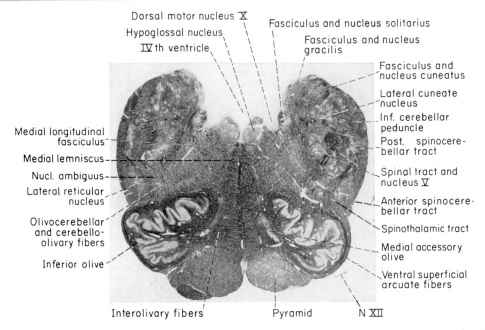

FIG. A-3. Photomicrograph of a transverse section of the medulla at the caudal part of the fourth ventricle. Note the reduced pyramid on the right which is due to partial degeneration of pyramidal tract fibers resulting from hemorrhage into the internal capsule (see Chapters 16 and 18). Weil stain.

Nucleus prepositus
Dorsal paramedian nucleus
Medial longitudinal fasciculus
Medial vestibular nucleus
Stria medullaris
Spinal vestibular nucleus and tract
Dorsal cochlear nucleus
Inf. cerebellar peduncle
Ventral cochlear nucleus
N. VIII
N. IX
Spinal tract and nucleus V
Medial lemniscus
Olivocerebellar and cerebello olivary fibers
Central tegmental (strio olivary) tract
Ventral superficial arcuate fibers
Pyramid
Arcuate nucleus

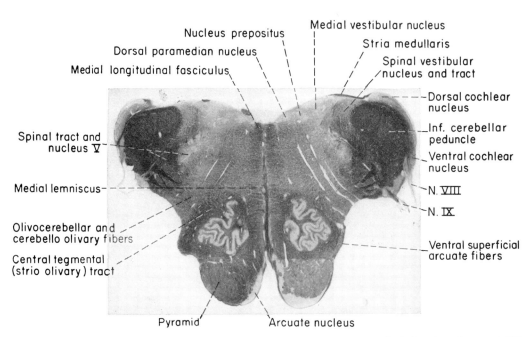

FIG. A-4. Photomicrograph of a transverse section through the medulla at the level of the glossopharyngeal (IX) and cochlear division of the vestibulocochlear (VIII) nerves. Note the reduced pyramid on the right. (See legend for Figure 52, which is a section from the same brain stem.) Weil stain.

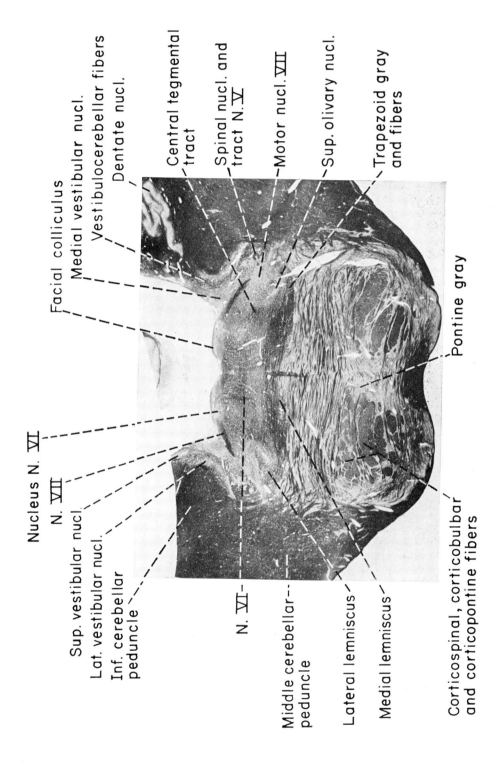

Facial colliculus

Medial vestibular nucl.

Vestibulocerebellar fibers

Dentate nucl.

Central tegmental tract

Spinal nucl. and tract N. V

Motor nucl. VII

Sup. olivary nucl.

Trapezoid gray and fibers

Nucleus N. VI

N. VII

Sup. vestibular nucl.

Lat. vestibular nucl.

Inf. cerebellar peduncle

N. VI

Middle cerebellar peduncle

Lateral lemniscus

Medial lemniscus

Corticospinal, corticobulbar and corticopontine fibers

Pontine gray

FIG. A-5. Photomicrograph of a transverse section through the caudal pons at the level of the nuclei of the facial (VII) and vestibulocochlear (VIII) nerves.

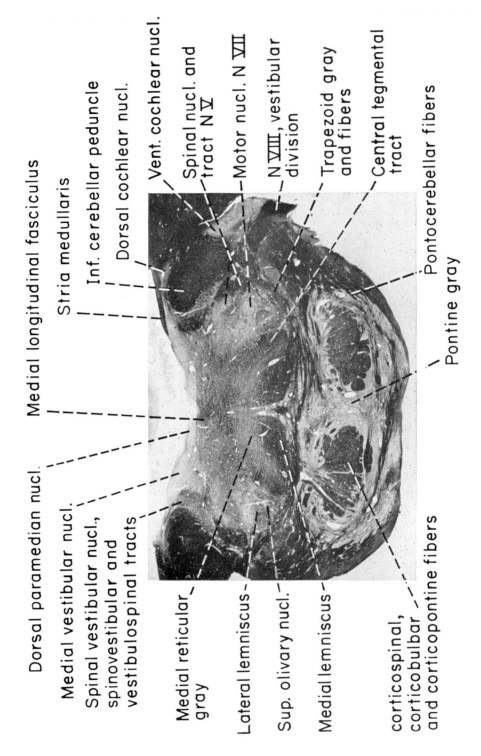

FIG. A-6. Photomicrograph of a transverse section through the caudal pons at the level of the motor nuclei of the abducens (VI) and facial (VII) nerves. Weil stain.

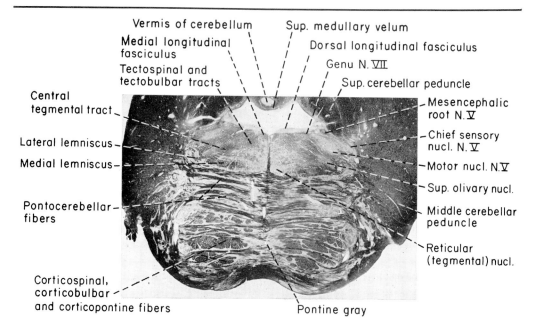

Vermis of cerebellum

Medial longitudinal fasciculus

Tectospinal and tectobulbar tracts

Sup. medullary velum

Dorsal longitudinal fasciculus

Genu N. VII

Sup. cerebellar peduncle

Central tegmental tract

Lateral lemniscus

Medial lemniscus

Pontocerebellar fibers

Corticospinal, corticobulbar and corticopontine fibers

Mesencephalic root N. V

Chief sensory nucl. N. V

Motor nucl. N. V

Sup. olivary nucl.

Middle cerebellar peduncle

Reticular (tegmental) nucl.

Pontine gray

FIG. A-7. Photomicrograph of a transverse section through the middle third of the pons at the level of the trigeminal (V) nerve. Weil stain.

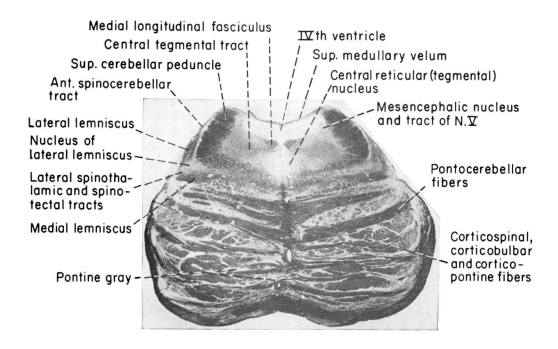

Medial longitudinal fasciculus

Central tegmental tract

Sup. cerebellar peduncle

Ant. spinocerebellar tract

Lateral lemniscus

Nucleus of lateral lemniscus

Lateral spinotha-lamic and spino-tectal tracts

Medial lemniscus

Pontine gray

IVth ventricle

Sup. medullary velum

Central reticular (tegmental) nucleus

Mesencephalic nucleus and tract of N. V

Pontocerebellar fibers

Corticospinal, corticobulbar and cortico-pontine fibers

FIG. A-8. Photomicrograph of a transverse section through the rostral third of the pons (Isthmus region). Weil stain.

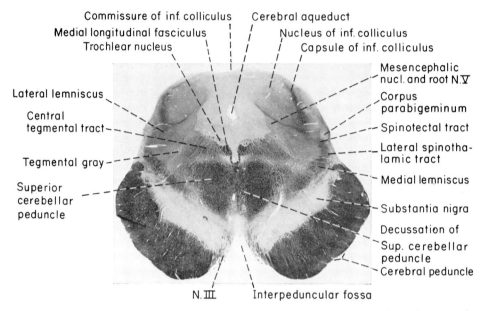

Commissure of inf. colliculus   Cerebral aqueduct
Medial longitudinal fasciculus   Nucleus of inf. colliculus
Trochlear nucleus   Capsule of inf. colliculus

Mesencephalic
nucl. and root N.V

Lateral lemniscus

Corpus
parabigeminum

Central
tegmental tract

Spinotectal tract

Lateral spinotha-
lamic tract

Tegmental gray

Medial lemniscus

Superior
cerebellar
peduncle

Substantia nigra

Decussation of
Sup. cerebellar
peduncle
Cerebral peduncle

N. III   Interpeduncular fossa

FIG. A-9. Photomicrograph of a transverse section through the inferior collicular level of the midbrain. Weil stain.

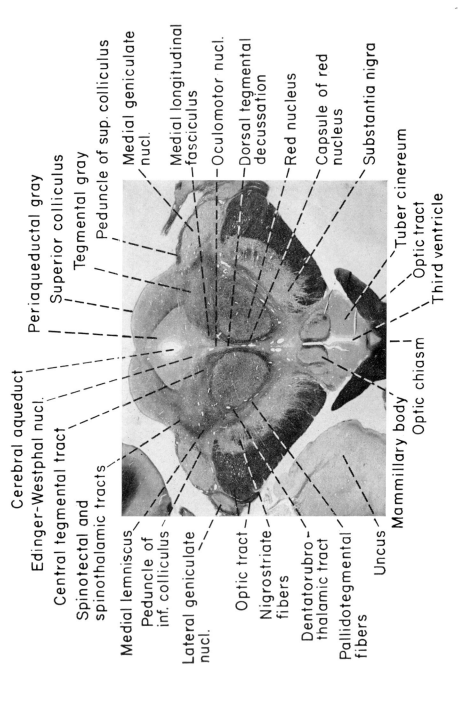

Cerebral aqueduct
Edinger-Westphal nucl.
Central tegmental tract
Spinotectal and spinothalamic tracts

Periaqueductal gray
Superior colliculus
Tegmental gray
Peduncle of sup. colliculus
Medial geniculate nucl.
Medial longitudinal fasciculus
Oculomotor nucl.
Dorsal tegmental decussation
Red nucleus
Capsule of red nucleus
Substantia nigra

Tuber cinereum
Optic tract
Third ventricle

Mammillary body
Optic chiasm

Medial lemniscus
Peduncle of inf. colliculus
Lateral geniculate nucl.
Optic tract
Nigrostriate fibers
Dentatorubro-thalamic tract
Pallidotegmental fibers
Uncus

FIG. A-10.   Photomicrograph of a transverse section through the superior collicular level of the midbrain. Weil stain.

Peduncle of sup. colliculus   Superior colliculus

Pulvinar   Commissure of sup. colliculus

Medial geniculate nucl.   Dorsal longitudinal fasciculus

Medial longitudinal fasciculus

Lateral genicu-
late nucl.   Medial lemniscus

Dentatorubro-
thalamic tract   Central tegmental
tract

Optic tract   Cerebral peduncle

Fasciculus   Oculomotor nucl.
retroflexus

Substantia   Red nucleus
nigra   Mammillothalamic
tract

Amygdaloid   Uncus   Ant. column of fornix
body   Tuber cinereum

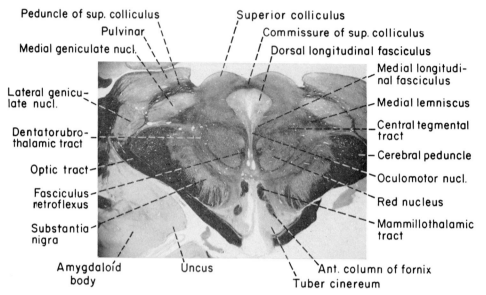

FIG. A-11. Photomicrograph of a transverse section through the rostral part of the superior level of the midbrain which passes through the posterior thalamic nuclei. Weil stain.

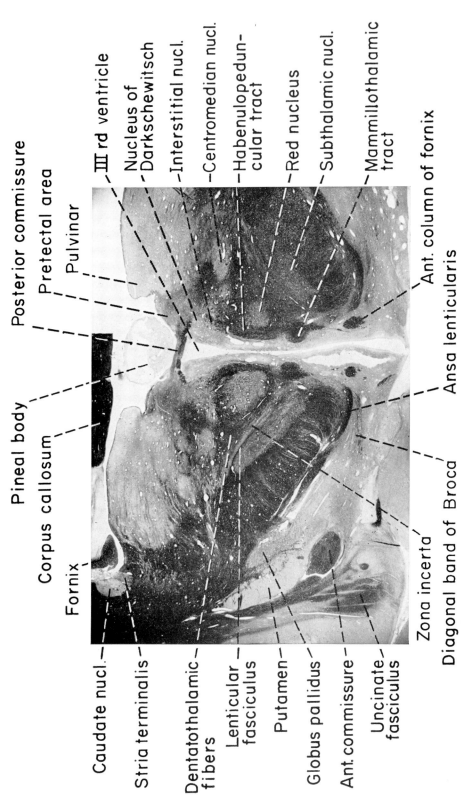

Posterior commissure
Pretectal area
Pulvinar
IIIrd ventricle
Nucleus of Darkschewitsch
Interstitial nucl.
Centromedian nucl.
Habenulopeduncular tract
Red nucleus
Subthalamic nucl.
Mammillothalamic tract
Ant. column of fornix

Pineal body
Corpus callosum
Fornix

Caudate nucl.
Stria terminalis
Dentatothalamic fibers
Lenticular fasciculus
Putamen
Globus pallidus
Ant. commissure
Uncinate fasciculus

Zona incerta
Diagonal band of Broca
Ansa lenticularis

FIG. A-12. Photomicrograph of a transverse section through the brain stem in the transition region between the diencephalon and midbrain. Several subthalamic structures are shown in addition to thalamic nuclei. Weil stain.

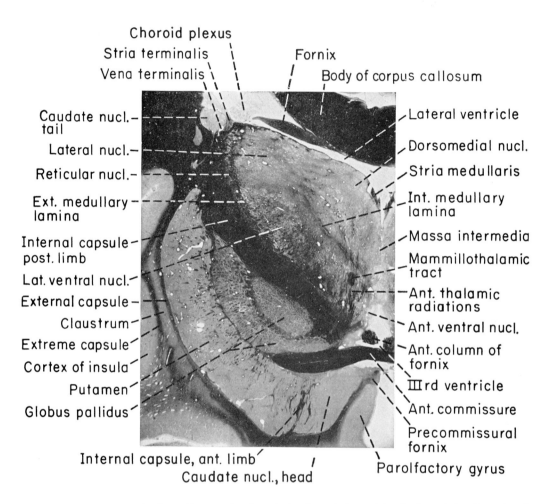

FIG. A-13. Photomicrograph of an oblique section through the diencephalon and basal telencephalon illustrating the thalamus and basal ganglia. Weil stain.

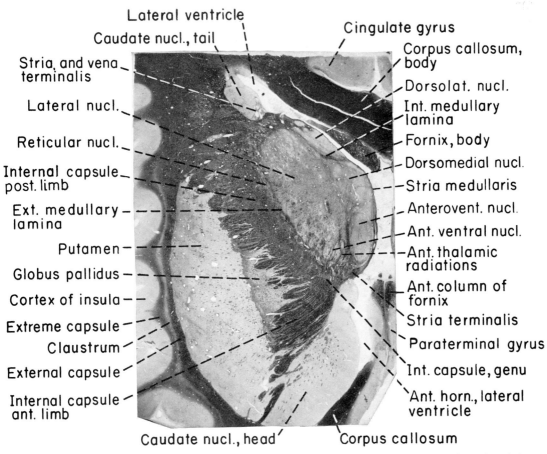

Lateral ventricle
Caudate nucl., tail
Stria and vena terminalis
Lateral nucl.
Reticular nucl.
Internal capsule post. limb
Ext. medullary lamina
Putamen
Globus pallidus
Cortex of insula
Extreme capsule
Claustrum
External capsule
Internal capsule ant. limb
Caudate nucl., head

Cingulate gyrus
Corpus callosum, body
Dorsolat. nucl.
Int. medullary lamina
Fornix, body
Dorsomedial nucl.
Stria medullaris
Anterovent. nucl.
Ant. ventral nucl.
Ant. thalamic radiations
Ant. column of fornix
Stria terminalis
Paraterminal gyrus
Int. capsule, genu
Ant. horn., lateral ventricle
Corpus callosum

FIG. A-14. Photomicrograph of an oblique section through the rostral third of the thalamus, which shows the relation of the thalamus to internal capsule, lentiform nucleus, and head of caudate.

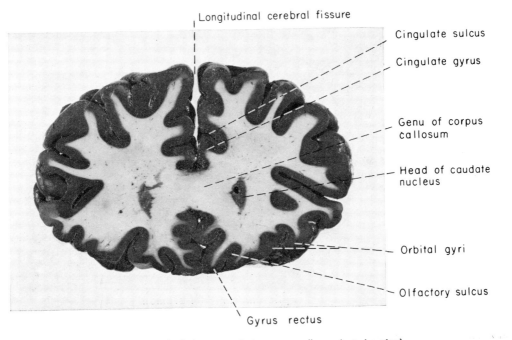

Longitudinal cerebral fissure

Cingulate sulcus
Cingulate gyrus
Genu of corpus callosum
Head of caudate nucleus
Orbital gyri
Olfactory sulcus
Gyrus rectus

FIG. A-15. Coronal section at the level of the genu of the corpus callosum (anterior view).

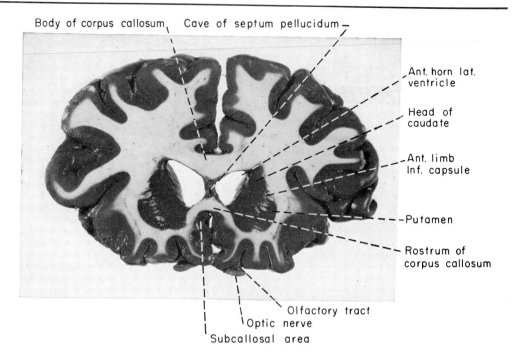

FIG. A-16. Coronal section at the level of the rostrum of the corpus callosum (anterior view).

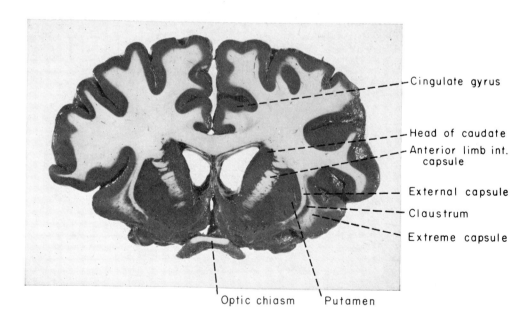

FIG. A-17. Coronal section at the level of the caudate nucleus (head) and putamen (posterior view).

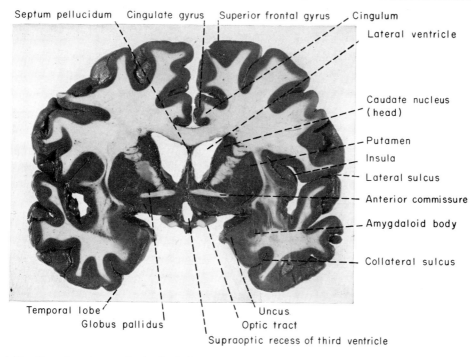

Septum pellucidum   Cingulate gyrus   Superior frontal gyrus   Cingulum

Lateral ventricle

Caudate nucleus (head)

Putamen

Insula

Lateral sulcus

Anterior commissure

Amygdaloid body

Collateral sulcus

Temporal lobe
Globus pallidus   Uncus
Optic tract
Supraoptic recess of third ventricle

FIG. A-18. Coronal section at the level of the anterior commissure (anterior view).

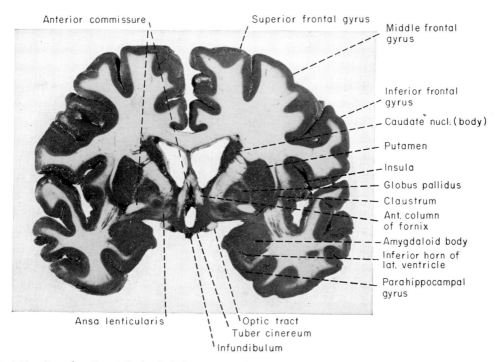

Anterior commissure   Superior frontal gyrus

Middle frontal gyrus

Inferior frontal gyrus

Caudate nucl. (body)

Putamen

Insula

Globus pallidus

Claustrum

Ant. column of fornix

Amygdaloid body

Inferior horn of lat. ventricle

Parahippocampal gyrus

Ansa lenticularis
Optic tract
Tuber cinereum
Infundibulum

FIG. A-19. Coronal section at the level of the anterior columns of the fornices (posterior view).

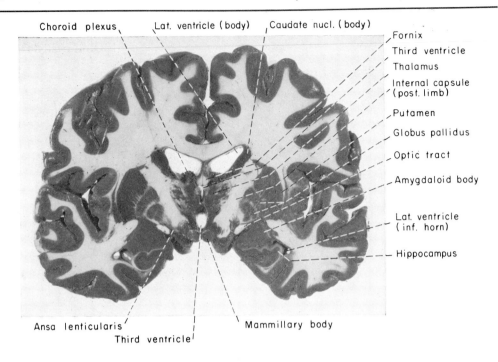

Choroid plexus   Lat. ventricle (body)   Caudate nucl. (body)

Fornix

Third ventricle

Thalamus

Internal capsule (post. limb)

Putamen

Globus pallidus

Optic tract

Amygdaloid body

Lat. ventricle (inf. horn)

Hippocampus

Ansa lenticularis   Mammillary body

Third ventricle

FIG. A-20. Coronal section at the level of the mammillary bodies (anterior view).

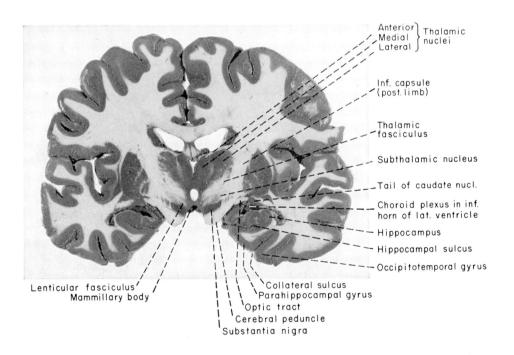

Anterior ⎫
Medial ⎬ Thalamic nuclei
Lateral ⎭

Inf. capsule (post. limb)

Thalamic fasciculus

Subthalamic nucleus

Tail of caudate nucl.

Choroid plexus in inf. horn of lat. ventricle

Hippocampus

Hippocampal sulcus

Occipitotemporal gyrus

Lenticular fasciculus
Mammillary body

Collateral sulcus
Parahippocampal gyrus
Optic tract
Cerebral peduncle
Substantia nigra

FIG. A-21. Coronal section at the level of the subthalamic area (posterior view).

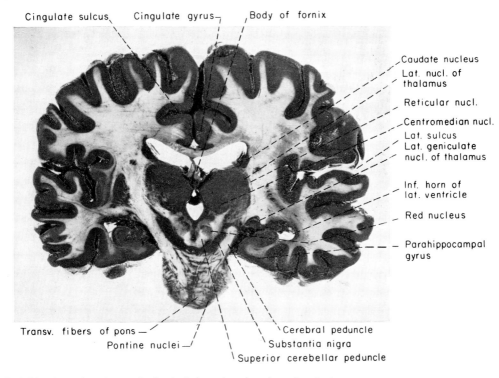

Cingulate sulcus   Cingulate gyrus   Body of fornix

Caudate nucleus
Lat. nucl. of thalamus
Reticular nucl.
Centromedian nucl.
Lat. sulcus
Lat. geniculate nucl. of thalamus
Inf. horn of lat. ventricle
Red nucleus
Parahippocampal gyrus

Transv. fibers of pons
Pontine nuclei
Cerebral peduncle
Substantia nigra
Superior cerebellar peduncle

FIG. A-22. Coronal section at the level of the red nucleus (posterior view).

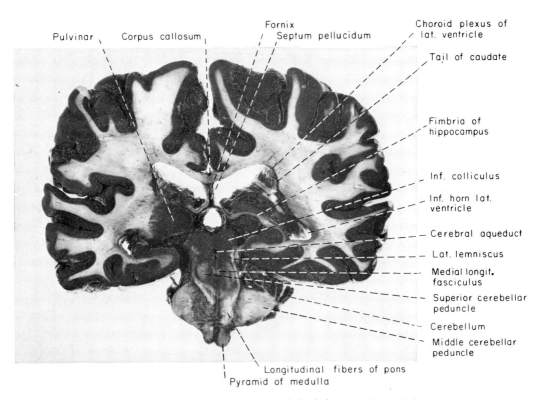

Pulvinar   Corpus callosum   Fornix   Septum pellucidum   Choroid plexus of lat. ventricle

Tail of caudate

Fimbria of hippocampus

Inf. colliculus
Inf. horn lat. ventricle
Cerebral aqueduct
Lat. lemniscus
Medial longit. fasciculus
Superior cerebellar peduncle
Cerebellum
Middle cerebellar peduncle

Longitudinal fibers of pons
Pyramid of medulla

FIG. A-23. Coronal section at the level of the posterior part of the thalamus (posterior view).

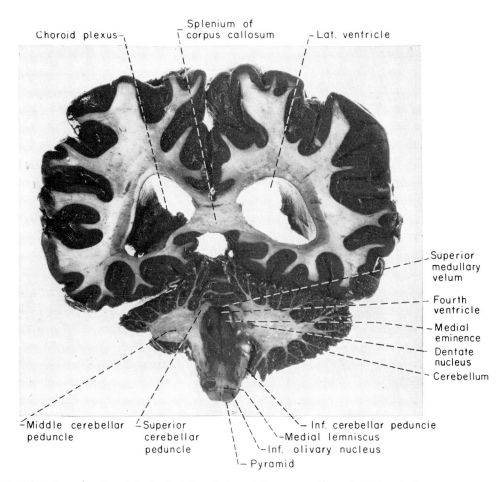

FIG. A-24. Coronal section at the level of the splenium of the corpus callosum (posterior view).

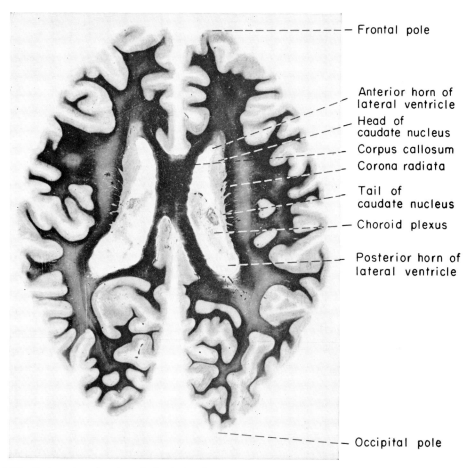

Frontal pole

Anterior horn of
lateral ventricle

Head of
caudate nucleus

Corpus callosum

Corona radiata

Tail of
caudate nucleus

Choroid plexus

Posterior horn of
lateral ventricle

Occipital pole

FIG. A-25. Horizontal section through the body of the corpus callosum.

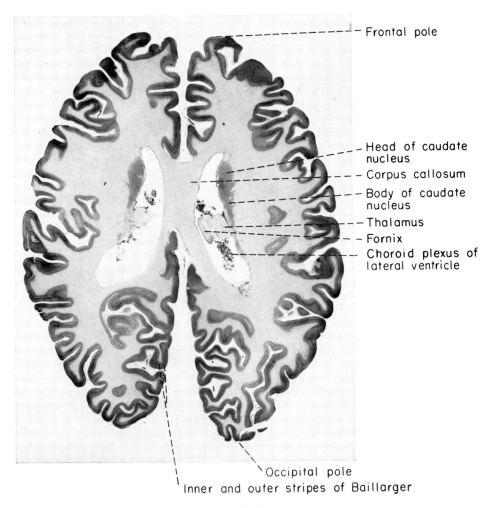

Frontal pole

Head of caudate
nucleus

Corpus callosum

Body of caudate
nucleus

Thalamus

Fornix

Choroid plexus of
lateral ventricle

Occipital pole

Inner and outer stripes of Baillarger

FIG. A-26.　Horizontal section through the head and body of the caudate nucleus.

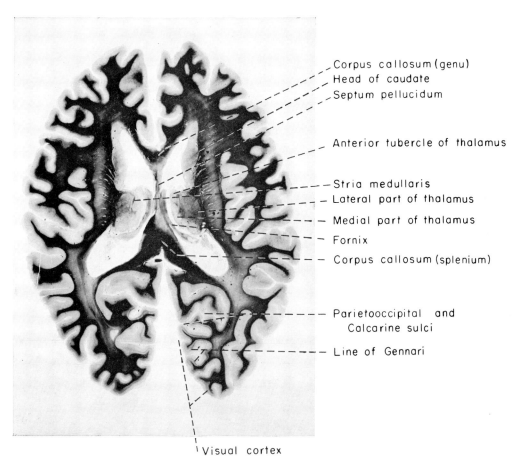

Corpus callosum (genu)
Head of caudate
Septum pellucidum

Anterior tubercle of thalamus

Stria medullaris
Lateral part of thalamus
Medial part of thalamus
Fornix
Corpus callosum (splenium)

Parietooccipital and
   Calcarine sulci

Line of Gennari

Visual cortex

FIG. A-27. Horizontal section through the genu and splenium of the corpus callosum.

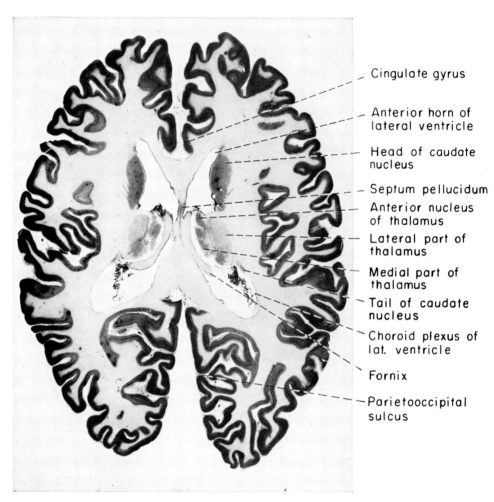

Cingulate gyrus

Anterior horn of
lateral ventricle

Head of caudate
nucleus

Septum pellucidum

Anterior nucleus
of thalamus

Lateral part of
thalamus

Medial part of
thalamus

Tail of caudate
nucleus

Choroid plexus of
lat. ventricle

Fornix

Parietooccipital
sulcus

FIG. A-28. Horizontal section through head of the caudate nucleus and upper part of the thalamus.

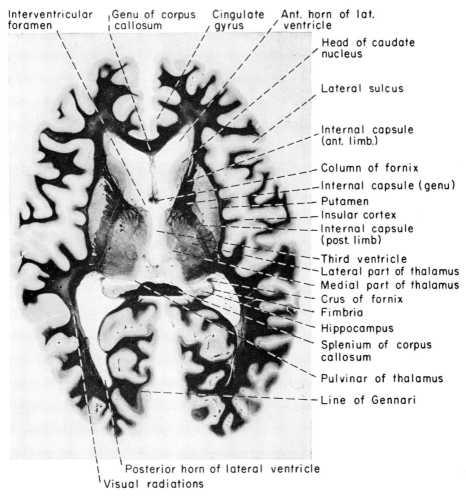

Interventricular foramen

Genu of corpus callosum

Cingulate gyrus

Ant. horn of lat. ventricle

Head of caudate nucleus

Lateral sulcus

Internal capsule (ant. limb.)

Column of fornix

Internal capsule (genu)

Putamen

Insular cortex

Internal capsule (post. limb)

Third ventricle

Lateral part of thalamus

Medial part of thalamus

Crus of fornix

Fimbria

Hippocampus

Splenium of corpus callosum

Pulvinar of thalamus

Line of Gennari

Posterior horn of lateral ventricle

Visual radiations

FIG. A-29. Horizontal section through the anterior limb, genu, and posterior limb of the internal capsule.

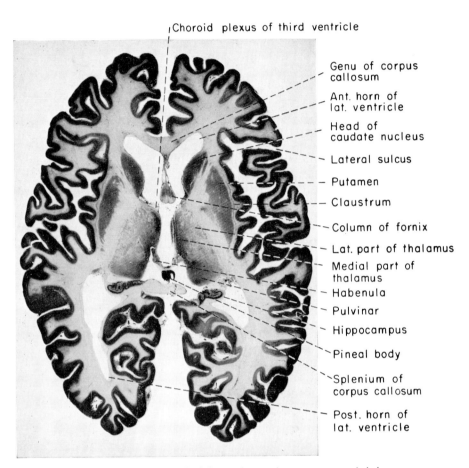

Choroid plexus of third ventricle

Genu of corpus callosum

Ant. horn of lat. ventricle

Head of caudate nucleus

Lateral sulcus

Putamen

Claustrum

Column of fornix

Lat. part of thalamus

Medial part of thalamus

Habenula

Pulvinar

Hippocampus

Pineal body

Splenium of corpus callosum

Post. horn of lat. ventricle

FIG. A-30.   Horizontal section through the head of the caudate nucleus, putamen, and thalamus.

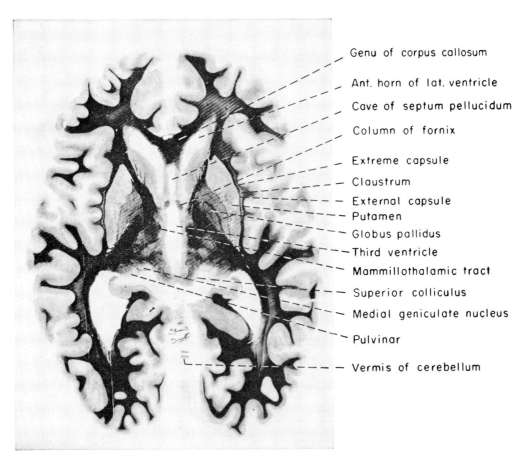

Genu of corpus callosum

Ant. horn of lat. ventricle

Cave of septum pellucidum

Column of fornix

Extreme capsule

Claustrum

External capsule

Putamen

Globus pallidus

Third ventricle

Mammillothalamic tract

Superior colliculus

Medial geniculate nucleus

Pulvinar

Vermis of cerebellum

FIG. A-31.   Horizontal section through the genu of the corpus callosum and superior colliculus.

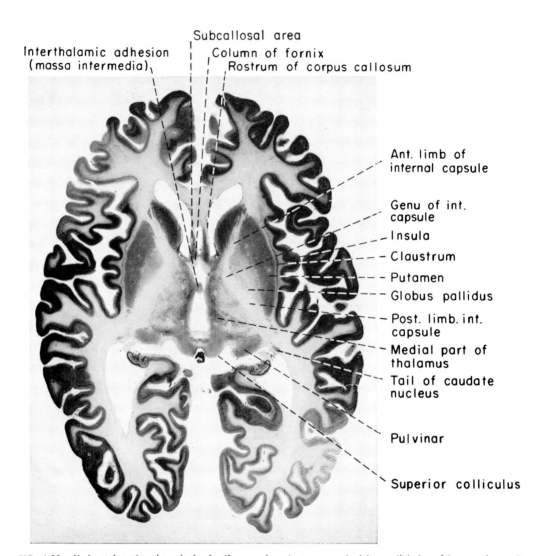

Interthalamic adhesion
(massa intermedia)

Subcallosal area
Column of fornix
Rostrum of corpus callosum

Ant. limb of
internal capsule

Genu of int.
capsule

Insula

Claustrum

Putamen

Globus pallidus

Post. limb. int.
capsule

Medial part of
thalamus

Tail of caudate
nucleus

Pulvinar

Superior colliculus

FIG. A-32. Horizontal section through the lentiform nucleus (putamen and globus pallidus), pulvinar, and superior colliculus.

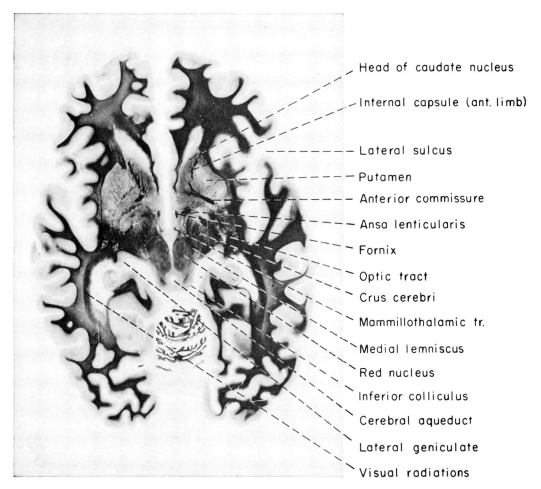

Head of caudate nucleus

Internal capsule (ant. limb)

Lateral sulcus

Putamen

Anterior commissure

Ansa lenticularis

Fornix

Optic tract

Crus cerebri

Mammillothalamic tr.

Medial lemniscus

Red nucleus

Inferior colliculus

Cerebral aqueduct

Lateral geniculate

Visual radiations

FIG. A-33.   Horizontal section through the anterior commissure, fornix, and mammillothalamic tract.

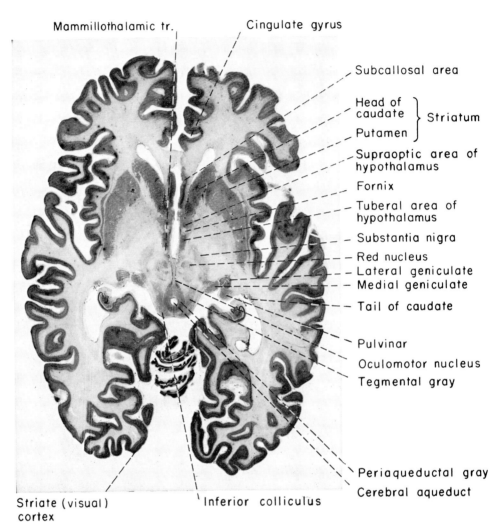

FIG. A-34. Horizontal section through the subcallosal area, red nucleus, and lateral geniculate nucleus.

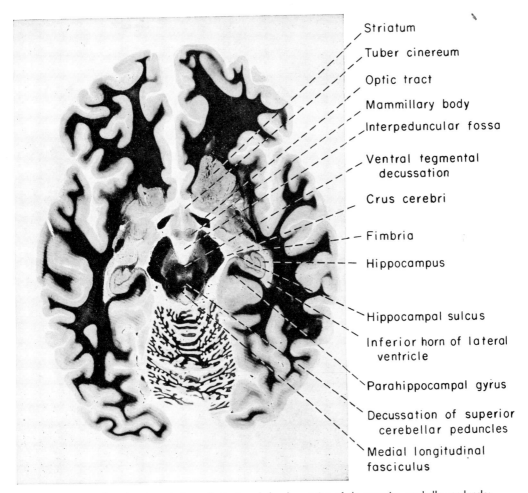

Striatum

Tuber cinereum

Optic tract

Mammillary body

Interpeduncular fossa

Ventral tegmental
decussation

Crus cerebri

Fimbria

Hippocampus

Hippocampal sulcus

Inferior horn of lateral
ventricle

Parahippocampal gyrus

Decussation of superior
cerebellar peduncles

Medial longitudinal
fasciculus

FIG. A-35. Horizontal section through the optic tract and the decussation of the superior cerebellar peduncles.

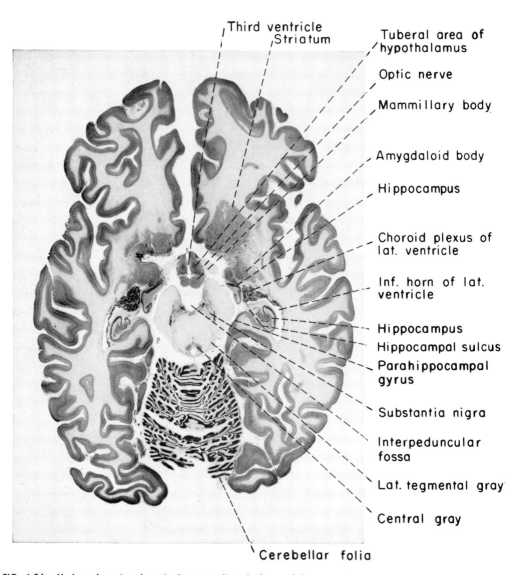

Third ventricle
Striatum
Tuberal area of hypothalamus
Optic nerve
Mammillary body
Amygdaloid body
Hippocampus
Choroid plexus of lat. ventricle
Inf. horn of lat. ventricle
Hippocampus
Hippocampal sulcus
Parahippocampal gyrus
Substantia nigra
Interpeduncular fossa
Lat. tegmental gray
Central gray
Cerebellar folia

FIG. A-36. Horizontal section through the mammillary bodies and hippocampi.

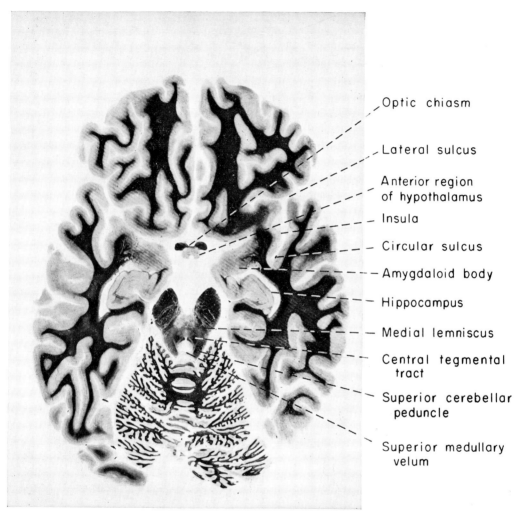

Optic chiasm

Lateral sulcus

Anterior region
of hypothalamus

Insula

Circular sulcus

Amygdaloid body

Hippocampus

Medial lemniscus

Central tegmental
tract

Superior cerebellar
peduncle

Superior medullary
velum

FIG. A-37.   Horizontal section through the optic chiasm and superior cerebellar peduncles.

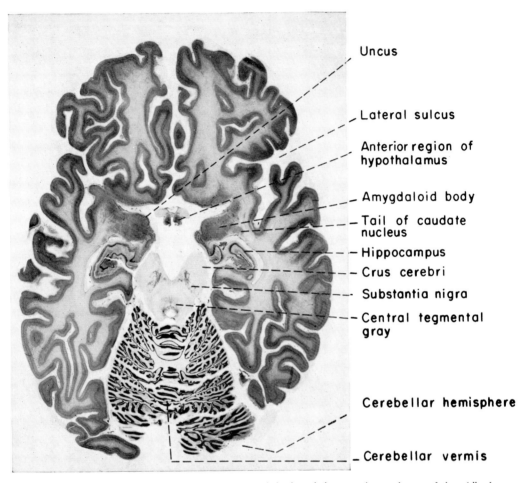

Uncus

Lateral sulcus

Anterior region of hypothalamus

Amygdaloid body

Tail of caudate nucleus

Hippocampus

Crus cerebri

Substantia nigra

Central tegmental gray

Cerebellar hemisphere

Cerebellar vermis

FIG. A-38. Horizontal section through the anterior region of the hypothalamus and central gray of the midbrain.

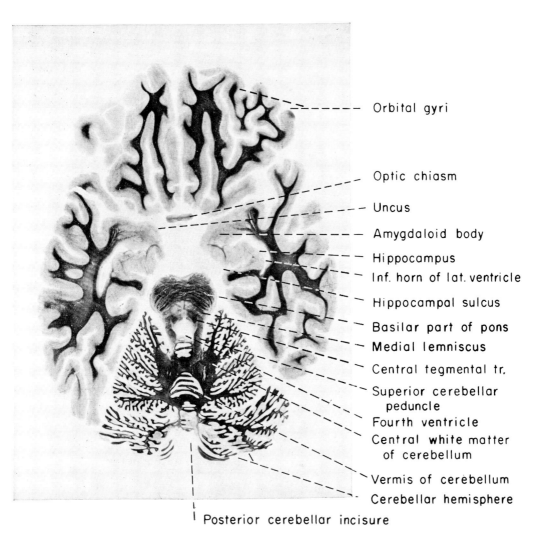

Orbital gyri

Optic chiasm

Uncus

Amygdaloid body

Hippocampus

Inf. horn of lat. ventricle

Hippocampal sulcus

Basilar part of pons

Medial lemniscus

Central tegmental tr.

Superior cerebellar
peduncle

Fourth ventricle

Central white matter
of cerebellum

Vermis of cerebellum

Cerebellar hemisphere

Posterior cerebellar incisure

FIG. A-39. Horizontal section through the optic chiasm and superior cerebellar peduncles.

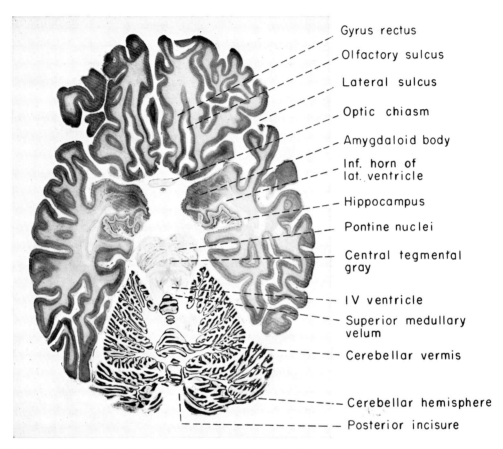

Gyrus rectus
Olfactory sulcus
Lateral sulcus
Optic chiasm
Amygdaloid body
Inf. horn of
lat. ventricle
Hippocampus
Pontine nuclei
Central tegmental
gray
IV ventricle
Superior medullary
velum
Cerebellar vermis
Cerebellar hemisphere
Posterior incisure

FIG. A-40. Horizontal section through the amygdaloid bodies and pons.

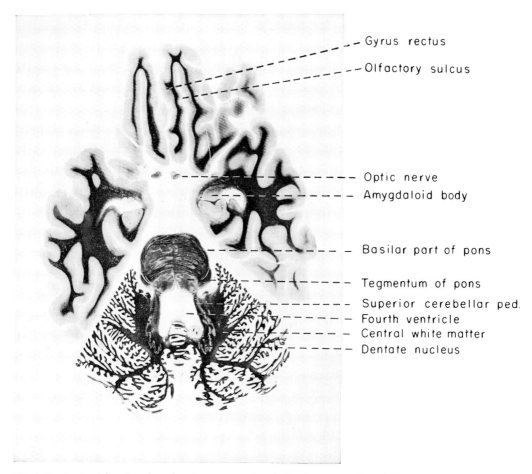

Gyrus rectus

Olfactory sulcus

Optic nerve

Amygdaloid body

Basilar part of pons

Tegmentum of pons

Superior cerebellar ped.

Fourth ventricle

Central white matter

Dentate nucleus

FIG. A-41. Horizontal section through optic nerves and central white matter of cerebellum.

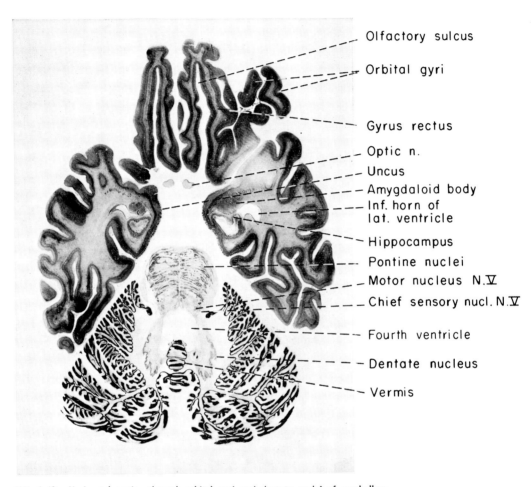

Olfactory sulcus

Orbital gyri

Gyrus rectus

Optic n.

Uncus

Amygdaloid body

Inf. horn of
lat. ventricle

Hippocampus

Pontine nuclei

Motor nucleus N.$\underline{\text{V}}$

Chief sensory nucl. N.$\underline{\text{V}}$

Fourth ventricle

Dentate nucleus

Vermis

FIG. A-42.   Horizontal section through orbital gyri and dentate nuclei of cerebellum.

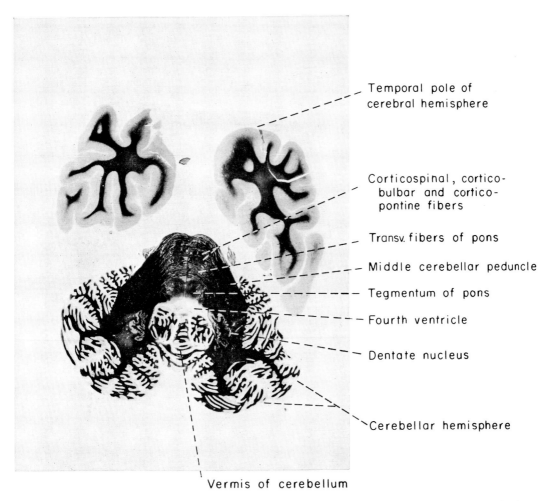

Temporal pole of
cerebral hemisphere

Corticospinal, cortico-
bulbar and cortico-
pontine fibers

Transv. fibers of pons

Middle cerebellar peduncle

Tegmentum of pons

Fourth ventricle

Dentate nucleus

Cerebellar hemisphere

Vermis of cerebellum

FIG. A-43.   Horizontal section through the temporal poles of the cerebral hemispheres and middle cerebellar peduncles.

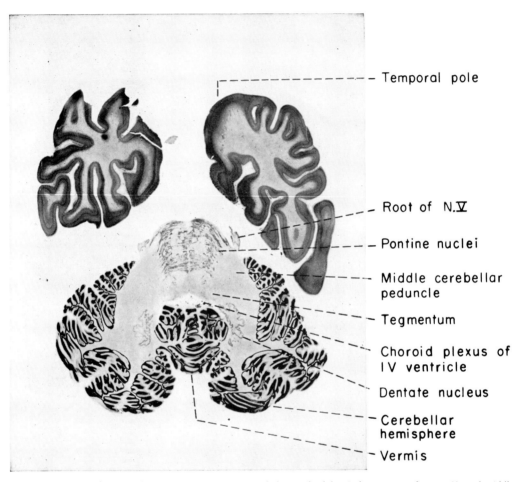

- Temporal pole
- Root of N. V
- Pontine nuclei
- Middle cerebellar peduncle
- Tegmentum
- Choroid plexus of IV ventricle
- Dentate nucleus
- Cerebellar hemisphere
- Vermis

FIG. A-44. Horizontal section through the temporal poles of the cerebral hemispheres, root of nerve V, and middle cerebellar peduncles.

Index

Boldface numbers indicate principal references; page numbers in *italics* refer to the Atlas.